Ego Identity

J.E. Marcia A.S. Waterman
D.R. Matteson S.L. Archer
J.L. Orlofsky

Ego Identity

A Handbook for Psychosocial Research

Springer-Verlag
New York Berlin Heidelberg London Paris
Tokyo Hong Kong Barcelona Budapest

James E. Marcia, Ph.D., Department of Psychology, Simon Fraser University, Burnaby, British Columbia, V5A 1S6, Canada

Alan S. Waterman, Ph.D., Department of Psychology, Trenton State College, Hillwood Lakes, CN 4700, Trenton, NJ 08650-4700, USA

David R. Matteson, Ph.D., Division of Psychology and Counseling, College of Education, Governors State University, University Park, IL 60466, USA

Sally L. Archer, Ph.D., Department of Psychology, Trenton State College, Hillwood Lakes, CN 4700, Trenton, NJ 08650-4700, USA

Jacob L. Orlofsky, Ph.D., Department of Psychology, University of Missouri, St. Louis, MO 63121, USA

Library of Congress Cataloging-in-Publication Data.
Ego identity : a handbook for psychosocial research / James E. Marcia . . . [et al.].
p. cm.
Includes bibliographical references (p.) and index.
ISBN-13: 978-1-4613-8332-1 e-ISBN-13: 978-1-4613-8330-7
DOI: 10.1007/978-1-4613-8330-7
1. Identity (Psychology) 2. Ego (Psychology) I. Marcia, James E. BF697.E475 1993
155.2 – dc20
93-2919

Printed on acid-free paper.

Production coordinated by Chernow Editorial Services, Inc., and managed by Christin R. Ciresi; manufacturing supervised by Jacqui Ashri.
Typeset by Best-set Typesetter Ltd., Hong Kong.

9 8 7 6 5 4 3 2 1

To our children,
Adam and Nicole,
(and to the memory of Sean),
Aaron and Jeremy,
Eric and Heather,
and Nicholas

Contents

Part I
Theory and Research in Identity and Intimacy

1 The Ego Identity Status Approach to Ego Identity

James E. Marcia

Ego Identity

The formation of an ego identity is a major event in the development of personality. Occurring during late adolescence, the consolidation of identity marks the end of childhood and the beginning of adulthood. Identity formation involves a synthesis of childhood skills, beliefs, and identifications into a more or less coherent, unique whole that provides the young adult with both a sense of continuity with the past and a direction for the future.[1] As an inner organization, identity may be compared with those psychological structures posited by cognitive developmental theorists, notably Piaget (Inhelder & Piaget, 1958). Identity differs from Piagetian structures, however, in that it is content- as well as process-based. Whereas Piagetian structures are primarily procedures for operating on experience, identity comprises both procedural styles and elements of content. More simply, identity, as a structure, refers to how experience is handled as well as to what experiences are considered important.

Erik Erikson's most substantial contribution to our understanding of identity has been placement of the concept within a scheme of normal personality development. The notion of identity, one's idea of who one is, how one defines oneself, has been a dominant theme in literature and the social sciences. Almost everyone, it seems, has something to say—or says something—about identity. But only Erikson has so placed the concept within a psychosocial developmental outline of the human life cycle that identity can be viewed in the context of an organizing theory (ego psychoanalytic) and its formation investigated empirically.

Identity may be considered in three aspects: structural, phenomenological, and behavioral. The structural aspect refers to the consequences identity has for the overall balance of psychodynamic processes. Identity

[1] These definitions of identity combine Erikson's and the author's.

Identity issue at Integrity Stage ↓ (column 4, row VIII)

CHRONOLOGICAL AGE		1	2	3	4	5	6	7	8
OLD AGE	VIII	T—M Intg.	A—S,D Intg.	I—G Intg.	Ind —I Intg.	Id —ID Intg.	Int —Is Intg.	G—S Intg.	**Integrity and Despair**
ADULTHOOD	VII	T—M G	A—S,D G	I—G G	Ind —I G	Id —ID G	Int —Is G	**Generativity and Stagnation Self-absorption**	Inty —D G
YOUNG ADULTHOOD	VI	T—M Int.	A—S,D Int.	I—G Int.	Ind —I Int.	Id —ID Int.	**Intimacy and Isolation**	G—S Int.	Inty —D Int.
ADOLESCENCE Genital Mature intrusion-inclusion	V	T—M Id.	A—S,D Id.	I—G Id.	Ind —I Id.	**Identity and Identity Diffusion**	Int —Is Id.	G—S Id.	Inty —D Id.
SCHOOL AGE Latent	IV	T—M Ind.	A—S,D Ind.	I—G Ind.	**Industry and Inferiority**	Id —ID Ind.	Int —Is Ind.	G—S Ind.	Inty —D Ind.
PLAY AGE Phallic (oedipal) Intrusion-inclusion Individuation	III	T—M I	A—S,D I	**Initiative and Guilt**	Ind —I I	Id —ID I	Int —Is I	G—S I	Inty —D I
EARLY CHILDHOOD Anal Eliminative-retentive Practising	II	T—M A	**Autonomy and Shame, Doubt**	I—G A	Ind —I A	Id —ID A	Int —Is A	G—S A	Inty —D A
INFANCY Oral 1. Passive-active Incorporative 2. Attachment 3.	I	**Basic Trust and Basic Mistrust**	A—S,D T	I—G T	Ind —I T	Id —ID T	Int —Is T	G—S T	Inty —D T

↑ (column 2, row I) Precursor to Autonomy at Trust Stage

1. Psychosexual zone
2. Related behavioral modality
3. Object relational phase

FIGURE 1.1 Erikson's eight stages of psychosocial (ego) growth.

is a stage of ego growth, hence its consolidation at late adolescence strengthens those aspects of personality having to do with judgment, delay, and efficacy. The phenomenological aspect of identity refers to the individual's experience of having or not having a sense of identity, as well as to the experience of one's particular style of identity formation. The behavioral aspect of identity refers to the observable components of the identity-formation process, what others can see of an individual's identity style. This approach touches on the social-interactional facets of identity. Following is a discussion of the three aspects of identity: structural, phenomenological, and behavioral.

The Structural Aspect

Erikson has posited eight stages of psychosocial (ego) growth, each stage reaching a crucial point during a specific chronological age. These ages, relevant age-specific crises, and corresponding psychosexual stages are presented in the Figure 1.1. Our focus in this book is on the "watershed" stage of Identity-Identity Diffusion occurring at late adolescence.

One advantage of studying identity within a psychosocial developmental framework, however, is that the theory in which the construct is embedded specifies antecedent and consequent conditions; hence, identity research has ramifications for ego developmental and ego psychoanalytic theory. Identity is not approached here as a free-floating construct, but as one that is an integral part of a larger developmental scheme. Here, then, are some comments on that scheme.

Looking at Figure 1.1, one sees that stage-specific crises are presented as being in a "versus" relationship. Unfortunately, this description can be misleading about the nature of the resolution of psychosocial crises, and Erikson has repeatedly cautioned against an either-or interpretation. Rather, the resolution of a psychosocial crisis takes the form of *predominance* by one characteristic over another, especially during pre-identity stages (e.g., more trusting than mistrusting during the infancy stage). The optimum resolution is a *combination* of these characteristics tilted toward the positive end, whose quality is captured somewhat by Erikson's schedule of virtues. For example, the positive resolution of Basic Trust-Mistrust yields the virtue, Hope. As the ability to become self-reflective increases, it is my opinion that this crisis-resolution process increasingly takes on the form of a dialectic. For example, at young adulthood, the "syntonic" pole, Intimacy, may represent the thesis; the "dystonic" pole, Isolation, may represent the antithesis; and a synthesis is achieved that represents the individual's unique way of "doing" Intimacy-Isolation. This unique individual style of resolving the Intimacy-Isolation dilemma is different from the Eriksonian virtue of that stage (viz., Love), although the resolution may be, in any individual, sufficiently positive to yield Love. The idea of a dialectical resolution process, different for each individual, combines the concept of a sequence of common life-cycle stages with an existential emphasis on individual styles of resolution. There is probably progressive growth in the synthetic quality of the resolution of stage-specific crises from infancy to old age. The greater the sense of one's identity, and the greater its importance to the individual, the more likely it is that one will put one's own stamp on psychosocial crises in the form of individually fashioned resolutions. Hence, after an identity is formed, the possibility for self-fashioned resolutions becomes greater because identity provides a more or less fixed reference point.

Another observation about the diagram is that each issue arises at every stage, although not with equal importance. There are sixty-four squares in the diagram, not eight. Hence, there are precursors to adolescent identity at toddlerhood, and subsequent identity issues in middle age. Each stage-specific crisis dominates its stage and colors or influences the other psychosocial issues occurring with it. For example, during adolescence when the predominant crisis is that of Identity, the issue of Basic Trust-Mistrust takes on identity characteristics (viz., trust of time). Similarly, during infancy, when Basic Trust-Mistrust is the predominant crisis, Identity takes on the characteristics of that period (viz., mother-child differentiation). This occurrence of every issue at every stage has implications for remediation (e.g., via psychotherapy) (Marcia, 1988b) and also captures the complex unity of personality.

Turning back to identity in Figure 1.1, we see it as the fifth life-cycle stage, preceded by school-age Industry-Inferiority and followed by young-adult Intimacy-Isolation. It is at this stage in ego growth that the accrued strengths of childhood are organized by the late adolescent into a sense of self and a direction for the future. This development has implications for balance among the major personality structures: id, ego, and superego (i.e., the imperative, executive, and judgmental processes indicated by these metaphors). Erikson's theory builds upon, and does not supplant, classical psychoanalytic theory. Hence, a change in ego growth affects those personality structures not specifically dealt with by psychosocial theory. A stronger ego, relative to other structures, emerges from adolescence as a result of identity formation and the ties to the superego figures of childhood are loosened as they are replaced by new ego ideals (Blos, 1962, 1974; Josselson, 1980). As identity is developed, ego functions other than those specifically implicated in identity development will be strengthened, an assumption in the initial research projects.

This assumption of continually accruing ego strength is built into the form of Erikson's theory, for the successful resolution of each stage is predicated on the successful resolution of foregoing stages. So that if one succeeds in forming an identity, it may be assumed that the earlier stages of Trust, Autonomy, Initiative, and Industry have also been resolved successfully. Moreover, the assumption is built into the theory, via the epigenetic principle, that given "an average expectable environment" each stage will arise and will be more or less successfully resolved.

To summarize, the formation of an identity, from a structural or intrapsychic perspective, betokens an increase in overall ego strength, so that other ego functions (e.g., delay of gratification, thinking under stress, mutuality of interpersonal relationships) should show heightened development concomitant with identity development.

The Phenomenological Aspect

Identity formation is, as Erikson says, the result of "the silent doings of ego synthesis" (1959), and "happens" given an average expectable environment. The formation of an identity is different, however, from the construction of an identity. In experiential terms, one becomes progressively aware of one's basic characteristics and one's position in the world. For example, one comes gradually to realize that one is separate from one's mother, the child of one's own parents, the possessor of specific skills and needs, a pupil in a particular school, a member of certain social and religious groups, the citizen of a specific country. This list describes a given or *conferred* identity, of whose elements an individual becomes progressively aware.[2] In contrast, identity begins to be *constructed* when the individual begins to make decisions about who to be, with which group to affiliate, what beliefs to adopt, what interpersonal values to espouse, and what occupational direction to pursue. Most, though not all, individuals "have" an identity in the original Eriksonian sense. Only some, however, have a *self-constructed* identity that is based upon superimposition of a decision-making process on the given or conferred identity. Later on, when discussing the identity statuses, those with conferred identities will be referred to as Foreclosures; those with constructed identities will be called Identity Achievement individuals. Persons with no firm identity will be called Identity Diffusions. Those who are in transition from no sense of identity or from a conferred to a constructed identity will be called Moratorium.

The experience of having an identity is that one has a core, a center that is oneself, to which experience and action can be referred. One can trace one's history in a meaningful way to one's present situation and can extend that line into probable futures. Individuals with *either* a conferred or a constructed identity have this sense of inner coherence. However,

---

[2] Another alternative (Waterman, 1984) is a "eudaemonic" identity, an organically emerging sense of one's identity, which arises out of introspection and leads to the "discovery" of who one already is. A similar issue has been discussed by Baumeister (1986) and Baumeister et al. (1985) in describing identity crises as ones of "motivation" or of "legitimation."

individuals who construct their identity, modifying or rejecting some conferred elements, also possess a sense of having participated in a self-initiated and self-directed process. They know not only who they are, they know how they became that, and that they had a hand in the becoming. Furthermore, they have developed skills useful in the adaptive process of further self-construction and self-definition.

One way of attempting to capture the personal experience of identity is to describe the outlook toward the future of different identity variants (see also Rapaport, 1985). Those lacking a coherent identity, the Identity Diffusion status, have little future sense. They are primarily present-oriented, with some regrets about a disappointing relationship with their parents. Having no central sense of self, they are subject to the vicissitudes of fortune, and feel, whether optimistically or pessimistically, somewhat out of control of their futures. Those individuals with conferred identities, the Foreclosure status, have adopted a lifelong "game plan," set out for them by their parents or similar authority figures. As they look to the future, they see themselves trying to live up to a prearranged set of ideals, occupational plans, and interpersonal forms. Their self-esteem is contingent upon the extent to which they "fulfill" the tasks given them. Individuals with constructed identities, the Identity Achievement status, also have game plans, but these tend to be their own, not their parents', and are subject to revision. They see the future as something to be shaped, a period of identity creation or realization rather than a time to meet preset standards. Individuals in the process of constructing their identity, the Moratorium status, are rather like trapeze performers, holding on to the bar of the past while swinging toward that of the future, often with much of the vacillation, fear, intensity, and excitement connoted by the circus image. At some times, all things seem possible to them; at other times, they can be so totally self-preoccupied that their whole phenomenological world is consumed with their present struggle.

To summarize, identity is experienced as a core or center that gives meaning and significance to one's world. This core may be conferred (given by one's childhood caretakers) or constructed (built by oneself out of conferred elements). Those with conferred identities experience their future as the fulfilment of expectations; those who have constructed identities experience their futures as the creation of self-relevant forms.

The Behavioral Aspect

Some of what has been said thus far about identity has been said, in some form, in other places by other theorists. What is unique about the identity status research is the attempt to go beyond the intrapsychic and phenomenological into the empirical realm. To accomplish this undertaking, identity had to be brought out into the open. There must be something that can be seen with relative clarity by observers who are relatively easy to train. Thus, it became necessary to leave the intrapsychic and phenomenological levels of description and to search for those observable behaviors which could serve as indicators of the presence or absence of the presumed underlying identity structure, knowing that the structure itself would never be observable. What follows is a description of the behavioral aspects of identity as they were identified in order to measure them.

The question to be answered was: "How does identity manifest itself in behavior?" Turning to Erikson's writings, the two areas that seemed paramount in adolescents' identity formation were occupation and ideology. About occupation, Erikson has written, "In general, it is primarily the inability to settle on an occupational identity which disturbs young people" (1963, p. 252). Of ideology, he said:

> To envisage a future, the young adult may also need something which Shaw called "a religion" and a clear comprehension of life in light of an intelligible theory . . . we would call this something-between-a-theory-and-a-religion an ideology. Whatever else ideology is and whatever transitory or lasting social forms it takes, we will tentatively view it here and discuss it later *as a necessity for the growing ego* which is involved in the succession of generations and in adolescence is committed to some new synthesis of past and future: a synthesis which must include but transcend the past, even as identity does. (1963, p. 97)

The differentiating behavioral quality within these areas that indicated presence or absence of identity seemed to be commitment. If one "had an identity" one would have to have commitments in these areas. One who did not have such commitments would be difficult to see as having an identity.

Hence, in looking for behavioral aspects of identity formation within the theory of identity formation, we identified, initially, two domains in which identity might manifest itself: occupation and ideology; and we recognized one process variable, commitment, within these areas to determine presence or absence of identity. Both the domain criteria of occupation and ideology, as well as the process criterion of commitment, were later expanded. These expansions will be discussed in the following section on identity status. Here we must recognize the translation of a complex theoretical construct into an empirical one. Identity is not just commitment in certain important life areas. But if identity is present, then it should be manifested in those observable criteria.

Hypothetically, identity could be present without commitments in the domains above; and such commitments might appear to exist without there being an underlying identity structure. Regarding the first possibility, at one time during the late 1960s and early 1970s a significant number of young people had ideological commitments that precluded occupational ones. They wanted no part of an "establishment" that they felt was sending them off to an unjustifiable war. We still saw these individuals as having an identity, albeit an alienated one. About the second possibility, one could conceive of an essentially identity-diffuse individual who might form a "shell" of an identity by allying him or herself with a large corporation (or controlling partner!) that dictates what one believes, how one dresses, where one lives, and the correct form of one's domestic arrangements. For the "alienated Achievements," occupational commitment was not present, but strong ideological commitment was; hence, an underlying identity structure could be assumed. For the Diffuse "shell," although occupational and ideological commitment seemed to be present, close questioning would reveal their superimposition on an essentially identity-vacant personality. In short, the assumption is that without commitment, we have no evidence for identity; however, the areas in which that commitment may be manifested can change with social conditions and historical eras.

The Identity Statuses

Defining Criteria

This research in identity began in about 1964 with fairly unstructured, but focused, interviews of about twenty male college students at Ohio State University. Since that time, the number of identity status interviews given runs into the thousands. Although these initial interviews confirmed the notion that occupation and ideology were important topics for late adolescent male identity development, they also made it apparent that there were two kinds of committed and two kinds of uncommitted subjects, rather than just the committed–uncommitted dichotomy. One type of committed subject seemed to have gone through "crises" or exploratory periods, when he questioned seriously his late childhood or early adolescent plans and values. His current commitments were either quite different from his earlier ones, or represented variations on previous themes. The other type of committed subject seemed not to have undergone much exploration of alternatives. He was firmly committed to life directions and values existing in relatively unmodified form since childhood. Furthermore, the former type of committed individual seemed different from the latter not just in his identity formation process, but also in the nature of his identity organization and in his approach to the world. In a few words, he was more flexible, less rigid. Reasoning that this was a difference worth recording, the criterion of commitment alone was expanded to include crisis (or "exploration of alternatives") as it was later, and more accurately, named by David Matteson (1977a, p. 356).

Just as we found two types of committed individuals, so we found two kinds of uncommitted ones. One group was concerned about their lack of specific commitments and was struggling to achieve some coherent

TABLE 1.1. Defining criteria of the identity statuses.

	Identity achievement	Moratorium	Foreclosure	Identity diffusion
Exploration of alternatives	Present	In process	Absent	Present or absent
Commitment	Present	Present but vague	Present	Absent

direction. The other group was relatively unconcerned with their directionlessness, either despairing of being able to impose any direction on their lives or insouciantly denying the need to. The former group seemed to be in the middle of what has become known popularly as an "identity crisis"; the latter group looked like Erikson's "Identity Confusion."[3] Again we needed to modify our criteria—this time in terms of the process preceding commitment, rather than just presence or absence of commitment.

After these initial criteria-refining interviews, it looked as if there were least four major variants in resolving the identity issue that we could expect from our late-adolescent males. These modes of identity resolution, called the identity statuses, and their defining criteria, are presented in Table 1.1.[4] Further descriptions of the identity statuses' defining and empirically determined characteristics occupy a significant portion of this handbook.

Construct Validity

Cronbach and Meehl (1955) proposed an investigatory paradigm, construct validation, to study complex constructs with essentially unobservable referents. Identity is certainly such a construct, and the first ten years of

[3]Erikson changed his label for the negative pole of the identity crisis from "Diffusion" to "Confusion." We have retained the "Diffusion" term for our subjects because those to whom it applies seemed to be more "spread out" and unclear than "mixed up."

[4]The reader familiar with the rich descriptiveness of Erikson's writings on identity may feel that very complex material has been squeezed into rather circumscribed form. There was a distinct purpose in this compression, and it was not to diminish the breadth of the construct. Rather, the purpose was to avoid, insofar as possible, socially desirable responding. Asking a subject whether he or she experienced a "sense of invigorating sameness and continuity," "a feeling of being at home in one's body," "inner assuredness of anticipated recognition from those who count" (just a few of the aspects of identity listed by Erikson), seemed to be begging for socially desirable responding. We thought it was important to keep the identity-defining questions as value-neutral as possible and to cast the more richly descriptive aspects of identity as dependent variables. For example, the manual for scoring the Incomplete Sentences Blank, designed as a concurrent validity measure for the new identity status interview, includes almost all Erikson's descriptions of identity concomitants.

identity research were devoted primarily to establishing its construct validity. A semistructured interview was designed to assess crisis (degree of exploration) and extent of commitment in the areas of occupation and ideology (comprising religious and political views). A manual with empirical examples and theoretical descriptions was provided for rating the interviews. The manual's content and interview structure were modified until interscorer reliabilities of about 80 to 85 percent could be predictably attained. Having developed a fairly reliable categorization scheme, the problem then became establishing predictive validity for the identity statuses, and, by extension, construct validity for the notion of identity.[5]

A first step in this procedure was constructing an alternative measure of overall identity to establish concurrent validity for the identity status interview. Although some measures of identity had been developed at about this time (Block, 1961; Bronson, 1959; Dignan, 1965; Gruen, 1960; and Rasmussen, 1964), they were limited either in content, tapping only aspects of Erikson's theory, or in form, being questionnaire methods allowing subjects little freedom of expression. We wanted a more broadly inclusive measure of Erikson's descriptions of the results of identity formation than the identity status interview that we were trying to validate. That is, we wanted to include as many facets of the outcome of identity development as possible. Also, we wanted a measure that allowed freedom of response while being objectively scorable. A sentence-completion test, the Ego Identity Incomplete Sentences Blank (EI-ISB) was constructed including identity-relevant stems. As with the structured interview, a scoring manual was written comprising theoretical criteria drawn from Erikson's writing and empirical examples from pilot subjects' responses. The EI-ISB and its accompanying manual were revised until interscorer reliabilities reached about $r = .90$.[6]

Our dependent variables were chosen with three objectives in mind. We wanted measures that would tap the more obvious aspects of identity resolution, some that would indicate hypothesized variation in underlying ego strength, and some that would show not just high–low identity differences, but differentiation among the individual identity statuses. For investigating the more obvious aspects of identity, we chose to employ a "change in self-esteem" condition. Subjects were given disguised and apparent self-esteem measures, exposed to negative and positive self-relevant information about a recently completed task, and then reassessed on the self-esteem measures. Absolute amount of change was the variable of interest here. Our reasoning was that subjects who had formed an identity would have a more internal locus of self-evaluation (be more

[5] The studies reported here represent six projects, descriptions of which are found in more detail in Marcia (1966, 1967).

[6] The EI-ISB yields only a continuous score on identity. It does not differentiate among the four identity statuses.

resistant to self-esteem manipulation) than would subjects who had not formed an identity. This hypothesis followed from Erikson's (1968) description of changes in superego functioning, viz., the growing importance of the ego ideal, concomitant with the formation of identity at late adolescence.

Our measure of differences among the statuses in underlying ego strength concerned the relative ability of subjects to perform a difficult cognitive task under anxiety-provoking conditions. Subjects were given Weick's (1964) modification of the Bruner, Goodnow, and Austin (1956) concept attainment task with accompanying stressful evaluation-apprehension conditions. By this method we hoped to determine whether or not nonidentity-specific ego functions, viz., thinking under stress, would be more advanced among subjects who had successfully resolved the psychosocial issue of identity than among those who had not successfully resolved this issue. Reasoning behind this hypothesis was based upon Erikson's (1959) description of identity development as one aspect of more generalized ego growth.

Finally, to establish separate characteristics for the different identity statuses, we administered several measures of personality variables: level of aspiration (i.e., realistic vs. nonrealistic reactions to success and failure); authoritarianism (relying on a strong source outside oneself to take over responsibility for one's decisions); and anxiety. Our results in these early studies are presented graphically in Figure 1.2.[7]

It is apparent from this diagram of dependent variable scores that differences were found between high and low identity statuses as well as among individual statuses with college males. Subjects high in identity (Identity Achievement and Moratorium) scored higher on the concurrent measure of identity (the EI-ISB) than did subjects low in identity (Foreclosures and Identity Diffusions), with Identity Diffusions being notably lowest. ("High" and "low" here refer to chronological proximity to Identity Achievement, for example, because Moratoriums are undergoing an exploratory period, they are considered "higher" in identity than are Foreclosures, even though the latter "have" an identity.) Identity Achievement subjects did best on the measure of thinking under stress (CAT)—in the absence of tested significant differences among the identity statuses in intelligence. Foreclosure persons had relatively high level-of-aspiration scores; that is, they consistently, perhaps rigidly, refused to lower their goals after failure experiences on the CAT. Level-of-aspiration scores of the other subjects were within normal limits. Identity Achievement and Moratorium subjects were more resistant to self-esteem manipulation, as reflected in change scores, than were Foreclosures and Diffusions. Moratoriums, characterized as being in the identity crisis, had

[7] Only results significant beyond the $p < .05$ level are graphed.

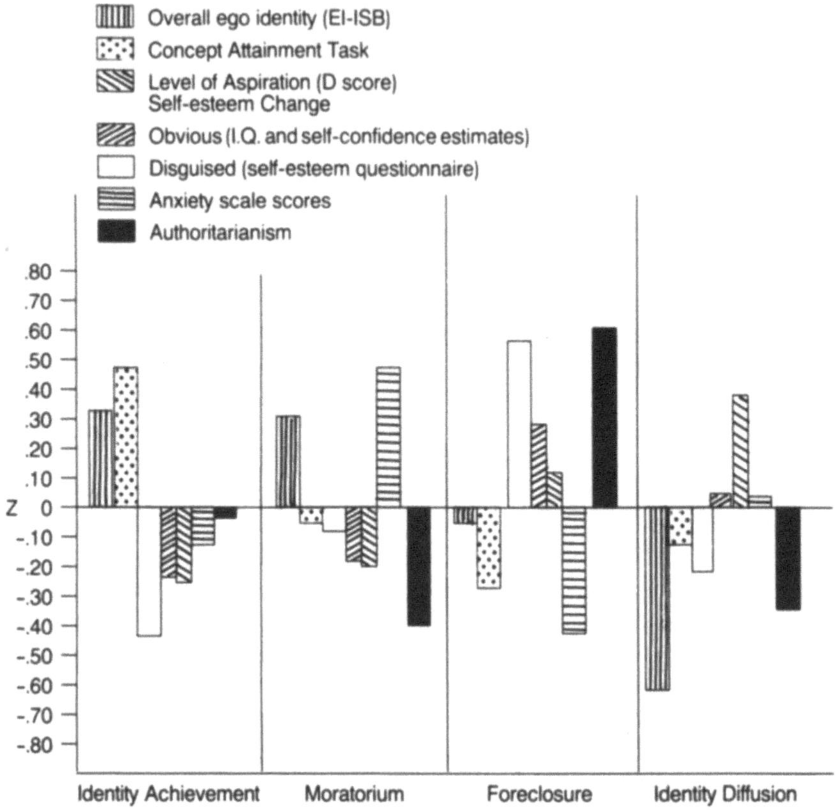

FIGURE 1.2 Summary of current findings on ego identity statuses. (Originally published in Marcia, J.E. (1967). Ego identity status: Relationship to self-esteem, "general maladjustment," and authoritarianism. *Journal of Personality*, *35*, 118–133.)

higher anxiety scores than did other subjects. And, finally, as expected, Foreclosures had the highest authoritarianism scores of all the subjects. At the conclusion of this series of studies, we had made a beginning in establishing construct validity for the identity statuses, at least among college males, both in terms of a high–low identity sense, and as representatives of separate modes of resolution of the identity issue.

Changes in Criteria for the Identity Statuses

The most significant change in identity status criteria has been addition of the interpersonal–sexual domains to the other two areas of occupation and ideology (religion plus politics). There have been essentially three phases to the addition of this new area. The first began with attempts to extend the identity status paradigm to women. Based upon Erikson's (1968) politically controversial, but nonetheless psychologically relevant, notion of the importance to women of coming to terms with their reproductive and nurturant capacities, we decided to include "attitudes toward premarital intercourse" as an additional area in determining identity status in women. Several studies (Marcia & Friedman, 1970; Schenkel & Marcia, 1972; Toder & Marcia, 1973) using this new area both established the relevance of the area for categorizing women's identity status, and established the predictive validity of the identity statuses for women, albeit, initially, with somewhat different meaning. (See Chapter 2.) The second phase in the addition of the new interpersonal–sexual domain came with David Matteson's suggestion that interpersonal issues, in general, were important to both men and women, and that an interview area covering this issue should be incorporated into men's identity interviews as well. Most recently, Harold Grotevant and his coworkers (Grotevant & Cooper, 1985; Grotevant et al., 1982) have included such interpersonal issues as dating, friendship, and sex roles in interviews with middle adolescents. Sally Archer (1981b, 1982, 1985c) has included sex-role preferences in interviews with all age groups; and Archer, Waterman, and Owens (1988) have included interpersonal relationship issues in their adult identity status interviews. In addition, Archer (1985a,b) focused on the family–career conflict as an identity domain and also on the spouse and parenting issues. Currently, the domains used for the identity status interview include *at least* occupation, ideology, and interpersonal issues.

Selection of Content Domains

The addition of the interpersonal domains for the identity status interview raises the general question of the criteria for selecting content areas. Because we are interested primarily in processes underlying identity (viz., exploration and commitment), there is some flexibility in choice of domain content. Two criteria for selecting content have been applied. First, the content should be that which can be assumed to be important during a particular chronological period. For example, dating issues are more important to early and middle adolescents than they are to adults, for whom attitudes toward extramarital relationships would have more relevance. The second criterion is variability of response. In searching for issues directly relevant to women's identity, we first tried out the area of "career–marriage conflict" (Marcia & Friedman, 1970). However, we were unable to elicit much variability of response among junior and senior college women and, so, we changed to "attitudes toward premarital intercourse."

This flexibility of interview content area, bearing in mind the foregoing criteria, is an advantage of the identity status approach. So long as the process variables of exploration and commitment can be assessed, and the guidelines of personal relevancy and variability of response are followed, there is a wide latitude of content area that can be used according to the chronological, cultural, or sexual characteristics of a population An especially prominent example is the rapidly growing body of work of Jean Phinney and her associates (Phinney, 1990, 1992; Phinney & Alipuria, 1990; Phinney & Tarver, 1988) studying the importance to distinguishable ethnic groups of the issue of their ethnicity. Her conclusion that "Examination of important areas [e.g., ethnicity] may yield greater insight into overall identity development than . . . traditional identity areas" (Phinney & Alipuria, 1990, p. 180) was supported by Saulnier (1990) in a study of identity development in homosexual men.

The proliferation of content areas, the age-related questions used to tap them, and the different shades of meaning given to them, have provided some of the stimuli for writing this book. A significant beginning on standardizing the identity status interview was made in a series of scoring workshops given by Waterman and Archer in 1980. Now, investigators in various countries are studying different age ranges, using somewhat different identity interviews. One of our goals here is to provide fairly standardized interview questions and criteria covering age ranges from early adolescence through adulthood. Although this presentation will not be exhaustive, it should provide a useful basic structure for undertaking identity status research.

Alternative Measures of Identity and Identity Status

Since the development of the original identity status interview (Marcia, 1964), several alternative procedures and measures have been developed. These appear to fall into three categories: (a) Measures of overall ego identity based upon the Ego Identity–Incomplete Sentences Blank (EI-ISB); (b) Scaling techniques applied to the identity status interview (ISI) itself; and (c) Questionnaire measures of identity status.

As previously discussed, the EI-ISB was developed to determine the concurrent validity of the identity statuses. Scores on the EI-ISB have been found to be related to the identity status categories (Marcia, 1966; 1967); androgyny (Deldin, 1977); ego development (Adams & Fitch, 1981; Adams & Shea, 1979); and the effects of parental divorce (Grossman et al., 1980). Simmons (1970) developed a multiple-choice form of the EI-ISB, the Identity Achievement Scale (IAS). Scores on the IAS have been found to be related to: Shostrom's Personal Orientation Inventory and scales on the Edwards' Personal Preference Inventory (Simmons, 1970); identity development in Nigerian adolescents (Jegede, 1976); parental influences on adolescent identity (Enright et al., 1980); women's attitudes toward women (Stein & Weston, 1982; and axiological maturity (Simmons, 1985)). A revision of the IAS was undertaken by Tan et al. (1977), who freed the measure from its contamination by social desirability factors and the admixture of Achievement and Foreclosure persons at the high end of the scale. They established some construct validity for their Ego Identity

Scale by correlating it with measures of internal locus of control, intimacy, and female college students' perceptions of parents (Kendis & Tan, 1978).

Matteson (1977a) introduced a scaling technique for rating each interview domain on a four-point scale according to the criteria of commitment, current exploration, past exploration, and involvement. This tool provides an overall score for each status for each subject, total scores for the four identity formation criteria above, and identity status scores for each interview domain. This scaling approach was expanded by Bosma (1985), who developed a method prefacing the administration of a scaled ISI with an initial questionnaire, thus ensuring the personal relevancy of the ISI domains to a particular subject. These are the advantages of these approaches: they provide measures of the separate aspects of the identity formation process; interscorer reliability is increased; and they furnish continuous measures of the statuses, yielding both identity status "profiles" for an individual and interval scores that facilitate use of parametric statistical analyses. Some disadvantages are: the identity assessment process, already rather lengthy, becomes even more time-consuming; it is not altogether clear how to combine the separate criteria to determine a clear identity status; and the opportunity for a sophisticated interviewer to exercise an informed judgment, independent of adding up numbers, is lost.

The most highly developed and validated group-administered questionnaire form assessing identity status is the Extended Objective Measure of Ego Identity Status (EOM-EIS2) developed by Adams and his colleagues (Adams et al., 1979; Adams et al., 1987; Craig-Bray & Adams, 1986; Grotevant & Adams, 1984; and Jones & Streitmatter, 1987).[8] This measure comprises statements reflecting characteristics of the different identity statuses. These are presented to subjects in multiple-choice format. Scores are obtained representing the relative standing of a subject on each identity status and an overall status is determined based upon cut-off scores. Three distinct advantages of this procedure over the interview method are: ease of group administration; elimination of interscorer reliability problems; and provision of continuous scores for each subject for each identity status. A disadvantage of this, or any other, questionnaire measure is that there is no opportunity to probe subjects' responses where further information might be important; e.g., depth or meaningfulness of exploratory period and extent of commitment. Also, because of

[8]Two measures of occupational identity status have been developed and some predictive validity established for each (Dellas & Jernigan, 1987; and Melgosa, 1987). Dellas and Jernigan (1990) have also recently obtained validity for newly developed objective scales of identity status in the religion and politics domains. Côté (1986) has constructed a scale for "identity crisis modality." This measure might be usefully administered in conjunction with other questionnaires because it provides a fairly detailed picture of an individual's identity crisis.

EOM-EIS scoring rules, some subjects have to be either discarded or classified, somewhat dubiously, as "low-profile" Moratoriums. Finally, the correspondence between the EOM-EIS and the ISI, with which the preponderance of identity status research has been conducted, is not as high as one would wish (see Craig-Bray & Adams, 1986). There are now, however, a fairly large number of studies (e.g., Adams & Jones, 1983; Adams et al., 1984; Bennion & Adams, 1986; Craig-Bray et al., 1988; Kamptner, 1988; Streitmatter, 1987; and many others) that demonstrate predictive validity for the EOM-EIS.

The choice of which measure to use depends upon what the investigator wishes to study. If a continuous measure of overall ego identity is desired, then the Tan et al. (1977) measure is the most efficient. If one wishes to obtain a scaled measure of aspects of the identity formation process, then either the Matteson procedure or the even more detailed Bosma one are useful. The Matteson technique is better for arriving at an overall identity status; the Bosma measure provides interview material more personally relevant for a particular subject. Where a screening measure, prior to ISI administration, is desired, where continuous scores are needed, or where one wants measures on a large group of subjects, and discarding some is no problem, then the EOM-EIS is the measure to choose. Clearly, if the authors thought these measures were sufficient to replace the ISI, we would not be writing this book. Although research should, and does continue on finding a more expeditious and reliably scorable alternative to the ISI, the interview remains the most flexible and, it is likely, the most valid measure we have for determining identity status. Some of these methodological issues have been discussed further by this author (Marcia, 1989c).

Other measures of psychosocial development are available that incorporate measures of identity (e.g., Constantinople, 1969; McClain, 1975; Ochse & Plug, 1986; Rosenthal et al., 1984), as are other measures of identity per se (e.g., Erwin & Schmidt, 1981; Hauser, 1971, 1972; Tzuriel, 1984; Tzuriel & Klein, 1977; see also the measures listed at the beginning of this chapter, most of which have been reviewed by Bourne, 1978a). Because this book is primarily about research conducted using an identity status or intimacy status approach, these measures will be discussed only in passing.

The Theoretical Basis of Identity Statuses

Ego psychoanalytic theory was the conceptual origin of the identity status approach to the study of ego identity. Although Erikson's stages of psychosocial development have sometimes been read and presented as a sort of theoretically disembodied scheme of personality formation, they are clearly rooted in psychoanalytic theory. One can trace a more or less direct line from Freud's initial concern with libidinal determinants of psychological functioning to his later emphasis on the role of the ego (Freud, 1923); to Anna Freud's description of ego defense mechanisms (1936); to Hartmann's (1964) and Hartmann, Kris, and Loewenstein's (1946) concepts of autonomous (nonlibidinally determined) ego functioning, creative (nonpathological) regression, and the epigenetic notion of a ground plan for ego development; to Rapaport's attempts to reconstruct psychoanalytic theory as psychological theory (1959); to White's concept of competence as a unique ego motive (1959); and, finally, to Erikson's description of specific stages of ego growth throughout the life cycle (1963; 1982). This process has been one of construction and reconstruction, not of supplanting. Hence, if one discusses Erikson's concept of identity, it rests within the theoretical context of other notions such as psychosexual developmental eras, unconscious determinants of behavior, the dynamic interplay of personality processes, and so on.[9] Erikson's concept of identity development presupposes all the more classical psychoanalytic clinical and theoretical material summarized and expanded in Blos's *On Adolescence* (1962). In addition, much of the current research on life-span development, especially the work of researchers such as Levinson (1978) and Vaillant (1977), incorporates Erikson's description of life-cycle growth. The work presented here on identity (and intimacy) statuses represents an attempt to investigate a portion of Erikson's ego developmental theory relying heavily upon empirical methods discussed in Cronbach and Meehl's (1955) article on construct validation of psychological theory. Hence, our approach to adolescent development differs from the traditional case-history method of psychoanalysis, the in-depth longitudinal approaches of the life-span researchers mentioned above, and the survey methods used by Douvan and Adelson (1966) and by Offer et al. (1981). Also, the focus of our research has been more on the validity of the construct of identity (and intimacy) than on the nature of adolescence. However, because of Erikson's valuable contribution in pinpointing identity formation as the primary ego developmental task of adolescence, we have also been able, in studying identity, to say something about adolescence.

The identity status labels themselves are not Erikson's, nor has he ever advocated or approved a status approach. The labels were taken from Erikson's writings to connote characteristics of identity formation men-

---

[9] Having said this, it is clear that this author's fantasy—that the identity status research would always be carried out within the context of psychoanalytic theory —is a reality not shared by a large number of other identity researchers, even the majority of authors of this book, who do not subscribe to psychoanalytic theory. The foregoing is a statement about the breadth of appeal of the statuses, a suggestion that they tap process dimensions underlying a number of psychological developmental lines (Marcia, 1988), and an acknowledgment of the difficulty of tying in the results of some identity status studies with psychoanalytically derived theoretical propositions.

tioned by him, but not necessarily emphasized or used in the same way by him. For example, Erikson uses the term "moratorium" to apply to a time period provided by societies during which its youth are freed from demands of production in order to integrate their identities. First, this period varies widely in different societies, being almost nonexistent in those where daily survival precludes the luxury of a time-out for youths to "find themselves," to our Western technological society, wherein the length of such institutionalized moratoria seems to increase in proportion to the complexity of technological demand and the wealth of the society, extending in many cases from puberty to young adulthood (25 to 30 years of age)—and, for some academics, a lifetime. Second, it has been clear from our interviews that, even though an institutionalized moratorium may be furnished by a society, individuals vary greatly in the degree to which they avail themselves of this opportunity. Some seem to ignore it completely (Foreclosures); others seem to luxuriate in it ("characterological" Moratoriums). Hence, when we speak of "Moratorium," we refer specifically to an individual who is exploring actively, on a cognitive and/or behavioral level, aspects of themselves and their world to make some integration.

A similar issue arises with the term "foreclosure." Although Erikson (1980) did use the term to describe a foreshortened Moratorium period, he tended to focus on the commitment aspect of identity formation, and did not differentiate clearly between the characteristics of an identity formed without an exploratory period and that formed subsequent to an exploratory period. Our interviews indicated quite clearly to us that these were different identity patterns with different developmental implications; hence, we labeled the relatively unexamined committed identity, Foreclosure, and the self-constructed committed identity, Achievement.

Historical Overview of the Identity Statuses

In the initial research the identity statuses were seen as various outcomes of the adolescent moratorium period described by Erikson (1968). The developmental origin or fate of these mattered little compared with the necessity for establishing their validity. When their validity had been accomplished, though, attention began to shift to the childhood antecedents of the identity statuses and their adult consequences. Correspondingly, the statuses became seen less fixed as outcomes and more in terms of their underlying process variables of exploration and commitment. (A good example is Bosma's {1985} Groningen Identity Scale, based entirely on measuring these two dimensions and developed out of an interest in describing more directly the identity formation process). It also became clear to researchers that few persons were "just" Achievements or Foreclosures, but rather a mixture of status designations, usually with one predominating. (This realization is reflected in the EOM-EIS measure yielding status profiles developed by Adams {Adams et al., 1979} with Grotevant {Grotevant & Adams, 1984}). Identity status within content domains, as contrasted with overall identity status, also became a subject of investigation as researchers grew more interested in teasing apart various components of identity development (Waterman, 1982). As the statuses began to be examined in a more developmental, longitudinal manner, it was apparent that individuals changed statuses, so that no status was a once-and-for-all description of one's identity—although some changes (e.g., from Achievement to Diffusion or Foreclosure) were less likely than others (e.g., from Foreclosure to Moratorium, from Moratorium to Achievement) (Waterman, 1982). The current approach to identity is a life-span developmental one, in which the identity integration at late adolescence is seen as an initial formulation, to be subject to reformulation and reintegration throughout the life cycle (Stephen et al., 1992; Waterman & Archer, 1990). In this context, identity statuses move from being descriptions only of late adolescent resolutions of a stage-specific psychosocial task to being also descriptions both of adult identity patterns (Archer, 1989b; Waterman, 1980) and, perhaps, of childhood identity antecedents (Marcia, 1986a).[10]

Prologue

In Chapter 2, the results of the past twenty-five years of identity status research are reviewed. An interesting aspect of this research is that it has been carried out by geographically diverse and, for most of the period, personally unrelated investigators. A disadvantage of this approach has been a nonprogrammatic quality; an advantage is that the method and the results have extraordinary generalizability. Unrelated researchers in differing geographic areas have been able to use the identity status interview, obtain reliable ratings, and achieve comparable experimental results. The major purpose of this book is to expedite that investigative endeavor by gathering in one place relevant theory, established findings, standard interview procedures, and scoring criteria.

---

[10] The dynamic quality of the identity statuses suggested by the research outlined above is not reflected in the identity names, which in addition to having a distinct capitalistic ring, as the author and literary critic, Leslie Fiedler, remarked at an informal symposium at the State University of New York at Buffalo in 1968, also have a "static" quality. Even though they represent process variables, they sound like fixed categories, especially "Identity Achievement." Perhaps an increase in connotative accuracy would be attained if Identity Achievement were to be subscribed; e.g., IA_1, IA_2, and so on, representing sequential identity reformulations throughout the life cycle. For better or worse, identity researchers have opted for consistency rather than aesthetics in retaining the original status labels.

2
The Status of the Statuses: Research Review

JAMES E. MARCIA

Identity status research has spanned more than twenty-five years and more than 300 studies. Although not all are reviewed in this chapter, the ones that are covered give a fairly coherent picture of what has been determined with some certainty and what is questionable. The issues raised in the four extensive reviews of identity status research (Bourne, 1978a,b; Marcia, 1980; Matteson, 1975; and Waterman, 1982) suggest the structure for this chapter, which is divided into four sections: (a) Personality characteristics of the different identity statuses, emphasizing "the internalization of self-regulatory processes"; (b) Developmental aspects; (c) Gender differences and sex roles; and (d) Cross-cultural studies.

Personality Characteristics of the Identity Statuses: The Internalization of Self-Regulatory Processes

"Internalization" is a concept shared by these theories: drive-oriented classical psychoanalytic, adaptation-oriented ego psychoanalytic, relationship-oriented object relations, and cognitive developmental. Bourne (1978b) writes from a psychoanalytic perspective:

> This process involves the development of an increasingly stabilized and internalized capacity for . . . homeostatic control of internal functioning, particularly in the realms of (1) the regulation of self-esteem (Kohut, 1971), (2) the exercise of self-calming functions and containment of affective fluctuations in response to stress, and (3) the autonomous organization of motives and resources to anticipate and meet adaptive demands. (Blos, 1974, p. 389)

Similarly, both Piaget's (1965) stages of cognitive development and Kohlberg's (1976) stages in the development of moral thought involve progressive internalization, self-representation, and self-construction of the world and of values.

The personality variables discussed in this section have in common an emphasis on an internal (structurally mature) mode of control and valuation contrasted with an external (structurally immature) mode. These are the general patterns expected from the identity statuses: Identity Diffusions should be the least internalized; having no firm identity, they are defined by their circumstances. Foreclosures may appear to be more internalized than Moratoriums; however, their internalization is based upon introjected, unreconstructed authority figures, and reflects little "metabolism" or sophisticated syntheses of early identifications—life issues have not been reformulated in the individual's own terms. Moratoriums, who are in the process of synthesizing internal structures may, in times of crisis, appear less internalized than Foreclosures; in less acute periods they should appear more internalized than Foreclosures, and they should always appear more internalized than Diffusions. Identity Achievement persons, having constructed their own identities, should appear to be the most internalized of the statuses.

General Personality Characteristics

Authoritarianism and Stereotypical Thinking

One of the most consistent findings in identity status research has been that male and female Foreclosures, especially relative to Moratoriums, score highly on measures of authoritarianism and socially stereotypical thinking (Marcia, 1966, 1967; Marcia & Friedman, 1970; Matteson, 1974; Schenkel & Marcia, 1972; and Streitmatter & Pate, 1989). They show preference for a strong leader over a democratic process, obedience over social protest, and the "pseudo-speciation" described by Erikson (1987): firm conviction that "their" group and "their" way are right. A possible consequence of this position is the somewhat chilling finding by Podd (1972) that, more than any other in a Milgram obedience task who had delivered what they believed to be maximum electrical shock to a "victim," it was the Foreclosures who were willing to do it again; in fact, all Foreclosures who administered maximum shock levels were willing to repeat their performance.

Anxiety

The ability to bind anxiety, to perform effectively in the face of inner turmoil, is a characteristic associated with higher levels of ego functioning, such as would ensue from formation of an identity. One caution about interpreting studies of anxiety among the identity statuses is that most of these have used paper-and-pencil self-report measures, which yield the estimate of anxiety that a subject is willing to report. In general, Moratoriums, and to a lesser extent Diffusions, have been highest in reported anxiety among the statuses, and Foreclosures have been the lowest (Marcia, 1967; Marcia & Friedman, 1970; Oshman & Manosevitz, 1974; Podd et al., 1970; and Sterling & Van Horn, 1989). The differences in identity statuses' reported anxiety are likely to be obtained for differing reasons. Moratoriums score highly because they are in a stressful, in-crisis state, and because they tend to be excruciatingly honest. Foreclosures may score low both because it may be a particularly adaptive status in some groups in certain historical periods, and because they are reluctant to admit pathology. The latter is reflected in their high social desirability scores (Orlofsky et al., 1973).

Self-Esteem

Although differences among statuses in stability of self-esteem were established in early studies, findings have not been clear on absolute levels of self-esteem. For example, Marcia (1967) and Orlofsky (1977) found no self-esteem differences in males; but Bunt (1968) found high identity males to be high in self-esteem. Foreclosure[1] and Achievement women had higher self-esteem than Moratorium and Diffusion women, according to Marcia and Friedman (1970) and Schenkel and Marcia (1972); but Prager (1982) and Read et al. (1984) found that only Identity Achievement women had high self-esteem scores; and Orlofsky (1977) reported no differences among women. One problem in this research area is the differing theoretical definitions of self-esteem. Within the ego psychoanalytic theoretical context of the identity statuses, self-esteem ought to refer to the similarity experienced between one's personal attributes and one's ego ideal standards, a match that should improve in adolescence as the unrealistically high goals of childhood introjects are modified (Blos, 1962; Josselson, 1980; Marcia, 1983). The identity formation process of questioning, exploration, and commitment is central to this modification. Foreclosures, who have not undergone the differentiation process, should have unrealistically high ego ideals and correspondingly low self-esteem. Identity Achievement persons should have a more realistically reconstructed ego ideal and higher resultant self-esteem. Some evidence for this description was found in Foreclosures' tendency to maintain and even raise their goals in the face of failures on a concept attainment task (Marcia, 1966) and their tendency toward underachievement (Berzonsky, 1985; Hummel & Roselli, 1983; Streitmatter, 1989). However, a definitive answer to the identity-self-esteem relationship awaits the construction of a more theoretically relevant measure.

[1] On a number of variables an Achievement-Foreclosure grouping emerges for women, contrasted with the expected Achievement-Moratorium grouping. This result seems due to social–historical factors, described in the Gender Differences section of this chapter.

Independence of External Pressure

Locus of Control

Locus of control refers to one's assignment of responsibility for what befalls oneself either to an external (luck, fate) or an internal source (Rotter, 1966). Because they have undergone a self-constructive identity formation process, individuals high in identity (Achievements and Moratoriums) are expected to be more internal, and Foreclosures and Diffusions are expected to have a more external orientation. These results were found for men (C.K. Waterman et al., 1970), for women (Howard, 1975), and for men and women (Dellas & Jernigan, 1987). Matteson (1974), studying Danish youths, found no differences on this variable. Ginsburg and Orlofsky (1981) and Adams and Shea (1979) found Achievement and Foreclosure women to be somewhat more internal than the other statuses. Matteson (personal communication) suggests that the Foreclosures' apparent internal orientation reported here may be due to socially desirable responding. In summary, Achievements tend to have an internal locus of control and Diffusions are external; the placement of Moratoriums and Foreclosures is intermediate, and their relative positions are variable.

Autonomy

Studying autonomy and self-directedness in males, Orlofsky et al. (1973) found Foreclosures to be lowest, and Matteson (1974) found both Foreclosures and Diffusions to be low. Similarly, C.K. Waterman and Waterman (1975) and Waterman and Goldman (1976) described Foreclosure men as reliant on their families for making life decisions, and Andrews (1973) reported male subjects high in identity to be independent and achieving, contrasted with low identity subjects' more passive, affective stance. Chapman and Nicholls (1976), studying New Zealand boys, reported the highest field independence among Achievements. Schenkel (1975) found Identity Achievement and Foreclosure women to be the most field independent of the statuses. Among men, then, it appears that Foreclosures and Diffusions are the least autonomous, but among women there is evidence for a high autonomy pattern for both Achievements and Foreclosures.

Change in Self-Esteem and Conformity

A direct way of looking at resistance to external pressure is to create social pressure experimentally and observe performance. This experiment was done in the first studies by Marcia (1966, 1967), described in Chapter 1. Toder and Marcia (1973), studying conformity in college women using an Asch type of task, demonstrated that Achievement persons conformed less and felt less discomfort than individuals in the other statuses. Foreclosure, not Moratorium, women were similar in their nonconformity to Achievements. Adams et al. (1984), though not directly replicating the Marcia and Toder study, did find among college men and women a greater tendency for Diffusions than for the other statuses to conform on a social peer-pressure measure. In summary, Identity Achievement individuals seem resistant to external pressures, and Diffusions are more compliant.

Ego Development

Loevinger and Wessler's (1970) measure of ego development describes progressively differentiated levels of "frameworks of meaning which one subjectively imposes on experience" (Hauser, 1976, p. 930). Individuals are categorized according to three levels of ego organization: Preconformist (impulsive to self-protective); Conformist (conformist to conscientious); and Post-conformist (autonomous to integrative). Contrasted with Erikson's psychosocial scheme, Loevinger's ego developmental theory is more general, refers more to underlying psychological structure, and is less specifically related to life-cycle stages. Loevinger's and Erikson's developmental notions have in common Werner's (1957) proposals of progressive differentiation, internalization, and hierarchical integration of ego functions.

The hypothesis that a certain level of ego development may be a necessary condition for identity formation and that this successful resolution should then contribute to further ego development was tested by Adams and Fitch (1981; 1982) in both cross-lag and cross-sequential design studies. Although they found a significant positive relationship between the two constructs, they were unable to demonstrate any causal connections. Another study confirming this relationship was that of Adams and Shea (1979), who found that among college males and females Achievements were at higher levels of ego development, that they were the only identity status present at the highest Post-Conformist (integrated) level, and that they never fell below the autonomous level. Also, Ginsburg and Orlofsky (1981), in a study of college women, found that Achievements and Moratoriums were located more frequently in the Post-Conformist stages, but Foreclosures and Diffusions tended to be Conformist and Pre-Conformist. Newman (1986), studying young noncollege women in an urban shelter, found a significant relationship between overall identity development and Loevinger's ego development. In summary, a positive relationship between identity status and ego development is well established; the exact nature of the relationship between the two and between the ego developmental stages and the psychosocial stages in general remains to be explicated.

One behavioral area in which to observe effects of ego development is impulse control—specifically, substance abuse. An investigation of nonprescription drug use in college showed that Foreclosures were predominant in, and Moratoriums notably absent from, the category of "adamant non-drug-user" (Dufresne and Cross, 1972), a finding consistent with Matteson's (1978) description of Danish Identity Achievement and Moratorium youths as freer in impulse expression than Foreclosures. Pack et al. (1976) reported a relationship between identity commitment (Achievement and Foreclosure) and the ability to stop using marijuana. Jones and Hartmann (1988), investigating the relationship between drug use and identity development in high school students, found Diffuse persons to be the most frequent users, Foreclosures least frequent, and Achievements and Moratoriums intermediate.

Cognitive Performance and Cognitive Style

An increment to ego strength in the form of a positive resolution of a psychosocial developmental stage such as identity should positively affect primary ego functions such as ability to think and plan. Hence, it was thought that the identity statuses should differ in measures of cognitive performance. A necessary precondition for investigating this relationship was the establishment of no significant differences among the identity statuses in general intelligence (Bob, 1968; Cross & Allan, 1970; Marcia, 1966; Marcia & Friedman, 1970; and Schenkel, 1975).

After Marcia's (1966) initial findings of a positive relationship between identity and cognitive performance under stress, Bob (1968), also studying college males, stated that as a cognitive task became more difficult, Foreclosures became cognitively constricted and Diffusions tended to withdraw. Waterman and Waterman (1972) found that Identity Achievement college students had better study habits than other statuses; unsurprisingly, Cross and Allen (1970) found them to have higher grade-point averages; and, finally, in an initial study on women's identity development, Marcia and Friedman (1970) reported that Achievements chose the most difficult, and Diffusions the least difficult, college majors. Similarly, studying high school girls, Raphael (1977) reported that Achievements had the highest grade-point averages.

Perhaps a more important issue than cognitive performance is cognitive style, the way in which one approaches cognitive tasks. One variable is the degree of complexity a person displays. Côté and Reker (1979) found that among college men the "unstable" statuses of Diffusion and Moratorium had more complex cognitive systems than did the "stable" Achievement status. (There were no Foreclosures in this study.) Likewise, Kirby (1977) found Foreclosures to be cognitively simple and Diffusions more complex. Tzuriel and Klein (1977), studying Israeli settlers, reported a curvilinear relationship between identity and complexity: high identity was associated with moderate complexity; low identity was related to either high or low complexity. Extrapolating somewhat from these three studies, it appears that Achievements and Moratoriums are moderately complex cognitively; Foreclosures are relatively simple cognitively; and Diffusions are extremely complex, some of them, perhaps, disorganized. Attempting to be more precise about the issue of cognitive approach, Berzonsky and Niemeyer (1988), using Kelly's (1955) Role Repertory Grid, have identified different information-processing styles among the identity statuses (e.g., Achievements as information-oriented and self-exploring foreclosures as normative, and Diffusions as diffuse and ad hoc).[2]

Another aspect of cognitive style is an attribute that could be described as thoughtfulness or creativity, one's ability and willingness to go beneath the surface of things and perhaps to come up with new ideas or syntheses. The following studies considered this depth or openness quality of cognitive style. Waterman et al. (1974) and Waterman and Goldman (1976) reported that college students high in identity were more culturally sophisticated than those low in identity; and Waterman et al. (1977) and Waterman and Archer (1979) found that high identity males and females in high school and college were more frequent poetry writers than low identity persons. This tendency for high identity persons to be more creative has been attributed by Gombosi (1972) and by Bilsker and Marcia (1991) to their capacity for adaptive regression. Studying college males, C.K. Waterman and Waterman (1974) reported that Achievement and Moratorium persons, compared with Foreclosures and Diffusions, were more reflective than impulsive; a finding replicated by Shain and Farber (1989) studying college women. Finally, Tesch and Cameron (1987), extending the study of identity development into young adulthood, remarked that openness to experience correlated positively with identity exploration (Moratorium-like), and negatively with intense commitment (Foreclosure-like).

Formal Operational Thinking and Identity Development

The possibility that attaining formal operational thought is either a condition necessary for, or an accompaniment of, identity resolution has been suggested by Chandler (1987), Erikson (1952), Marcia (1980), and Kohlberg and Gilligan (1972), who stated: "... the relativistic questioning of conventional morality and conventional reality associated with logical and moral stage development is also central to the adolescent's

[2] Recently, a very promising research area concerning decision-making and information-processing styles characteristic of the identity statues has expanded considerably (Berzonsky, 1988, 1989, 1990; Berzonsky, Rice, & Niemeyer, 1990 Berzonsky & Sullivan, 1992; Blustein & Phillips, 1990; Neimeyer & Rareshide, 1991).

identity concerns" (p. 171). On the other hand, Blasi and Hoeffel (1974) have argued persuasively against this position; they are supported by Berzonsky and Barclay (1981) and Kurfiss (1981).

The preponderance of evidence supports an intermediate position. Wagner (1987), studying college males and females, found a positive relationship between one of two measures of formal operations and one of two measures of identity. Rowe and Marcia (1980) obtained a positive relationship between identity and formal operations with college males and females; however, their study included only three Achievements. Finally, Leadbetter and Dionne (1981) reported a positive relationship between the two variables among male high school students. Among those who have failed to confirm such a relationship are Afrifah (1980), Berzonsky et al. (1975), Cauble (1976), and Leiper (1981). Clearly, the strong case for the identity–formal operations relationship, that the latter is a necessary condition for the former, cannot be supported.

As one moves from physical–mathematical indices of formal operational thought to social–moral ones, the picture changes. Using a broader, more socially oriented measure of cognitive sophistication, integrative complexity, Slugoski et al. (1984) found that, among college males, Achievements and Moratoriums were clearly more cognitively advanced than Foreclosures and Diffusions, with Moratoriums scoring higher than Achievements. Boyes and Chandler (1992), employing a measure of levels of skeptical doubt, found that high identity high school students were at more sophisticated levels than low identity students.

In development of moral thought, assumed to depend upon levels of cognitive development (Kohlberg, 1976), the theoretical link with identity is clear and the empirical relationship is well established. Both identity and moral reasoning are assumed to involve the cognitive developmental processes of disequilibration (questioning, exploration) and accommodation (resolution, commitment). Only one study (Cauble, 1975) has not found a relationship between identity and levels of moral reasoning. Among those who have demonstrated this relationship are Lieper (1981) and Podd (1972) with college males; Hult (1979) and Poppen (1974) with women; and Rowe and Marcia (1980) with college men and women. Interestingly, like the Slugoski et al. (1984) study, Moratoriums frequently score more highly than Achievements. Skoe and Marcia (1991) have extended these findings to include the establishment of a relationship between identity in women and "care-based" moral developmental thought as described by Carol Gilligan (1982). Among these college women, the relationship between the care-based measure and identity was greater than was that between the justice-based measure and identity.

Using non-Piagetian measures of moral development, Hogan (1973) found high identity individuals to be more empathic, ethical, and socialized than low identity persons. Simmons (1985), using the IAS (see Chapter 1), reported that persons high in identity were more compassionate and had a more balanced concern both for their own freedom and for the well-being of others than did low identity persons.

Interactive Styles

The foregoing sections dealt primarily with those personality characteristics of the identity statuses reflecting internalization of self-regulatory processes. This portion reviews studies describing the ways in which different identity status individuals interact with their peers and how they are perceived by them.

In a study of patterns of cooperation and competition in a Prisoner's Dilemma game, Podd et al. (1970) reported that Moratoriums emerged as the distinctive group, displaying less cooperation with an authority opponent than with a peer, yet matching their opponents' responses more than the other statuses—seen as a Moratorium tendency toward both rebellion and conformity. Adams et al. (1987) wrote that adolescents in the higher identity statuses were less self-conscious than those in lower statuses. Read et al. (1984), studying identity status and social influence style among college women, found that Foreclosure women perceived themselves as less analytic, less philosophical, and less able to integrate ideas from multiple perspectives. Behaviorally, they were the most interpersonally manipulative (least self-revealing), and, together with Diffusions, most likely to use bribes and deception to exert social influence. Achievement and Moratorium women said that they enjoyed being alone with their own thoughts and that they were able to process extensive stimulus information. Interacting with others, they used more direct, assertive social influence techniques, thus risking social disapproval. Among college men, Slugoski et al. (1984) stated that Foreclosures displayed two predominant styles in small-group discussions of moral issues: aggressive assertion or submissive compliance. Both strategies were viewed as their defenses against changing preformed opinions. Clinical psychology graduate students who were Identity Achievement were found to have more facilitating counseling styles than non-Achievements (Genthner & Neuber, 1975; Neuber & Genthner, 1977). Finally, Goldman et al. (1980) solicited reactions to persons described according to their identity status. Achievements and Moratoriums were most liked, and seen as intelligent, knowledgeable, and well adjusted. (They also reported more satisfaction with peer support in a study by Caldwell et al., 1989). Diffusions were least liked, and generally evaluated lowest. Subjects who were themselves non-Diffusions preferred identity-committed targets, but Diffusions preferred noncommitted targets. The authors wrote: "If you have undergone a crisis, you are judged by all as being more likeable, intelligent, knowledgeable, and adjusted" (p. 161).

Two persons have completed noteworthy descriptive studies of identity statuses' interactional style: James Donovan (1970; 1975) and Ruthellen Josselson (1972; 1973; 1988). Both investigators used the results of a number of psychodynamic-based measures as well as classroom and interview observations to describe their subjects. Because no brief summary could do justice to the richness of these descriptive presentations, we recommend the original material. Of special interest is Josselson's (1988) book describing, longitudinally, women's pathways of identity development, with much-needed emphasis on the connection as well as the separation component of individuation.

Developmental Aspects of the Identity Statuses

The greatest volume of research since Marcia's (1980) literature review has considered developmental issues and a chapter in this book is devoted to this subject. It is to be expected that, in the course of establishing construct validity, once concurrent and predictive validity are ascertained, antecedent and consequent conditions can be determined.

Two studies investigating age boundaries of initial identity resolution are those of Meilman (1979) and Archer (1982). Meilman, studying males in age groups from 12 to 24 found no Achievements or Moratoriums among 12-year-olds and only 4 percent among 15-year-olds. The appearance of significant numbers of Achievements and Moratoriums began at age 18 and increased until age 24, with a corresponding decrease in Foreclosures and Diffusions throughout this age span. The most noticeable change from lower to higher identity statuses occurred around age 21–22. Archer investigated change in identity status in specific interview domains among 11- to 17-year-old boys and girls. She found 19 percent Achievements and Moratoriums among 17-year-olds, corresponding closely to Meilman's 24 percent among 18-year-olds. The occupational domain was the area in which most junior and senior high school students were Identity Achieved. Raphael (1975) reported no high school senior females in the Identity Achievement status. The conclusion that may be drawn from these studies is that when the overall identity status category system is used, Moratoriums and Achievements do not appear much before the senior year in high school, although persons may be high in identity in specific domains. Also, if one uses a continuous scale of identity development such as the EOM-EIS (see Chapter 1), scores can be obtained for all statuses beginning in junior high school (see, e.g., Jones & Streitmatter, 1987; Streitmatter, 1989). Matteson (personal communication) states that the age boundaries cited above might not hold across socioeconomic settings (e.g., in areas where future college attendance was not a reasonable expectation).

Childhood Antecedents

The relationship between identity formation at late adolescence and the resolution of prior psychosocial stages has been the subject of a number of studies, most of them using either Constantinople's (1969) or Rasmussen's (1964) measure. In general, positive relationships have been found between earlier stage resolution and subsequent identity formation with Identity Achievements showing most, and Diffusions showing the fewest, positive resolutions of previous stages (Waterman, 1982).

Contrasting with the psychosocial approach are the studies of several researchers who have investigated more psychoanalytic-based concepts. Josselson (1982) found that Moratorium and Achievement women reported early memories at the highest psychosexual developmental level (post-oedipal and blended memories) and that Foreclosures and Diffusions reported memories at lower levels (pre-oedipal and oedipal). These findings were replicated in a study with an improved design by Orlofsky and Frank (1986), who reported that among college males and females, Achievements and Moratoriums again had more blended or integrated (early plus later psychosexual stage) memory content than did Foreclosures and Diffusions. Early memories in both of these studies were treated as salient life-organizing themes, not as veridical accounts of events. Orlofsky and Frank's conclusion, that "mature identity resolution during late adolescence may be hindered by lack of resolution . . . of basic issues of nurturance and security" (p. 20) was echoed in two studies by Kroger on attachment style among the identity statuses (1985, 1988). Attachment style refers to the nature of resolution of the separation–individuation phase of early childhood development as described by Bowlby (1969) and Mahler et al. (1975). Studying male and female college students in New Zealand, Kroger found high identity persons to be more secure and less anxiously attached than those in low identity statuses, and that the identity attachment relationship was, in general, maintained over a two-year period. Interpreting Early Memory findings as reflecting ego structuralization in adolescence, Kroger (1990) supported the results of Josselson and Orlofsky and Frank. She found that Achievements' themes involved moving alone contentedly or alongside others; Moratoriums spoke of moving against others; Foreclosures sought security and support; and Diffusions' themes were marked by a desire for relatedness.

Middle and Late Adolescence

Family Characteristics

Family studies on identity statuses have not been longitudinal; rather, they have consisted of current perceptions of past and present family interactions, or direct measures of present family interactions; hence, it is difficult to make valid causal statements. Bearing this caveat in mind, we summarize how individuals in different identity statuses characterize their families (see Marcia, 1980; Waterman, 1982; and Chapter 3 in the present book). Foreclosures report their families as close, loving, and child-centered, with encouragement to conform to family values. Diffusions see their families as somewhat distant and rejecting; in particular, they see their same-sexed parent (whom they may admire greatly [Cella et al., 1987]) as nonaccepting and nonemulatable. Moratoriums are ambivalent about their parents and are engaged in push-pull oedipal battles, attempting to please while struggling for autonomy. Achievements have families who support their differentiation and with whom they can maintain rapprochement; the ambivalence of the Moratorium period seems to have given way to mutuality, to a balanced and realistic appraisal of similarities and differences, likes, and dislikes.

Two noteworthy findings on parent variables pertain to the father's role in identity development and the equivocal effects of parental separation and absence. Father variables seem especially important in identity formation for both males and females (Bary, 1978; Enright et al., 1980; Kendis & Tan, 1978; and LaVoie, 1976). This finding bears somewhat on the importance of masculine values for identity formation (see the Sex Roles portion of this chapter). On parental separation, early studies showed that father absence (Oshman & Manosevitz, 1974) and broken homes (Jordan, 1970) were related to Identity Diffusion. More recent research suggests, however, that for high school girls high identity is positively related to being in a single-parent home (St. Clair & Day, 1979), and among college males is associated with parental divorce (Grossman et al., 1980). The effects of parental separation on identity formation are not simple, and specific determination is likely to involve research as complex as that undertaken by Grotevant and Cooper.

These investigators, studying patterns of family interaction and their effects on adolescent identity formation via a direct, observational method, have contributed the following insights into identity formation: (a) Both connectedness to and separateness from family (individuation) are important (see also Kamptner, 1988); (b) Differentiation between father and mother contributes to successful identity development of offspring; and, (c) Father–son interaction is important for boys' identity, and all family interactions are important for girls' identity (Cooper et al., 1983; Grotevant & Cooper, 1983, 1985, 1986). In partial support of these findings, Campbell et al. (1984) reported that Diffusions were least attached to parents; among Achievements and Moratoriums, mother factors (especially a moderate level of affection) were important for connectedness, and father factors (especially reasonable independence from) were important for individuality (see also Papini et al., 1989); and, finally, high connectedness and low independence characterized Foreclosures, but low connectedness and moderate or low independence was characteristic of Diffusions. Similarly, in an observational study in Holland, Bosma and Gerrits (1985) reported that Achievement adolescents and their families discussed issues more actively than did Foreclosure and Diffusion families, supporting an earlier finding of Matteson's (1974) in Denmark that Achievements, contrasted with Foreclosures and Diffusions, were more nearly equal participants in family decision making. Finally, Adams (1985) reported a positive relationship between parents' and daughters' identity status, interpreting it within a social-learning, symbolic-interactionist framework.

College

For three reasons, many identity status studies have used college populations: most researchers work in university settings; the age of identity resolution, around 18–22, is the age of most college students; and college is a definable social institution within which identity formation may be expected to take place. Seven longitudinal studies of identity development in college have been carried out (Adams & Fitch, 1982; Costa & Campos, 1988; Dellas & Jernigan, 1987; Kroger, 1988; Kroger & Haslett, 1987; Waterman et al., 1974; and Waterman & Goldman, 1976). These studies are discussed in more detail in the chapter on development. Very general conclusions are that Moratoriums tend to be the most unstable status (except in the Dellas & Jernigan study) and most of them become Identity Achievement in their later college years. About 50 percent of subjects change their identity status from the freshman to the senior year, the general direction being toward the higher identity statuses. In addition, there is a strong suggestion from the majority of these researchers, following the initial emphasis on this point by Waterman, that longitudinal investigations of identity development proceed by separate domains, rather than by overall identity status.

The effects of college environment on identity development have been examined in two studies. Adams and Fitch (1983) reported committed (Achievement and Foreclosure) males and females to be in departments having high scholastic emphasis (echoing Marcia & Friedman, 1972), with females considering especially the employment opportunities associated with a particular department. Once in a department, that department's emphasis on social awareness appeared to facilitate identity stability and development for both men and women; in the absence of this emphasis, both sexes regressed in identity status. In Portugal, Costa and Campos (1986) found more high identity persons in the faculties of Law and Arts, and more Foreclosures in Engineering and Medicine. They attributed these differences to opportunities in the former faculties for discussion (and possible disequilibration) and the emphasis in the latter faculties on rote memory.

Examining differential effects of the college experience on the identity statuses, Waterman and Waterman (1970) reported that individuals who were Moratorium in the occupational domain were the most dissatisfied with their college experience, and occupational Foreclosures were the most satisfied. In another study, Waterman and Waterman (1972) wrote that Moratoriums changed college major more frequently than did other statuses. Also, among college-leavers, Achievements did so for self-initiated reasons but Foreclosures and Diffusions left in the face of negative external pressure (e.g., low grades). Rothman (1984) stated that Achievements and Foreclosures tended to be goal-oriented, but Diffusions got caught up in trivial obsessive-compulsive routines.

Non-College Youths

In two studies of identity development in noncollege settings, both Munro and Adams (1977) and Morash (1980) found more Achievements among working than among college youths. These investigators attributed this difference to the absence of an institutionalized psychosocial moratorium and the subsequent pressure to make life decisions. In a longitudinal study controlling for socioeconomic, age, and geographical effects, however, Archer and Waterman (1988) found that individuals attending college were more advanced in identity formation than those who were working or who were combining college attendance with work. These studies and those cited immediately above point to the need for describing contexts in terms of factors that facilitate or hinder psychosocial development.

Adult Consequences of Initial Identity Formation

Intimacy

An assumption in Erikson's theory is that successful resolution of one psychosocial stage ought to affect directly the resolution of the next one. Hence, identity achievement should lead to successful resolution of the intimacy–isolation stage. All studies reviewed suggest that it does (Constantinople, 1969; Craig-Bray et al., 1988; Hodgson & Fischer, 1979; Kacerguis & Adams, 1980; Kahn et al., 1985; Kinsler, 1972; Schiedel & Marcia, 1985; and Tesch & Whitbourne, 1982). Several of these researchers report that identity appears to precede intimacy for men, as Erikson assumed, but that identity and intimacy appear to codevelop in women. A more thorough review of intimacy research is in Chapter 5 in this book.

Longitudinal Studies After Late Adolescence

Marcia (1976) reported that 43 percent of Achievement and Moratorium males interviewed six to seven years later were still in these same statuses, whereas 84 percent of Foreclosures and Diffusions remained in the low identity statuses. Josselson (1987, 1988), in her informative account of the histories of women interviewed first in college and then fifteen years later, also saw a tendency for Diffusion to persist. Kroger, in a series of studies (1986, 1988, unpublished ms., and Kroger & Haslett, 1987), has examined identity status transition pathways and change rates across interview domains.

Identity Statuses in Adulthood

Both Amstey (1977) and Archer, Waterman, & Owens (1988) found that adult women who had returned to college to complete their education were more frequently Achievement or Moratorium than Foreclosure. Archer (1985b) and Owens et al. (1987) concluded that both identity and intimacy generally increased with age (see also Freilino and Hummel, 1985) and early, *nonreflective* commitments tended to lead to subsequent disruptive life experiences among the statuses. (This finding may bode ill for the more numerous Foreclosure college marriages reported by Lutes [1981].) In addition, Identity Achievement women had liberated ideas about women's role and were high in masculinity; Moratorium women expressed some dissatisfaction with marriage; Foreclosures were traditional in attitudes toward women's role and high in femininity; and Diffusion women were high in masculinity and generally dissatisfied with marriage and parenting.

Identity Development in Adulthood

Having formed an initial identity at late adolescence (Identity Achievement), an individual might be expected to undergo subsequent Moratorium-Achievement (MAMA) cycles. As is clear in Marcia's (1976) follow-up study, however, not all adults do so. Some proceed through adulthood with their initial identity resolution unreconstructed and seem like Foreclosures. Studying identity development in adulthood, Whitbourne (1986) found that "openness to experience" predicted identity flexibility in adult men and women. Thinking along similar lines, Stephen et al. (1992) described two variables thought to predict to life-span identity development: dialectical reasoning and an experiential (as opposed to instrumental) outlook. Among university students, Moratoriums and Achievements tended to have a more experiential outlook and to be higher in dialecticism than Foreclosures and Diffusions. Significantly, Moratoriums were the highest of the statuses on both of these measures. Whether or not these variables will predict for adult development remains to be seen.

Gender Differences in Identity Formation

Content Areas of the Identity Status Interview

The foremost issue here is whether or not men and women differ in the relative importance of interview domains to their identity formation, and, specifically, whether interpersonal issues are more important to women's identity formation than to men's. That they are important to women has been established by Archer (1985a), Kroger (1983), Marcia and Friedman (1970), Schenkel and Marcia (1972), and Josselson, (1988). That interpersonal concerns may be more important for women's identity than for men's is suggested by a fairly impressive number of studies (Archer, 1989c; Bilsker et al., 1988; Craig-Bray et al., 1988; Douvan & Adelson, 1966; Hodgson & Fischer, 1979; Josselson et al., 1977b; Kahn et al., 1985; Mellor, 1989; Poppen, 1974; Thorbecke & Grotevant, 1982; and C.K. Waterman & Nevid, 1977). The foregoing does not mean, however, that interpersonal issues are not important for men's identity (Matteson, 1977; Mellor, 1989; and Rogow et al., 1983). In his summary Mellor (1989) states: "[There may be] a connectedness theme in self–other development that is nonspecific to gender and that is useful for both males and females in generating relational self-definitions to resolve the identity crisis" (p. 372). Likewise, that interpersonal issues seem to have some predominance for women's identity formation does not mean that occupational and ideological issues are not important to them. Hopkins (1980, 1982), having constructed an "inner-space" interview to assess women's identity, had to conclude: "It is very clear from the present study that outer space concerns are no longer peripheral to female identity formation" (1982, p. 565). Confirming this result, Kroger (1986) found occupation to be the most highly ranked issue in importance for both male and female New Zealand university students, as did Bilsker et al. (1988) among a similar group in Canada. Although Archer (1989c) found more Foreclosures among men than women (more women tending toward Achievement and Moratorium, especially in the family roles domain), she found few other gender differences in process, domain, or timing. Hence, Marcia's (1980) hypothesis that women's identity formation, because of its complexity, might take longer than men's was not supported. In fact, as Adams and Gulotta (1983) suggested and Streitmatter (1988) demonstrated, females may be chronologically ahead of males in the identity formation process. Following are, perhaps, the best summaries of this research to date. On women's identity development, Kroger (1983) states: "Rather than decisions about individual content areas, meta-decisions about how to balance competing identity contents and at the same time consider the implications for significant others seemed to capture identity concerns for many women from this sample"

(p. 15). Investigating gender differences in identity development in high school students, Thorbecke and Grotevant (1982) concluded, "... it appears that for young men, vocational and interpersonal identity achievement proceed independently.... For young women, it appears important to negotiate identity achievement in the interpersonal domain in order to be engaged in occupational identity formation" (pp. 488–489).

The Meaning of the Identity Statuses for Men and Women

Based upon many of the studies reviewed by Marcia (1980), it appeared that Foreclosure women were performing quite similarly to Identity Achievement women on a number of dependent variables. This finding led to the possibility that the Foreclosure status might have some adaptive significance for women that it did not have for men. From the perspective of ten more years of research, however, it appears that the earlier conclusions were erroneous. Out of eight studies with women conducted before 1977 in which a grouping of statuses could be ascertained, seven showed the Achievement-Foreclosure, Moratorium-Diffusion pattern. Since 1977, out of sixteen studies with discernible patterns, only four show the earlier grouping; the remaining twelve conform to theoretical expectations underlying the identity statuses. Of the two explanations for this change in pattern, the first is articulated by Orlofsky and Ginsburg (1981): "If Moratorium women are in fact developing beyond the conventional adjustment attained by Foreclosure women, we would expect them to excel on measures which go deeper than the surface level of functioning assessed by self-report and behavioral measures utilized in previous studies" (p. 299). When such "deeper," ego-structural measures are used, Moratorium women do perform positively, like Achievement women (Adams & Shea, 1979; Ginsburg & Orlofsky, 1981; Kroger, 1988; Orlofsky & Frank, 1986; and Josselson, 1982).

The second reason for changes in status ordering has to do with changes in social conditions: there has been a pattern of increasing support for women undergoing the choice and struggle involved in the identity development process (Morgan & Farber, 1982). Identity research has not been isolated from the concerns of feminism. Stein and Weston (1982) found non-Traditional women to be more advanced in identity than Traditional women; and Prince-Embury and Deutchman (1981) reported that pro-ERA (Equal Rights Amendment) women scored higher on an identity measure than anti-ERA women. One variable in particular, fear of success, highlights the impact of social values on women's identity development. Studying college women, Howard (1975) found Identity Achievements' greater fear of success compared with the other statuses. In a definitive study on this variable, Orlofsky (1978b), comparing college men and women, found that Identity Achievement and Moratorium women had higher achievement scores than did Foreclosures and Diffusions and also greater fear of success. He concluded:

> . . . the high Fear of Success scores obtained by Achievement and especially Moratorium women are understandable as reflecting the conflicts which these more ambitious achieving women probably experience as they pursue . . . less traditional, more achievement-oriented goals. Since Foreclosure and Diffusion women are less motivated for academic vocational achievement, they experience less conflict between achievement strivings and traditional feminine role behaviors. . . . (p. 60)

The effects of growing social support for women's achievement and identity formation is indicated in the post-1978 studies on fear of success by Freilino and Hummel (1985), who found Diffusion women to have the greatest fear of success, and Owens, et al. (unpublished ms.), who found a negative relationship between identity achievement and fear of success.

In summary, whether because of more sophisticated measurement or for sociopolitical reasons, or both, the issue of the grouping of the identity statuses for women is no longer problematical. Moratorium women resemble more closely Identity Achievement women than they do Foreclosure women. Also, even though the genders may arrive at identity via somewhat different pathways, the meaning of the identity statuses, as reflected in gender x status standings on dependent variables, seems similar. As Archer and Waterman (1988) conclude in an article on psychological individualism summarizing gender differences in sixteen identity studies: "Taken together, the results do not warrant concluding that gender differences exist with respect to this [identity] variable" (p. 69).

Sex Roles and Identity

Although one's gender is a given with which one must come to terms in constructing an identity, the degree to which one subscribes to the roles and values socially assigned to one's gender varies. Hence, one can be morphologically male, yet masculine, feminine, androgynous, or undifferentiated in endorsement of sex-role attitudes. The following group of studies take up the differential effects of sex-role subscription on identity and intimacy development.

The first studies in this area were by Deldin (1977), who found masculinity important for identity formation in college males, and Orlofsky (1977), who reported masculinity and androgyny important for Identity Achievement in both college men and women and sex-role undifferentiated persons to be Diffuse. Schiedel and Marcia (1985) replicated and extended these findings. They report that masculinity was important for identity development, especially for women, and that femininity was important for intimacy development, especially for men. Androgynous persons tended to be high in both identity and intimacy. Studies using the identity statuses and other identity measures and various sex-role inventories have replicated the results above (Crown, 1985; Della Selva & Dusek, 1984; Fannin, 1979; Grotevant & Thorbecke, 1982; Tzuriel, 1984; and Waterman & Whitbourne, 1982a). Except for Lamke and Peyton (1988), who found only weak support in a study of high school students, across various measures of identity, intimacy, and sex-role typing, the relationships among androgyny, high intimacy, and high identity, as well as between masculinity and identity and femininity and intimacy are fairly well established.

Cross-Cultural Research

Two emphases are discernible in the cross-cultural studies reviewed. The first is the establishment of validity for the identity statuses (and, by extension, Erikson's theoretical concept) in societies other than that

TABLE 2.1. Cross-cultural studies on identity.

Author(s)	Sample	Description
Matteson, 1974	Denmark	Family interaction
Chapman & Nicholls, 1976	New Zealand	Maori and Pakeha boys
Jegede, 1976	Nigeria	Comparative IAS scores
Muto, 1979	Japan	Validation of ISI
Kumar et al., 1980	India	Managerial styles
Afrifah, 1980	Ghana	Formal operations
Arora, 1981	India	Marital dyads
Bosma, Graafsma, 1982, et al.[A]	Holland	Development and GIDS
Kato, 1983	Japan	Validation of ISI
Kroger, 1983, et al.	New Zealand	ISI, personality
Huh, 1984	South Korea	ISI domain importance
Owen, 1984	Cuban-American	ISI, IPD, self-esteem
Park, 1984	South Korea	Religiosity
Rall, 1984	South Africa	Identity-intimacy
Abraham, 1986	Mexican-American	Comparative patterns
Costa, Campos, 1986, et al.	Portugal	Identity contexts
Streitmatter, 1988	Hispanic, Native American, Asian	Comparative
Phinney, 1989, et al.	Black, Hispanic, Asian-Americans	Comparative
Rotheram-Borus, 1989	Black, Puerto Rican, Filipino	Comparative
Mohammed, 1990	Egypt	Validation of ISI
Mayeseless, 1990	Israel	Identity in army
Flum, 1990	Israel	High school identity

[A] Et al. following a date, as here: "1982, et al." means that the same author(s) have produced, similar works.

of North America. Validity, here, does not mean identical behavior. Foreclosures in a "foreclosed" setting ought not to be found behaving exactly like Foreclosures in a setting that encourages moratoria. Rather, cross-cultural validity means that, taking into account the processes underlying an identity status, one ought to be able to make verifiable predictions about that status's behavior in a given cultural context. The second emphasis has been on extending our knowledge about identity development itself. Most of these studies are reviewed in the foregoing text. Table 2.1 lists studies involving other than Caucasian, North American populations. We recommend the original sources, for a review would be too lengthy for this chapter.

3
Developmental Perspectives on Identity Formation: From Adolescence to Adulthood

ALAN S. WATERMAN[1]

The construct of ego identity was introduced and elaborated within an explicitly developmental framework (Erikson, 1959, 1963, 1968). It is therefore not surprising that one of the earlier directions of research work on identity was an assessment of its changes over the life span. Because Erikson's conceptualization of identity was formulated for clinical analysis, however, whether of individuals or of cultures, he did not delineate readily testable hypotheses about identity formation. This chapter, therefore, is intended to provide a theoretical analysis of the nature of identity formation, including the direction and timing of development, sex differences, and antecedents of change, and to review research data that bear on developmental hypotheses.

Developmental Hypotheses

The Direction and Timing of Development

At its simplest, the basic hypothesis of identity development is that the transition from adolescence to adulthood involves progressive strengthening in the sense of identity. Because the identity status interview developed by Marcia (1966) involves categorizing individuals according to their strategy for handling the task of identity formation and does not yield a continuous measure, more complex developmental patterns can be identified. A schematic presentation of the pathways of identity status formation consistent with Erikson's theory is given in Figure 3.1.

A person who is in the Identity Diffusion status may (a) become a Moratorium by beginning to seriously explore a variety of identity alternatives (D $\rightarrow$ M); (b) become a Foreclosure by latching on to the

[1]This chapter is an updated version of an article originally published as Waterman, A.S. (1982). Identity development from adolescence to adulthood: An extension of theory and a review of research. *Developmental Psychology*, *18*, 342–358. Copyright 1982 by the American Psychological Association. Adapted by permission of the publisher.

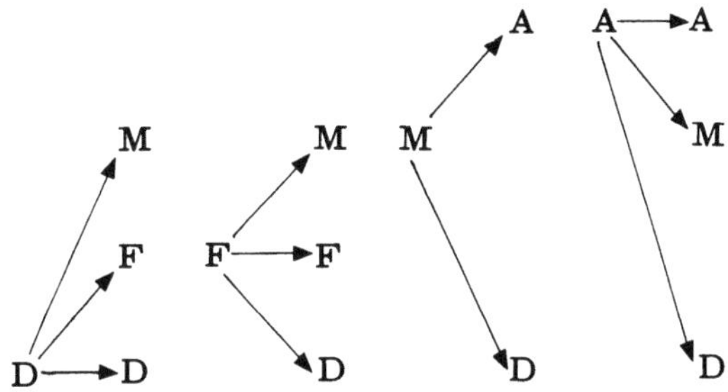

FIGURE 3.1. A model of the sequential patterns of ego identity development (D = Identity Diffusion; F = Foreclosure; M = Moratorium; A = Identity Achievement).

first real possibility that is presented, without ever evaluating other courses of action (D → F); or (c) continue indefinitely in the Diffusion status, never making a serious effort to work out identity issues (D → D).

A person who is in the Foreclosure status may (a) become a Moratorium if the early commitments are challenged in a way that requires considering alternative possibilities (F → M); (b) continue as a Foreclosure, carrying into adulthood commitments to the goals and values that were developed prior to or during adolescence (F → F); or (c) become an Identity Diffusion if the initial commitments gradually become less meaningful without steps being taken to revise or replace them (F → D).

A person who has entered the Moratorium status may (a) become an Identity Achiever by establishing firm, meaningful commitments to specific goals and values (M → A); or (b) become an Identity Diffusion by giving up on efforts to find something worthwhile to which to become committed (M → D).[2]

A person who has become an Identity Achiever may (a) continue as an Achiever, maintaining the commitments to the goals and values that were worked out during the identity crisis (A → A); (b) again become a Moratorium, reentering crisis if the earlier resolution proves unsatisfactory in some way (A → M); or (c) become an Identity Diffusion if the commitments that were established gradually lose their vitality without triggering a new crisis (A → D).

Of the changes in status just described, the following constitute progressive developmental shifts: from the Identity Diffusion status into either the Foreclosure or Moratorium statuses; from the Foreclosure into the

[2] Maintenance of the Moratorium status (M → M) is not included here because it is considered unlikely that an individual would continue indefinitely in an identity crisis. The level of anxiety associated with the lack of closure on personal goals, values, and beliefs makes it probable that the task of identity formation will eventually be put aside if the individual does not successfully resolve an identity crisis.

Moratorium status; and from the Moratorium into the Identity Achievement status. Each represents movement involving either initiation of reflective consideration of identity alternatives or development of personally meaningful commitments. A change into the Identity Diffusion status from any of the others can be considered developmentally regressive because it involves putting aside identity concerns, at least temporarily, without having established a satisfactory resolution. The shift from the Identity Achievement to the Moratorium status might more appropriately be considered the resumption of a crisis rather than a developmental regression. In this regard, Stephen, Fraser, and Marcia (1992) have referred to MAMA (Moratorium–Achievement–Moratorium–Achievement) cycles. Such cycles reflect continuation of the identity formation process; an attempt to make more rewarding choices, not a renunciation of identity concerns.

The model described above is descriptive rather than a theory of development because virtually no patterns of identity status change are inconsistent with it. The utility of the model rests in the opportunity it affords to study the relative frequency of the different developmental paths and the circumstances that influence their adoption. It thus becomes possible to compare the patterns of development among various groups within a population (and between populations) and to identify the influence of sociohistorical conditions on identity formation.

The basic hypothesis of identity development may now be phrased: Movement from adolescence to adulthood involves a preponderance of changes in identity status, which can be characterized as progressive developmental shifts.

On two questions related to the direction of identity development, little a priori work has been done. One is the relative stability of the various identity statuses. It can be anticipated that the Moratorium category will be the least stable of the statuses because it is associated with an expressed desire to make changes in one's life. Further, it is difficult for individuals to sustain the subjective discomfort usually associated with identity crises. If a successful resolution cannot be achieved, the person is likely to eventually renounce the task as unresolvable. However, which status will be the most stable is unclear. Both the Foreclosure and Identity Achievement statuses involve commitments, but the stability of either type of commitment may be influenced by a wide variety of life events. The lack of commitment characteristic of the Identity Diffusion status may or may not prove to be a relatively stable developmental quality. Further, it is possible that the relative stability of the various statuses will vary by the domain in which identity is considered.

The other question best approached empirically concerns the timing of identity changes. In discussing the epigenetic principle, Erikson (1959) refers not only to a proper sequence of stage development but also to a proper rate. Stage 5 in his theory can be assumed to cover much or all of the period from puberty through the college years. He does not, however, suggest a timetable for the ages at which particular identity issues are most likely to arise, become a focus of development, and reach eventual resolution. Wide individual differences in the timing of identity development may be expected, but it should be interesting to determine if characteristic times (or settings) are associated with the greatest probability of change.

Sex Differences in Identity Development

Because Erikson (1963, 1968, 1975) has written extensively on the differences in psychological functioning between the sexes, it might be expected that he would anticipate gender differences in the patterns of identity formation. Whether he intended such a hypothesis is questionable, however. Before addressing that issue, it will be helpful to look at the differences he does describe.

Working from his experiences with the play constructions of preadolescent participants in a long-term developmental study, Erikson (1963) discussed differences between the sexes in the real and symbolic use of space. He drew an association between the play constructions and anatomically based genital modes. Males, with external genital organs, erectable and intrusive, developed play constructions characterized by height and downfall, strong motion and its channelization or arrest. Females, with internal genital organs having vestibular access, constructed static interiors that were open, simply enclosed, and peaceful or intruded upon. Erikson did not, however, conclude that intrusion and enclosing were the exclusive prerogatives of males and females, respectively. Rather, he saw these differences as ones of "predisposition and predilection." He wrote that where cultural and historical conditions permit, each sex may be led "to make use of, to share, and at times to imitate, the configurations most typical of the other sex" (Erikson, 1975, p. 233).

The emphasis Erikson (1975) placed on the presence of anatomically based gender differences in behavior reflects an effort to counter the assertions some have made that *all* gender differences are learned. He has not postulated different developmental processes for males and females. Thus, although biological predispositions may be expected to play some role in the *content* of identity choices, they would not necessarily be involved in the *processes* by which identity elements are selected. Both genders may undergo comparable experiences of crisis and commitment. Any gender differences in the frequency of presence in the different identity statuses could be interpreted as a function of cultural influences, not as a result of the unfolding of different developmental capabilities.

Several hypotheses reflect the cultural influences on the identity development of males and females. Frieze et al. (1978) have described the role conflicts, role overload, and role changes that confront women in contemporary American society. Any of these aspects of role functioning may contribute to increased identity concerns. For women, a conflict is generally perceived between fulfilment of family responsibilities and career objectives, but such a conflict for men is not seen as occurring frequently. Thus, identity crises over the relative priorities to be assigned to family and career may be expected to occur more often for women than for men.

The current societal attention to gender-role issues has focused more on a changing role for women than for men. This emphasis may be reflected in an increased probability of women going through a Moratorium and becoming Identity Achievers in this area. Similarly, for identity questions relating to sexual expression, the sexual double standard, the risks of pregnancy, and such issues as birth control and abortion, all would tend to stimulate greater consideration of alternatives among women than men.

Two other areas of identity concern frequently studied are religious beliefs and political ideology. We offer no hypothesis about gender differences in either area. Although it has been assumed that women have had greater involvement in religion, and men in politics, it is doubtful that this preponderance holds true for recent generations.

Antecedent Conditions Relating to Identity Development

The choice of a developmental pathway for identity formation may be influenced by a variety of interrelated variables, including: (a) the extent of identification with the parents prior to and during adolescence; (b) the parenting style(s) with which the person has been reared; (c) the availability of model figures perceived as successful; (d) social expectations about identity choices arising within the family, the school, and the peer group; (e) the extent to which the person is exposed to a variety of identity alternatives; and (f) the extent to which the preadolescent personality provides an appropriate foundation for coping with identity concerns. These variables differ in importance and effect at different points in the developmental process. Next, we summarize the variables that may contribute to determining the course of development identity.

Identity at the Start of Adolescence

As adolescence begins, a person is likely to be in either the Foreclosure or the Identity Diffusion status. The presence of Foreclosure commitments is most likely to occur under circumstances where there is a strong identification with one or both parents and where the expectation has been strong that a child will follow family traditions about vocation, religion, politics, and so on. In such conditions, the Foreclosure status is the result of incorporating a parent's identity or aspirations as one's own.

However, if parents are dissatisfied with their work roles, do not practice their religion, or are apathetic about political issues, they are models for *not* having commitments. Identification will then result in increased likelihood that a son or daughter will be Diffuse rather than Foreclosed.

Parenting styles may also be expected to influence the initial identity status, perhaps because of differences in the expectations conveyed to children or because of effects on identification. Parents with an authoritarian style often have relatively specific aspirations for their children and the power they evidence in the household should facilitate identification. Thus, such parents should foster development of early Foreclosure commitments. (These commitments may prove to be unstable if the son or daughter later rebels against parental authority.) In contrast to authoritarian parents, those using permissive, neglecting, or rejecting techniques are likely to provide a context in which a child enters adolescence as an Identity Diffusion. Such parents neither serve as effective models nor do they expect their children to develop any particular goals, values, or beliefs.

It is unclear what effect a democratic parenting style may have on early identity development. The caring such parents evidence toward their children, and the psychological support they give, provide a good foundation for identification and hence for early development as a Foreclosure. Democratic parents, however, are likely to place only mild pressures on a son or daughter to adopt their life-style, undercutting the need to have early commitments. As a consequence, the child may develop early preferences and interests but feel that the act of decision can wait until later.

Beyond the family, the community in which a person lives should affect the initial phases of identity formation. If an individual lives in a homogeneous community with established traditions, the likelihood is greater that he or she will develop as Foreclosure. When one's friends and acquaintances come from similar backgrounds and seem headed in similar directions, it is easy to accept that this is the way things should be. If the shared community expectations are reinforced by the school system, the probability of early Foreclosure commitments is further increased. Thus, children who attend relatively homogeneous parochial schools or prep schools would be expected to be initial Foreclosures more frequently than children who attend the more heterogeneous public schools. The friends and acquaintances one develops in heterogeneous schools and communities represent a wider variety of life-styles and belief systems. When alternatives are seen as readily available, the preadolescent is less likely to feel certain about whether or not to follow the family's traditions and expectations. The result will be a somewhat higher probability of being an initial Diffusion.

Another probable determinant of a person's identity status at the start of adolescence is the personality structure that emerged during the early stages of development. According to the epigenetic principle discussed by

Erikson, children who have been reasonably successful in establishing the personality components associated with the first four stages in the life cycle (i.e., basic trust, autonomy, initiative, and industry), will have a firmer foundation for developing a sense of identity. In contrast, intense feelings of mistrust, shame and doubt, and so on generally preclude forming strong commitments about one's future. Thus, where early development has proceeded smoothly, individuals may initially be in either the Foreclosure or Identity Diffusion statuses, but under less fortunate circumstances, adolescents should fall predominantly into the Diffusion category.

The Initiation of Identity Crises

Some of the adolescents who initially are in the Foreclosure status will enter an identity crisis; others will remain stable. Similarly, some Diffusions will enter a crisis and others will not. Because the Foreclosure and Diffusion statuses differ in the presence of commitments, differences would be expected about the events that will precipitate a crisis.

Among initial Foreclosures, one of the most important determinants of entering a crisis or of continued stability is likely to be the extent to which the commitments formed early are accepted by peers, parents, and other adults. If the initial commitments are challenged, an identity crisis is the probable result. The confirmation or disconfirmation of the person's expectations about the chosen identity elements should be another influence on the likelihood of entering a crisis. For example, if one finds the work in one's chosen vocation to be substantially different from what had been anticipated, the resulting disillusionment may trigger an occupational identity crisis. A crisis may also be initiated if one's academic performance is not adequate to permit entry into the chosen field.

Even when the initial identity choices made by Foreclosures continue to be perceived as attractive, exposure to information about interesting alternative goals or beliefs never previously considered may bring about an identity crisis. The greater the exposure to new possibilities, the more likely it is that a person will reevaluate his or her original commitments. Thus, the probability of a crisis occurring should be higher among individuals from heterogeneous, cosmopolitan communities than for those from homogeneous communities; higher among those who attend college than among those who enter the work force directly from high school; and higher for those with a high level of curiosity and wide-ranging interests than for those whose interests run in a narrow range.

Although mere exposure to new ideas can move a Foreclosure into the Moratorium status, seeing one's friends and acquaintances undergoing such a crisis may exert an even more powerful effect through modeling. Further, if the adolescent comes to believe that an identity crisis is expected of someone of his or her generation, the result may be a self-fulfilling prophecy.

Family variables may also influence the probability with which a Foreclosure enters a crisis. The parents' approach to decision making may serve as a model for handling identity-related questions. Where parents show little evidence of having questioned their own beliefs and/or when they show reliance on the view of authorities, the likelihood of entering a crisis may be less than when the parental models show reflective questioning of their personal values and consequent independence of thought. Parental encouragement of adolescents to think for themselves should further facilitate consideration of identity alternatives.

Another family variable relevant here is the relationship between parents and adolescents. If adolescents become disillusioned with the life-style adopted by the parents, the effect will be to undermine identity elements developed through identification. Similarly, when adolescents rebel against parental authority, identity crises may be the consequence. Rebellion is not in itself an identity crisis, but efforts to break away from family control may lead to actively choosing a new, independent life-style.

Among initial Identity Diffusions, a primary cause of identity crises is likely to be societal expectations that an individual will work out personal goals, values, and beliefs during the high school and college years. Although most initial Diffusions are subjected to similar expectations, however, not all strive to form commitments. If the person anticipates that it will be possible to find an expressive life-style, then a positive value will be placed on going through an identity crisis. Alternatively, if the person does not believe it is possible to achieve personal gratification in today's world, there is no incentive for considering identity alternatives. In addition, exposure to new ideas, peer modeling, and family variables may be expected to contribute to movement from the Identity Diffusion status into the Moratorium category.

The Outcomes of Identity Crises

Once an identity crisis has begun it may end either by forming personally meaningful commitments (i.e., entering the Identity Achievement status) or by renouncing the task as unresolvable (i.e., becoming Identity Diffuse). In line with the epigenetic principle, it would be expected that the personality structure established during the early stages will influence the outcome of an identity crisis. A person who has been successful in meeting the demands of the early stages has a developmental foundation that can facilitate the resolution of identity crises. A sense of basic trust may be experienced as confidence that answers to identity questions can be found. A sense of autonomy contributes to a feeling that one will find his or her own identity rather than have to submit to choices imposed by authority figures. A sense of initiative leads both to more total activity and more varied activity in the search for a meaningful identity. Finally, a sense of industry underlies confidence in one's ability to follow through on whatever commitments are established. In contrast, negative outcomes on the components of the early stages are likely to be associated with pessimism about the outcome of an identity search. Feelings of hopelessness will reduce the willingness to endure the pressures of an identity crisis and consequently will increase the likelihood of becoming Identity Diffuse.

The success of adult models in a person's family and community should influence the outcome of an identity crisis. The presence of successful models is likely to increase the Moratorium's optimism about finding meaningful commitments in his or her own life. They may serve as examples for coping with identity concerns and may suggest content alternatives that can be profitably explored. If the only adult models available lack commitments and are frustrated with their lives, then those seeking commitments may begin to feel little hope of ever finding a successful resolution to their own crises. Unsuccessful models demonstrate only what does not work, not what is necessary to establish meaningful commitments.

The availability of psychological support, or the lack of it, may be another important influence on the course and outcome of an identity crisis. Meaningful commitments may be more likely to develop if the significant others in a Moratorium's life encourage the exploration of a variety of alternatives. The individual then has the psychological space necessary to work out personal choices. In contrast, criticism given for considering particular alternatives, or undue pressure brought to bear to reach some immediate conclusions, are likely to diminish the prospect of a successful resolution to the crisis. Such circumstances may generate feelings of psychological reactance and lack of control over the direction of one's life.

Reentry into the Crisis

The successful resolution of an identity crisis does not mean that the commitment established will remain an enduring aspect of a person's identity. Many of the same variables that can lead to initiation of an identity crisis among Foreclosures and Identity Diffusions can lead to reentry into crisis among Identity Achievers, that is, initiate a potential MAMA cycle. An established identity resolution may give way because, in practice, it turned out to be different from what was expected, or sufficient social support was not received, or its implementation was blocked. Also, continued exposure to alternatives may lead to identifying a more attractive possibility than the established commitment and result in a new crisis over whether or not to make the change. It can be hypothesized that renewed identity crises will be somewhat easier to resolve than an initial crisis because the person will already have learned techniques that facilitate resolution of crises. When the reentry into crisis is repeated on numerous occasions, though there may also develop the belief that any choices made will be temporary, that is, the commitments formed will be tenuous.

Regressive Changes

When individuals move into the Identity Diffusion status, the change may be labeled regressive. Changes out of the identity statuses characterized by commitments may occur with or without going through a renewed identity crisis. In the former instance, there is a failure to successfully resolve the new crisis. In the latter, an established commitment gradually loses its importance and vitality. The person may continue activities in a particular area but does so without the feeling that they are personally expressive or satisfying.

The movement from commitments to Diffusion may result from stagnation or "burnout." Performing the same activities over a long period without creating new challenges or developing new skills may result in progressive loss of interest and increasing boredom. Also, the frustrations of work or other activities may build up over time so that identity elements that were once personally expressive now are a source of dissatisfaction. These are the events often associated with a "midlife crisis." Yet, for any of a variety of situational or psychological reasons, a person may choose not to alter established ways of living. Changes here reflect the interrelationships between the components of Stage 5 (identity vs. identity diffusion) and Stage 7 (generativity vs. stagnation) in Erikson's theory. The regression involved in becoming Diffuse is not one of a return to an earlier level of functioning. The stagnating adult is not behaving like an adolescent who is drifting along some path of least resistance. Rather, the regression is implied in the weakening of qualities once associated with more successful or rewarding psychosocial functioning.

Research Evidence

The Direction and Timing of Development

Development Prior to and During the High School Years

Prior to the high school years interest in identity related questions appears to be slight. Ciaccio (1971) used a TAT type of storytelling projective instrument to assess the extent of concerns indicative for each of the first five stages described by Erikson. His samples consisted of males at ages five, eight, and eleven. The results of a "unit utterance" scoring procedure indicated that the eleven-year-old boys were beginning to evidence identity concerns but the frequency of these was far lower than those associated with the earlier stage components of initiative and industry. Similarly, in studies using the identity status interview with eleven- and twelve-year-olds (Archer, 1982, 1985b; Meilman, 1979), few instances of identity exploration for either sex have been found. The earliest age at which movement toward the more sophisticated form of identity processes has been shown involved a cross-sectional comparison of seventh- and eighth-graders on the Extended Objective Measure of Ego Identity Status (EOM-EIS), a paper-and-pencil instrument (Streitmatter, 1988). Seventh graders were found to more strongly endorse statements reflecting the Identity Diffusion status and eighth-graders more strongly endorsed statements associated with the Moratorium and Identity Achievement statuses. Strength of endorsement of items is not in itself, however, equivalent to placement in those statuses.

The results of cross-sectional studies of development during the high school years using paper-and-pencil instruments have revealed small differences, occasionally statistically significant. Pomerantz (1979) found twelfth-grade females to score significantly higher than eighth-grade females on the Rasmussen Ego Identity Scale, but the difference for males, though in the expected direction, was not significant. Wagner (1987), using Marcia's Ego Identity Incomplete Sentences Blank with age groups ranging from ages ten to twelve and sixteen to eighteen, found significantly higher identity ratings with increasing age for both males and females. LaVoie (1976), however, working with high school sophomores, juniors, and seniors of both sexes, found only a nonsignificant increase with increasing grade level on the same instrument. In another cross-sectional study of high school sophomores, juniors, and seniors, Markstrom (1987) found that females decreased in use of the Foreclosure and Identity Diffusion statuses, as measured by the EOM-EIS. No significant pattern of changes was found for males. Jones and Streitmetter (1987), also employing the EOM-EIS, found no significant grade effects, from grades seven to eight and eleven to twelve, although the pattern of means was in the expected direction. Similarly, Howard (1960), comparing sophomore and senior high school females, found a nonsignificant increase in scores on her own identity questionnaire.

Three cross-sectional studies of identity formation prior to and during the high school years have involved the identity status interview (Archer, 1982, 1985b; Meilman, 1979). Meilman (1979) interviewed college-bound males aged twelve, fifteen, and eighteen for the domains of vocation, religion, politics, and avocation. Archer (1982, 1985b), in her two studies interviewed sixth-, eighth-, tenth-, and twelfth-graders of both sexes without regard to future plans. In her first study the interview covered the domains of vocation, religion, politics, and sex-role attitudes, and in the second study the domains of vocation, sex-role attitudes, and family roles were used.

In all three studies at the youngest level virtually all participants were in the Foreclosure and/or Diffusion statuses, with the probability of being in a particular status differing by the interview domain. The Foreclosure status was more often observed for the domains of religious beliefs (Meilman, 1979), sex-role attitudes (Archer, 1982), and avocation (Meilman, 1979), and the Diffusion status was more frequent in the domains of political ideology (Archer, 1982; Meilman, 1979), and vocation (Meilman, 1979).

A significant increase in the frequency of the Identity Achievement with increasing age was found in all three studies (Archer, 1982, 1985b; Meilman, 1979), with the increase distributed across all content domains of the interview. Corresponding decreases in use of the Identity Diffusion status were found in two studies (Archer, 1985b; Meilman, 1979), decreases that were also distributed across the various content areas. Age and grade effects were not found for either the Foreclosure or Moratorium statuses, except for a grade by sex interaction for the Moratorium status reported in the second study by Archer (1985b). In that study the frequency of the Moratorium status held relatively steady for males across the four grade levels, but twelfth-grade females were notably higher in use of this status. This interaction was attributable almost entirely to the inclusion of the domain of family roles.

In the only reported longitudinal study with this age group, Hauser (1971) combined interview and Q-sort procedures to assess identity formation in samples of Caucasian and black male high school students from lower socioeconomic status backgrounds over a three-year period. He found that Caucasian adolescents showed a pattern of "progressive identity formation," characterized by frequent changes in self-concept during the early high school years, followed by increasing consistency and stability as the person approached high school graduation. In contrast, black adolescents showed general stability in their identity elements over the entire study period; a pattern Hauser (1971) labeled "identity foreclosure." He interpreted this lack of change as reflecting a problem in development, in that important developmental issues had been dodged rather than resolved. Many of the stable identity elements were defined in the negative; that is, the adolescent knew what he did not want to become rather than what alternative he actively wanted to pursue. The result was a rigid and impoverished self-definition.[3] Hauser speculated that these racial differences may have resulted from greater discrimination directed toward blacks than toward whites from the same background.

Development During the College Years

It is during the college years that the greatest gains in identity formation appear to occur (Waterman, 1985). College environments provide a diversity of experiences that can both trigger consideration of identity issues and

[3] In Marcia's (1966) classification system, such individuals would probably have been called Identity Diffuse.

suggest alternative resolutions for identity concerns. The results of numerous studies confirm that, in general, senior men and women have a stronger sense of personal identity than do their freshman counterparts and that identity commitments held as seniors are more likely to have been arrived at by successful resolution of identity crises.

Cross-sectional studies using paper-and-pencil measures of identity yield a consistent pattern of findings, with high scores associated with advancing age and/or year in college. Such results have been found for the Dignan Ego Identity Scale (Dignan, 1965; Stark & Traxler, 1974; Thompson, 1963) and the Stage 5 scale of the Inventory of Psychosocial Development (Constantinople, 1969; Whitbourne, Jelsma, & Waterman, 1982), though the effects were not always statistically significant. Longitudinal studies using the Inventory of Psychosocial Development provide further evidence of identity development during the college years (Constantinople, 1969, 1970; Whitbourne et al., 1982). Fry (1974) found significant gains on the Stage 5 components for a sample of college students from rural backgrounds but a retrogressive shift for those from urban backgrounds.

In addition, Dellas and Jernigan (1988) conducted a short-term longitudinal study of male and female cadets entering the U.S. Air Force Academy using the Dellas Identity Status Inventory–Occupation (DISI-O). For male cadets there was a significant decrease in the frequency of the Identity Achievement status in the occupational domain over the period of basic training, but no significant change in frequency during the first semester. No characteristic pattern of changes was observed for the female cadets. The results of the Dellas and Jernigan (1988) study appear attributable more to the circumstances of a military career choice for the sexes than to generalized normative trends.

Three longitudinal studies have traced identity development among American college students using the ego identity interview procedure. Adams and Fitch (1982) interviewed males and females from different college classes at a state university in succeeding years. In other studies, changes from the freshman to the senior year were assessed among male students at a technological institute (Waterman & Waterman, 1971; Waterman, Geary, & Waterman, 1974) and at a private liberal-arts college (Waterman & Goldman, 1976). In each of the studies the interview covered vocational choice, religious beliefs, and political ideology. The results from the three schools were quite similar:

1. College appeared to facilitate identity development in the domain of vocational plans. Both studies covering the freshman to the senior year found significant increases in the frequency of the Identity Achievement status and decreases in the frequency of the Moratorium status. In addition, there was a decrease in the frequency the Identity Diffusion status at the liberal arts college. In the one-year study there was a significant decrease in the frequency of Identity Diffusions and a nonsignificant increase in Identity Achievers.

2. College experiences appear to undermine traditional religious beliefs without necessarily helping the students establish alternative belief systems. At all three colleges there were significant decreases in the frequency of students in the Foreclosure status. At the state university there was an increase in the frequency of Identity Diffusions.
3. Although the development of new, clearer commitments in political ideology was observed during the college years, a substantial proportion of the students demonstrated little interest in the topic. Significant increases in the frequency of Identity Achievement status were observed over one year at the state university and over four years at the technological institute. At the state university there was also a significant increase in the frequency of the Moratorium status. Significant decreases were found for the Identity Diffusion status at the state university and for the Foreclosure status at the technological institute. No systematic changes were found for the students at the private liberal-arts college. In both four-year studies, more than half the participants were approaching graduation without clear beliefs in this area and without trying to form commitments.

Although the patterns of identity development observed were relatively consistent across the three studies, some differences were observed. The differences may have been due to the distinctive characteristics of the student populations at the three schools. Differences in the timing of the studies may also have affected the results, particularly in political ideology. For example, the first four-year study was conducted at the technological institute from 1968 to 1972 during the height of protest against the Vietnam war. The second study, conducted at the private liberal-arts college, took place from 1970 to 1975, with the senior-year interviews conducted after the issue of the Vietnam war had subsided, and following the Watergate scandal. Also, in all three studies, follow-up data were obtained only from individuals who continued at their respective school throughout the period of research. As yet, nothing is known about the patterns of continued development of those who withdraw from college. Data are needed not just on identity formation among college dropouts, but also on college women over the period from the freshman to the senior year and on individuals of both sexes of corresponding ages who do not pursue post-secondary education.

Development During the Adult Years

Since the time of the previous review of the research on identity development (Waterman, 1982), literature on identity development during the adult years had grown considerably. The conclusion tentatively advanced then that "it appears that the adult years are a period of strengthening of identity but not a time when many new identity issues are raised or novel possibilities considered" (Waterman, 1982, pp. 348–349) now needs modification. Stability in the sense of identity continues to be most evident, but there is now also substantial evidence of identity changes accompanying changes in an individual's life circumstances.

Research with the IPD has yielded mixed results on identity development during the adult years. In a cross-sectional study men and women ranging in age from 22 to 67 conducted by Tesch (1985), scores on the Stage 5 scale (Identity vs. Identity Diffusion) of this paper-and-pencil instrument were uncorrelated with age for either group. However, in a ten-year longitudinal study conducted by Whitbourne and Waterman (1979) of males and females first tested as college graduates, this IPD scale significantly increased when the participants were retested as alumni. In a second sample followed over an 11 year period beginning in college, a similar increase was observed (Whitbourne et al., 1992). Given the design of this study research, however, it is possible that all or most of the increase could have occurred while the participants were still in college. No further increase in IPD Stage 5 scale scores was found for the original sample during the adult years, with the assessment carried out at the point of second follow-up. At the time, the participants in the sample were between the ages of 40 and 44.

In cross-sectional research involving the identity status interview, the picture of adult identity formation formed does not suggest a normative trend. The earliest study of this type was conducted by Waterman and Waterman (1975) and compared the distribution of the identity statuses between college males and their fathers, many of whom had not attended college. They found the fathers (men between ages 40 and 65) were more frequently in the Foreclosure status in the three topic domains covered in the interview: vocational choice, religious beliefs, and political ideology. Their sons were more likely to be in the Moratorium and Identity Diffusion statuses. In the most comparable sample of women currently available, Archer, Waterman, and Owens (1988) found a similarly high frequency of women in the Foreclosure status. The women in that study ranged in age from 23 to 50 and were enacting one of three patterns of life activities: homemaking, college attendance, or full-time career. Age of the respondent was unrelated to frequency of use of the various identity statuses in each of the three subsamples.

Freilino and Hummel (1985) conducted a comparison of the frequency of the identity statuses between two samples of women attending college, one of the traditional college age (18 to 23) and the other adult returnees (over age 30). The adults were significantly more likely to be in the Identity Achievement and Moratorium statuses and the traditional-aged students were significantly more likely to be Identity Diffuse. The importance of returning to college as relating to identity formation for women was indicated in the findings of Archer et al. (1988), where the college-attending subsample was significantly more likely to be in the Identity Achievement status compared to the women in the homemaker group. Analyses of the content of the identity interviews revealed that many of the identity crises of the college-returning women precede their resuming their education and thus may have prepared them for changing their pattern of life activities. In an additional study employing a cross-sectional design, Whitbourne and Tesch (1985) compared college students (aged 20 to 22) with college alumni (aged 24 to 27) of both sexes for the frequency of the identity statuses. The alumni sample was significantly more likely to be Foreclosed, with the pattern of frequencies similar across the interview domains of vocation, religion, politics, and sex role.

Two longitudinal studies have been carried out with adult respondents involving use of the identity status interview. Caracelli (1988) conducted a one-year longitudinal study of women in either their first or second year of reentry into college. The age range of her sample was 22 to 55. Change in identity status was expected for these women because they were making a transition in their pattern of life activities. Although stability of the identity statuses was most evident across the five areas covered in the interview: vocation, role of spouse, role of parent, family and career priorities, and women's roles, approximately 14 percent of the identity status scorings had changed over the one-year period. For her entire sample across interview domains, there was a significant increase in the frequency of the Identity Achievement status and a significant decrease in the frequency of the Foreclosure status. Although the Moratorium status did not show a significant change in frequency, it showed both greatest movement into any status and the greatest movement out of any status. Of fifteen women who left the Moratorium status, all but two had successfully established identity commitments.

Marcia (1976) followed up on men who had originally been interviewed six years earlier while in college. All were living within a fifty-mile radius of the city in which their college was located. The results were reported in terms of change in overall identity status, a judgment arrived at by combining information from the vocational, religious, and political domains of the interview. The identity statuses, aside from the Moratorium status, were fairly stable (70 percent). The individuals in the Foreclosure and Identity Diffusion statuses were found to be more stable than were those in the Identity Achievement status. Six of the seven Identity Achievers at the time of the first interview were committed as well in the follow-up. Three of the men were now classified as Foreclosures, however. These must be considered anomalous changes because once a person goes through an identity crisis, he or she can no longer fit the technical definition of the Foreclosure status. Five of the seven Moratoriums in college had firm commitments at the follow-up, and two had become Diffuse. Only one of the sixteen participants who was Foreclosed or Diffuse at the beginning of the study became an Identity Achiever and two others were going through an identity crisis six years later.

Three studies have been conducted with adults using a retrospective methodology in which respondents reflect on their sense of identity at various times in their lives. O'Connell (1976), using her Sense of Identity Inventory, contrasted the reflections of three groups of married women with school-age children who differed in their pattern of life activities: *traditional* women who were full-time homemakers, *neotraditional* women who had resumed a career after an interruption for childrearing, and *nontraditional* women who were continuously committed to their careers. Women in all samples indicated they had experienced an increasingly strong sense of identity as they moved from adolescence, through the periods when they were first married, had their first child and their children were of preschool age, to the time where their children were of school age. O'Connell (1976) observed that after marriage, "traditional and neotraditional women's sense of identity seems to undergo a moratorium (i.e., a hiatus) which is not terminated until the school-children stage of the life cycle, but nontraditional women develop their senses of identity in a more straightforward progression" (p. 683).

Archer (1985a) interviewed a sample of divorced women, using their reflections to assess their identity statuses at four marker events in their lives: high school graduation, the time of marriage, the time of separation or divorce, and the present. She found a significant increase in use of Identity Achievement status, with the greatest increase occurring between the time of divorce and the present. For the Moratorium status a significant effect for marker events was also found, with an increase occurring between the time of marriage and the time of divorce and a decrease occurring between divorce and the present. In addition, a significant decrease in the frequency of the Foreclosure status was found, with the drop occurring between high school graduation and the time of divorce and leveling thereafter. Changes in the identity statuses were most notable in the domains of role of spouse, family and career priorities, and sex-role attitudes, and were not evident on vocational plans, religious beliefs, or political ideology.

Kroger and Haslett (1991) conducted a retrospective study of identity formation among New Zealand adults whose occupational level was either professional or managerial or who had a spouse at that level. They found that the probability of entering the Identity Achievement status increased throughout the adult years, with such movement occurring in all interview domains assessed (vocation, religion, politics, sex-role, and relationship values). The likelihood of entering the Achievement status did vary by domain, though, and by the life circumstances of the respondents in sex, education level, and employment status.

One additional study used a novel methodology, the results of which may contribute to understanding of identity development during the adult years. Mallory (1983) made use of Q-sort data from the Berkeley/Oakland Growth Study to assess identity status changes longitudinally over four times: junior high school, senior high school, age 30 to 37, and age 40 to 47. To use the data available, she first constructed composite profiles for each status for each sex in terms of the qualities appearing as items in the Q-sort. As expected, she found increasing congruence over time between the personality profiles conveyed by the Berkeley/Oakland Growth Study participants and the profiles representative of the Identity Achievement status. There was a corresponding decrease in congruence with the profiles associated with the Identity Diffusion status. No age effect was observed for the Foreclosure status. Perhaps the most surprising finding of the study was the timing of changes. Although it had been expected that the greatest movement toward the Identity Achievement status would occur between senior high school and age 30 to 37, the data revealed that the greatest changes occurred between 30 to 37 and 40 to 47. These data appear inconsistent with what has been found with other methodologies and might be dismissed as a product of a novel, thinly validated procedure. But the methodological differences between this study and other research give rise to an interesting speculation. The traditional identity status interview assesses the respondent's recollections of decision-making processes by which identity elements are formed. In contrast, the Q-sort composite profiles of the identity statuses employed by Mallory (1983) are based on psychological correlates of the statuses, not the decision-making processes themselves. It may be, therefore, that there is an important time-lag effect with respect to the impact of identity formation processes. During the high school and college years, particularly the latter, the sense of personal identity is most actively being formed, as evidenced by the normative changes in the identity statuses. However, the full influence of the decision-making style used then, particularly the Identity Achievement status, may not be felt until well into the adult years. This hypothesis is worthy of further investigation.

The Comparative Stability of the Identity Statuses During the College Years

The three longitudinal studies of identity development during the college years have also provided data on the relative stability of the identity statuses during the time when the most extensive changes are occurring. Comparisons of relative stability can be made for a one-year period at the state university (Adams & Fitch, 1981), and a four-year period at the technological institute (Waterman & Waterman, 1971; Waterman et al., 1974) and the private liberal arts college (Waterman & Goldman, 1976). Table 3.1 gives the percentage of instances in which an individual was in the same identity status at both the beginning and end of the study period in a particular content domain of the interview.

As expected, the Moratorium status was the least stable of the four statuses across the period from the freshman to the senior year, and was

TABLE 3.1. Stability of the ego identity statuses in longitudinal research.

Identity status	1-year stability at a state university[a]	4-year stability at a technological institute[b]	4-year stability at a private liberal-arts college[c]
Identity achievement	68%	59%	54%
Moratorium	50%	9%	0%
Foreclosure	61%	44%	46%
Identity diffusion	42%	50%	67%

[a] Data from Adams and Fitch, 1982.
[b] Data from Waterman & Waterman, 1971 and Waterman et al., 1974.
[c] Data from Waterman & Goldman, 1976.

the second least stable status in the shorter study. In the two four-year studies there were thirty-four instances of identity crises in particular interview domains found in the freshman year. Not one of these crises continued during the senior year. Of these crises, more than three-quarters ended in the formation of clearly defined, personally meaningful commitments. At the technological institute, 76 percent of the Moratoriums had become Identity Achievers and the corresponding figure at the private liberal-arts college was 85 percent. In the one-year study, considering only instances where the person had emerged from the Moratorium status, firm commitments had been developed in 85 percent of the cases. Thus, the probability is very high that identity crises experienced in college will be successfully resolved.

The stability of the other identity statuses was generally comparable and reflected considerable shifting about. It was evident that even where individuals had firm commitments at the start of the study, by the time of the follow-up, approximately one-third to one-half were no longer in the same identity status. This finding for the Identity Achievement status makes it clear that successful resolution of an identity crisis does not give permanence to the commitment formed. Although the Achievement status was slightly more stable than the Foreclosure status, the factors that lead to initiation of a crisis or to regression appear to apply to both statuses.

When the comparative stability data are analyzed separately for the different domains of the interview, some differences emerge. The Identity Achievement and Foreclosure statuses were more stable in vocational plans than in the other topic domains. Conversely, the Identity Diffusion status was more stable in religious beliefs and political ideology than in vocational plans. The Moratorium status was highly unstable in all interview domains.

Sex Differences in Identity Development

Although the topic of sex comparisons in identity functioning is addressed at length in Chapter 4, it should be noted that there appear to be few differences between the sexes in either the direction or timing of identity formation. On paper-and-pencil measures of identity, sex differences have not been found on the identity items of the IPD (Constantinople, 1969; Whitbourne & Waterman, 1979; Waterman & Whitbourne, 1982), the Identity Achievement Status Scale (Simmons, 1970), the Texas Psychosocial Identity Scale (Dunivant & Bieri, 1973), Rasmussen's Ego Identity Scale (Pomerantz, 1979), Marcia's Ego Identity Incomplete Sentences Blank (LaVoie, 1976), or the original Objective Measure of Ego Identity Status (Adams, Shea, & Fitch, 1979). In several studies employing the EOM-EIS with middle school and high school students (Abraham, 1986; Jones & Streitmatter, in press; Markstrom, 1987; Streitmatter, 1988), females were found to more strongly endorse items associated with the Identity Achievement and Moratorium statuses, whereas males more strongly endorsed items reflecting the Foreclosure and Identity Diffusion statuses. Dellas and Jernigan (1987) found females entering the U.S. Air Force Academy less likely than male cadets to be in the Foreclosure status about occupation, as measured by the DISI-O, and more likely to be in the Moratorium status. Finally, Dunivant and Bieri (1973) found that females scored higher than males on Gruen's Ego Identity Scale and Block's Role Consistency Index.

Comparisons of the frequency of the ego identity statuses assessed by the identity status interview have similarly revealed only limited differences between the genders on identity formation. No consistent patterns of sex differences have been found for the interview domains of vocational choice, religious beliefs, political ideology, or sex-role attitudes, at the middle school or high school years (Archer, 1982, 1985b, 1989c; Grotevant et al., 1982; Matteson, 1977), during the college years (Adams & Fitch, 1981; Hodgson & Fischer, 1979; Orlofsky, 1978b; Poppen, 1974; Rothman, 1978; Waterman & Nevid, 1977; Whitbourne & Tesch, 1985), or for adults (Whitbourne & Tesch, 1985). Comparisons of males and females on the frequency of the identity statuses in interview domains reflecting on values, beliefs, and goals in interpersonal context have yielded significant differences with fair consistency. Females are more often found in the Identity Achievement and Moratorium statuses, but males are more often Foreclosed or Identity Diffuse with respect to family roles (Archer, 1985b) and friendship (Grotevant et al., 1982) among high school students, and in the domain of attitudes toward premarital intercourse among college students (Orlofsky, 1978b; Poppen, 1974; Waterman & Nevid, 1977).

Taken together, the results from the research with paper-and-pencil instruments and the identity status interview indicate general comparability for males and females in both the direction and timing of identity formation. The findings also support the observation by Archer (1985b, 1989c) that the task of identity formation is more complex for females than for males in that they endeavor to work out for themselves their goals, values, and beliefs in more domains than do males. Not only do females experience the desire to establish their sense of identity in vocational choice, religious beliefs, political ideology, and sex-role attitudes in the same manner as males, but they engage in more active reflection and decision-making regarding identity in a relational context than do their male counterparts.

Antecedent Conditions Relating to Identity Development

Although many hypotheses were offered about variables that may contribute to determining the course of identity development, only a few have been investigated. The search for antecedent influences has focused on family and school variables, developmental characteristics believed to be hierarchically related to identity, and personal activities and interests.

Family Variables

Considerable attention has been directed toward identifying the nature of differences in family relationships and parenting styles characteristic of individuals in the various identity statuses. Because this literature has been reviewed in Chapter 2, only a brief summary of the findings is presented here.

As would be expected, Foreclosures have been found to have the closest relationships with their parents. Both sons and daughters evaluate their parents most favorably and describe their families as child-centered. The fathers of Foreclosures are seen as relatively possessive and intrusive toward their sons but more supportive and encouraging for their daughters. In turn, Foreclosure sons were the most willing to involve their families in making important life decisions. In contrast, Diffusions of both genders reported the most distance from their families. The parents of Diffusions were seen as indifferent, inactive, detached, not understanding, and rejecting. Both males and females in the Moratorium and Identity Achievement statuses were relatively critical of their parents and were likely to report themselves to be in conflict with their families. Sons in these statuses were not likely to turn to their families when making important life decisions. This tension within the family appears related to ambivalence of both parents and offspring over the latter's attempts at individuation. With successful resolution of an identity crisis, better family relationships may be established. Finally, there is evidence that, in general, the nature of the relationship with the parent of the same gender is more strongly related to identity status than is the relationship with the opposite-sex parent.

It is an attractive hypothesis that parental behavior contributes to identity formation and the pattern of research results obtained provides readily interpretable links between family functioning and the various identity statuses. For both methodological and conceptual reasons, however, it cannot be concluded that the family variables studied are actually influences on identity development. In most studies the researchers have relied solely on reports obtained from adolescent or youth respondents. These measures are subject to errors of memory, defensive distortion, and conscious impression management. The same problems afflict studies in which information was obtained from the parents. Even if the accuracy of the reports were assumed, it would still not be possible to reach a conclusion about any causal contribution of family variables. The type of behavior shown by an adolescent may well have elicited particular responses from the parents that could account for the observed relationships. It is easier to provide a supportive, child-centered environment when children identify strongly with the parents and follow family traditions without questioning. In contrast, the ambivalence and conflict found in the family backgrounds of Moratoriums and Identity Achievers may have been a response to the sometimes extreme shifts in behavior engaged in by a son or daughter going through a stressful, and stressing, identity search. Similarly, the lack of involvement shown by the parents of Identity Diffusions may have been partially the result of an adolescent providing few strongly directed behavioral stimuli to which the parents could respond. It is probably not possible to entirely unravel the complex causal effects in any relationship of long duration. Long-term, longitudinal, predictive studies appear necessary if any meaningful evaluation is to be made of the likelihood that parenting behaviors contribute to the process by which identity is formed.

Along another line, Waterman and Waterman (1975) hypothesized that parents serve as role models for the type of decision-making processes involved in identity formation. No relationship was found between the identity statuses shown by a sample of fathers and their college-attending sons. Adams (1985) did, however, find a relationship between parent and adolescent identity for a sample of college females. Mothers and fathers who were in the more sophisticated identity statuses, as assessed by the OM-EIS, were very likely to have daughters with equally sophisticated identities, but parents with less developed identities did not predict to the level of their daughter's development.

Variables relating to family stability have also been investigated as possible contributors to identity development, with conflicting results to date. Oshman and Manosevitz (1976) found that a sample of college males who experienced father absence from an average age of about ten had significantly lower full-scale scores on the Rasmussen Ego Identity Scale than did samples from intact families and families in which the mothers had remarried. The direction of differences was the same on all stage scales, but the effect for the stage 5 (Identity vs. Identity Diffusion) items was not significant. Jordan (1970) found that college males in the Identity Diffusion status were more likely to have come from broken homes than were those in the other statuses. In contrast, St. Clair and Day (1979) reported that in a sample of high school females, two-thirds of students in the Identity Achiever status came from homes disrupted by divorce or the death of one parent, but fewer than one-fifth of the students in each of the other statuses were from broken homes. Jones and Streitmatter (1987) reported that high school students of both sexes from intact families were more likely to endorse Foreclosure items on the EOM-EIS than were respondents from other family arrangements.

School Variables

Only a few studies have made comparisons made between individuals who did and did not continue their education beyond high school (Munro & Adams, 1977; Morash, 1980; Archer & Waterman, 1988). Because the college environment is generally believed to be particularly conducive to identity formation, both in stimulating consideration of alternatives and providing support for successful resolution of identity crises, differences in distribution of the identity statuses between the two groups would be anticipated. If such differences are found, however, they may be accounted for either by personality functioning arising prior to leaving high school predictive of future college vs. work activities, or to differential influences of college and employment arising after high school graduation. The data currently available have yielded inconsistent results on differences in identity formation of college and working youth.

Munro and Adams (1977) contrasted the identity statuses of male and female college students with those of working youths using the identity status interview. Their working sample was recruited from an urban location by approaching individuals passing a chosen location. Although no differences were found between the groups in identity statuses in the vocational domain, working youths were more likely to be in the sophisticated identity statuses on religious beliefs and political ideology than were their college-student age mates. Morash (1980) studied a group of noncollege youths attending night courses in an apprentice program and reported "that working class youth had . . . a higher frequency of diffusion and identity achievement statuses" (p. 316) than did the college students interviewed by Marcia (1966, 1967). Though the effect for the Identity Diffusion status was statistically significant, the effect for the Identity Achievement status was not.

As part of a larger longitudinal study, Archer and Waterman (1988) compared the distribution of the identity statuses one year after high school graduation for three samples: working youths, college youths, and youths combining work and school. The samples in this study were recruited during the junior year of high school, thus controlling for community of origin. The college youths were significantly more likely than working youths to be in the Identity Achievement status, and a trend in the same direction was found for the Moratorium status; they were also less likely to be in the Identity Diffusion status. The group combining work and school were in most respects more similar to the working sample than to the college-only sample. Because identity status data from the interviews conducted during the junior and senior year of high school did not predict whether the participants would continue on to college, enter the work force, or combine these activities, the findings of this study suggest the importance of post-high school contextual variables in stimulating thinking about identity issues and in aiding their resolution.

The working samples in the three studies were selected in quite different ways, which may have contributed to the different outcomes observed. Given the substantial proportion of individuals who do not pursue a college education, considerably more research attention should be directed toward understanding the direction and timing of identity formation among this segment of the population and to identifying variables influencing such development.

In a study addressing a different aspect of the question of school impact, Adams and Fitch (1983) examined the effects of the psychological environments of university departments on the identity status development of college students. They found that programs with more academic and scholastic emphasis attract students with a more highly formulated sense of identity. The perceptions by students of reinforcement by peers or faculty of a broad societal perspective were associated with stability or advancement in identity formation over a one-year period. Without encouragement of such an awareness, students were likely to regress to less mature identity statuses. Similarly, Costa and Campos (1989), studying Portuguese college students, found that developmental changes in identity status over three years occurred differentially among students in different major programs.

Developmental Characteristics

One test of the epigenetic principle, that the successful resolution of the crisis associated with each of the earlier stages of psychosocial development provides the foundation for the successful development of identity, is furnished by the pattern of intercorrelations among the stage scales of the Inventory of Psychosocial Development (Constantinople, 1969). This instrument is designed to assess the personality components associated with each of the first six stages of Erikson's theory. As expected, the scores on the stage 5 scale for Identity vs. Identity Diffusion have been shown to yield significant correlations with each of the earlier stage scales in samples of undergraduates drawn from five colleges and a sample of adult, college alumni (LaVoie & Adams, unpublished ms.; C.K. Waterman, Buebel, & Waterman, 1970; Waterman & Whitbourne, 1982). Marcia and Miller (1980), working with a sample of adult women, compared the identity statuses as assessed by the ego identity interview with regard to scores from the Inventory of Psychosocial Development. Women in the Identity Achievement status had the highest scores on each of the early stage scales and those in the Identity Diffusion status consistently had the lowest scores. Rothman (1978) conducted a similar study with a college-student sample but used the Rasmussen Ego Identity Scale instead of the Inventory of Psychosocial Development. Again the Identity Diffusion status was associated with the lowest scores on each of the early stage scales, but no clear pattern appeared among the other statuses. The stage components of autonomy and industry most clearly discriminated among the statuses.

Ego identity has also been assumed to rest upon a developmental foundation provided by aspects of ego functioning other than those Erikson focused on. Efforts have been made to relate progress in identity formation to Loevinger's ego stages, Kohlberg's stages of moral reasoning, and Piaget's stages of cognitive functioning. In each instance there is a possibility that a certain level of stage functioning may constitute a necessary but not sufficient condition for adopting a particular path of identity formation. The research bearing on the relationships among various stage schemes is discussed in Chapter 2. Overall, the findings indicate that although there is concomitant development of identity, ego processes, and cognitive functions, it has not been established that advances in one area are necessary as a foundation for movement in other areas.

Because virtually all the research on developmental characteristics has involved assessment at only one time, it has not been possible to determine what variables, if any, constitute antecedents of progress in identity formation. The associations observed could be operating in either direction, and changes may be occurring simultaneously rather than sequentially. Again, longitudinal research is needed to establish whether any of the stage constructs are predictive antecedents of identity development.

Interests and Activities

Although a large number of correlates of the identity statuses have been identified, any of which might contribute to identity development, in only a couple of instances is there reason to believe a sequential arrangement may exist. In the longitudinal studies conducted at the technological institute and the private liberal-arts college (Waterman & Waterman, 1971; Waterman et al., 1974; Waterman & Goldman, 1976), the College Student Questionnaire—Part 1 (Peterson, 1965) was given at the beginning of the freshman year. The "Cultural Sophistication" scale, tapping an interest in such areas as art, music, literature, and foreign films, was found to be predictive of identity formation. At both schools, freshmen who were Identity Achievers scored higher on the scale than did freshmen who were not Identity Achievers. More important, students who became Identity Achievers during their college years had more cultural interests as freshmen than did students who did not enter the status. Cultural interests may contribute either to creating identity crises and/or to their resolution. The exposure to new ideas through cultural media may challenge the views with which a person was raised and suggest more promising identity alternatives to which commitments can be formed.

A possibly related variable shown to be associated with identity development is expressive writing activity. Among samples of both high school and college students, males and females who wrote poetry were far more likely to be in the Identity Achievement status than were students who had never written poetry (Waterman & Archer, 1979; Waterman, Kohutis, & Pulone, 1977). No differences were found between students who had kept a personal journal or diary and those who had not. Because expressive writing was found to have started relatively early in adolescence, the poetry-writing activities were almost certainly antecedent to achieving a stable sense of identity.

It had been expected originally that poetry writing and journal keeping would yield similar results. The differences may be explained by the ways in which the students approached the two types of expression. Both groups saw their writing as helping to increase their self-understanding, but there were differences in the themes written about and in the perceptions of the functions the writing served (Waterman & Archer, 1979). Journal keeping appeared to be used primarily for making a record of current activities and for describing relationships with friends and parents. In contrast, poetry writing was seen as a vehicle for the creative expression of more abstract, emotional concerns. Further, poetry writers were much more likely to want to share their writings than were journal keepers. Thus, poetry writing may be a technique that is instrumental in working through an identity crisis by aiding in the exploration of possible identity alternatives and by serving as a means for gaining feedback from others.

Rather than there being a direct, facilitative connection among cultural interests, poetry writing, and identity formation, all three may derive from some common underlying psychological quality related to curiosity and exploration. The impetus to explore the realm of ideas and feelings through cultural media, and personal emotional states through poetry writing, may also be involved in the tendency to consider a variety of identity alternatives.

Conclusions

The basic hypothesis embodied in Erikson's theory of identity development, that movement from adolescence to adulthood involves changes in identity that can be characterized as progressive developmental shifts, fares very well in empirical studies. There is substantial evidence of an increased probability both that consideration will be given to identity alternatives and that personally meaningful commitments will be formed. On the timing of development, it appears that only limited changes occur prior to or during the high school years. The most extensive advances in identity formation occur during the time spent in college. (Not enough research has been conducted with noncollege samples of equivalent age to determine the relative contribution of ontogenetic and situational variables to such changes). The period immediately after college appears most often to involve a consolidation of the sense of identity, but continued exploration of identity alternatives was also evident. Specific situational changes in life activities during the adult years, such as divorce or resuming one's education, have been shown to be accompanied by reexamination of identity issues, whether in anticipation of, or following, such life changes.

Of the topic domains that may become the focus of identity concern, documentation is greatest for progressive developmental shifts in vocational choice. Though identity questions about sexual expression have not been studied longitudinally, the high probability of the Identity Achievement status among women indicates similar progress in this area. Less consistency has been observed for the patterns of identity change in religious beliefs and political ideology, perhaps as a function of differences in background characteristics of the participants in various studies or changing sociohistorical conditions.

Comparisons of the patterns of identity formation shown by males and females yield far more evidence of similarities than differences. About the *processes* of development, the genders show generally similar probabilities for consideration of identity alternatives and establishing commitments. Females, however, appear to have a more complex task in identity formation because more areas of their lives appear salient for identity formation. The similarities between genders in developmental processes employed do not contradict the substantial evidence from other research that males and females differ in the *content* of their identity choices (Frieze et al., 1978).

The research on identity formation has yielded increasing information on the antecedents of developmental change. Although findings on the relationship between parental behavior and the identity statuses of adolescents are consistent with theoretical expectations, the alternative explanations cast doubt on the hypothesized causal influence of parental variables. Similarly, we have extensive data consistent with a hierarchical arrangement of Erikson's psychosocial stages, but the methodological limitations of the research do not permit determination of the direction of effect. As yet, only a couple of personality or activity variables have been identified as predicting of the direction of future identity formation.

4
Differences Within and Between Genders: A Challenge to the Theory

DAVID R. MATTESON

Erikson's theory of adolescent identity is deeply challenged by the data comparing male and female identity development.

Though the original identity status interviews focused on areas thought to be important to male identity (occupation and ideology), interview schedules for new domains were developed as identity researchers began to pay attention to female identity development. Comparisons between genders were handicapped because early research generally used different interview formats for males and for females. It became clear that research with both genders needed to include interviews from both the "male" and the "female" schedules, with separate scoring by domains. Soon it was recognized that we needed to move beyond the assumption of gender differences to cover different styles of development within each gender (Matteson, 1975, pp. 182–185), such as the differences between "traditional" and "liberated" women. Historical changes in women's identity were included and some of us anticipated, in future decades, a change in men's identity styles as well. The purpose of this chapter is to compare and contrast the data on female and male identity development, including within-gender differences, and examine the implications for a general theory of identity formation. (See Matteson unpublished, 1988, for details on the history of these developments in the research.)

Identity Formation in Women: Impressionistic Data

Because most of the research on identity has focused on men and has been surveyed in preceding chapters; we need not survey men's identity process. Identity studies with women in the college years (Josselson, 1972, 1973) and in the middle years (Marcia & Miller, 1980), as well as direct observations of Danish youths in structured interactions with their parents (Matteson, 1974) suggested some strong parallels with the research on men.

Foreclosure women seemed to have close ties with their parents, parentally based superegos, and a desire to recreate their familial closeness in their current relationships (Josselson, 1972, 1973). They discount any unhappiness or discontent they feel as part of woman's role (Marcia & Miller, 1980). Direct observation of family interactions suggested that Foreclosures' glowing descriptions of their families of origin involved a coverup of the highest ratio of negative (compared to positive) expression of feelings (paralleling Donovan's 1970, 1975 findings in observing Foreclosure men in groups). Traditional gender roles, with mother deferring to father, prevailed in the Foreclosure families (Matteson, 1974).

College-age Diffusion women were characterized by fear, flight, and fantasy in extensive interviews (Josselson), and characterized their parents as "not really there." In family interactions, the parent of the same sex was the most passive member of the triad, and the triad as a whole had few interactions compared to the other types of families (Matteson, 1974). Even in middle age, Diffusion women were afraid of being hurt or betrayed, had doubts about femininity, and were preoccupied with infantile issues (Marcia & Miller, 1980).

Female Moratoriums seemed to show the intense style of relating that had characterized male Moratoriums, confirmed for both genders in the observations of family triads. These triads were the most active, and showed the least evidence of the parents following stereotyped sex roles, with father dominating. The high risk-taking and experience-seeking that evokes positive descriptions of young male Moratoriums was seen less positively in the study of middle-aged females:

> They are involved in a "yes-but" game wherein they "want to be themselves" but feel guilty, defiant, approval-seeking and afraid. They feel ambivalent about their wife-mother roles, and seem to want a guarantee of security. (Marcia & Miller, 1980)

In contrast, the college women who had attained Identity Achievement status demonstrated a personal autonomy not present in women of the other statuses. They were more concerned with their own goals, and who they might be, than by whom they might be loved (Josselson, 1973). And middle-aged women in this status viewed themselves as competent and assertive, looking back on their previous identities as "vicarious."

These parallels made it look, at first, as if the identity status categories were functioning similarly for women and for men, though the content may have been different.

Identity Formation: Standardized Measures

Comparisons Between Genders

Males in each of the identity statuses have been found to differ on measures of anxiety, self-esteem, and attitudes toward authority. These variables have been tested for females as well:

Anxiety

As might be expected from their "in-crisis" position, Moratorium women, like their male counterparts, are more anxious than those in committed statuses (Marcia & Friedman, 1970; Schenkel & Marcia, 1972; Romano, 1975). Foreclosure women are also like their male counterparts, showing the least anxiety. For women, however, the low anxiety scores do not appear to be due to defense; Foreclosure women perform adequately on cognitive tasks under stress, in contrast to male Foreclosures (Marcia & Friedman, 1970).

In men the anxiety appears to subside once the moratorium period has ended and an identity has been achieved. For women, when identity is assessed using the sexual ideology domain, those who have achieved identity have the lowest anxiety (Schenkel & Marcia, 1972). However, when identity is assessed using the earlier interview format (occupation, politics, and religion), female Identity Achievements appear more anxious than their male counterparts (Marcia & Friedman, 1970; Howard, 1975). It appears that anxiety in the women respondents is related not only to being in crisis, but to being accepted in "man's world."

Self-Esteem

The importance of the domains by which identity is assessed is attested to by results on this variable as well. Identity Achievement women have the lowest scores on self-esteem when identity is assessed using the original content areas (Marcia & Friedman, 1970). But when identity status is based on the sexual ideology interview (Schenkel & Marcia, 1972), women who have achieved identities have the highest self-esteem. Foreclosure women score high on self-esteem regardless of the identity content (Marcia & Friedman, 1970; Schenkel & Marcia, 1972; Gold, 1980).

Attitudes Toward Authority

For women in the various identity statuses, results on this variable directly parallel those for men. Foreclosures are the least critical, regardless of which interview format is used (Marcia & Friedman, 1970; Schenkel & Marcia, 1972; Matteson, 1974). Moratoriums are not only highly critical of authority (ibid.), but show greater anxiety when interacting with authority figures, and are less cooperative (Podd et al., 1970).

Other Variables

In the discussion of anxiety we saw that female Foreclosures perform adequately on cognitive tasks under stress, in contrast to male Foreclosures. In addition, female Foreclosures show some positive characteristics on variables that have not been tested in men. They are not particularly vulnerable to outside influence, and along with Achievements, show higher field-independence on perception tasks (Schenkel, 1975), conform less and show less discomfort in peer-pressure situations (Toder and Marcia, 1973), and have more internal locus of control (Howard, 1975; Marcia & Miller, 1980). Thus, for women, vulnerability to outside influence seems related to lack of commitment.

The locus of control variable has been tested in men; male Moratoriums and Achievements have more internal orientation than Foreclosures and Diffusions. Thus for men, autonomy appears to increase with exploration; men in Moratorium and Achievement statuses consistently score higher than Foreclosures and Diffusions, whether we measure autonomy directly (Matteson, 1974), through locus of control, or through critical attitudes toward authority. But for women, autonomy appears to increase with commitment, with or without exploration. It is women in the committed statuses (Foreclosure and Achievement) who seem to have the base of security that permits freedom from external controls (Howard, 1975). Additional evidence of this pattern comes from a study of high school women, showing greater personality integration and psychosocial maturity for women in the committed statuses (LaVoie, 1976).

Is Exploration Functional for Women?

Marcia (1980) was the first to interpret this pattern as an indication of the importance of stability in female development. Although for men, proximity to the Identity Achievement status is related to superior functioning, for women, commitment to an identity (whether Foreclosed or Achieved) emerges as the important variable.

Explanations for the superior performance of women in the stable statuses are elaborated in later sections of this chapter. Recognizing stability as a key factor for female identity development led Marcia and others to question the value of a period of exploration of alternatives for women.

Though some evidence shows that the Foreclosure status is more adaptive for women than for men, we cannot generalize that foreclosure of an identity has the same positive effects for women as achieving an identity. There are four problems with such a conclusion: (1) the data on which it is based, (2) data from other studies that contradict the generalization, (3) a tendency for more recent studies of women to show patterns closer to those of male populations, and (4) related research from other areas of adolescent psychology.

First, the data on which this interpretation was based are not totally persuasive. Female research participants drawn from one set of populations were compared to males drawn from different populations. In addition, the measures of the dependent variables were not always consistent between the studies of women and those of men.

Even more important, some of the results of studies with women did not show positive effects for Foreclosures. Marcia recognized this result, pointing out that Foreclosure women did seem to be more deferent to their boyfriends' wishes than Moratorium women, who developed clear tactics to assure themselves greater independence in their relationships (Greenhouse, 1975). This stereotypic feminine yielding seems to be part of a pattern that differentiates Foreclosure women from those achieving identity. Though Foreclosure women are not highly susceptible to external control exerted by strangers, they do yield uncritically to the influence of authorities (see preceding section). They appear to follow their mothers' model of yielding to male leadership (Matteson, 1974) when they relate to opposite-sex peers. The family interactions of Foreclosure youths were observed to be the least expressive. There is some evidence that creative expression (e.g., in writing poetry) is an important antecedent of Identity Achievement. Foreclosure women are less likely than Identity Achievement women to express themselves in poetry writing (Waterman & Archer, 1979). They are also less likely than Identity Achievement women to return to higher education once they marry and have children (Luria, 1980). In short, on certain variables Foreclosure women do not function like Achievements.

It is noteworthy that all the studies that have assigned identity statuses on the basis of the communal areas alone (sexual ideology or sex roles, see Table 4.1) have found significantly better functioning in Achievement women on some variables (see the "Anxiety" and "Self-esteem" sections above). It is also interesting that two recent studies have failed to replicate the earlier studies in which Foreclosure women functioned as well as Achievement women. Although an early study showed internal locus of control to be related to the stable statuses (Foreclosure and Achievement) in women, no such relationship was found in a later study (Orlofsky & Ginsburg, 1981).

TABLE 4.1. Identity and intimacy areas.

Abstraction		Operational
		Interview domains
	Agentic identity	Occupation
Sociocultural		Religion
	Ideological identity	Politics
		Values
		Sexual ideology
		Sex roles
	Interpersonal identity	Family roles
		Friendships
Communal		Dating
	Intimacy	Intimacy (Orlofsky)

Second, though early evidence suggested that female Foreclosures showed higher ego stability (Toder & Marcia, 1973), recent evidence using the same instrument has shown the contrary.

Third, some years ago, women did not seem to make clear progress from Diffusion to Identity Achievement during the college years, unlike men (Constantinople, 1969). However, more recent data generally suggest an increase in ego identity for both sexes as they increase in age (Protinsky, 1975; LaVoie, 1981; Prager, 1982; Archer, 1989c, though an exception is Schiedel & Marcia, 1985). Most persuasive, because of the cohort-sequential design (Schaie & Baltes, 1975), is a ten-year follow-up on Constantinople's original subjects (Whitbourne & Waterman, 1980). The results show that the trend of men toward higher identity statuses with increasing age held for the new cohort as well. The older sample of women, whose progress toward identity development during the college years was ambiguous, later showed the same age trend as the men. The new sample of young women was further advanced in identity formation than was the earlier sample at the same age. These are the most compelling data to date, suggesting that times are changing and that the progression of identity is important for today's college-educated women, whether in young adulthood or in middle age.

Finally, it is important to view identity status research in the context of other adolescent research. The extension of exploration into late adolescence (prolonging identity formation) has been shown in numerous developmental studies to be related in both sexes to humanizing of values, overcoming of prejudice and stereotyping, and acceptance of diversity and complexity (see Matteson, 1975, Ch. 11, 13). When we compare Foreclosure and Achievement women on the variables that have differentiated "protracted adolescence" from "abbreviated adolescence" (Blos, 1962), we find some important differences. Foreclosure women are not as sophisticated as Achievement women. Like male Foreclosures, they score significantly lower on moral reasoning (Poppen, 1974), on Piagetian cognitive tasks (Raphael, 1975), and somewhat lower on cognitive complexity (Matteson, 1974). The women who have gone through exploration of alternatives appear more sensitive (Josselson, 1972, 1973; Donovan, 1970, 1975) and better able to express impulses (Matteson, 1974). The differences among statuses just mentioned are consistent, regardless of sex, and do not appear to be attributable to differences in intellectual ability (Marcia, 1966, 1980). The evidence that Foreclosure women generally function like Identity Achievements is an illusion further challenged by findings from three studies using projective or deeper personality measures. In each case, Identity Achievement and Moratorium women were more advanced in their ego development than Foreclosure or Diffusion women (Orlofsky & Ginsburg, 1981; Josselson, 1987; Orlofsky & Frank, 1986).

Interestingly, the importance of exploration in female development was clear in the much earlier study of Danish females because, in addition to using the identity status categories, that study included direct ratings of the two process variables. The exploration scale discriminated on autonomy and "yea-saying" when the commitment scale did not (Matteson, 1974). To conclude, for personality differentiation and ego development, exploration of identity appears as important for women as for men.

Social Support for Identity Development

Assuming that exploration is important to women's identity as well as men's, the difficulty women have in achieving identity in our society (Marcia, 1979) must be recognized. The recognition is especially due if identity is defined using the occupation, religion, and politics (ORP) interviews; recall that women who achieved identity in ORP had the lowest self-esteem (Marcia & Friedman, 1970; Howard, 1975). Women who return to exploring identity in midlife may have a particularly difficult time, as suggested by their longing for "a guarantee of security" (Marcia and Miller, 1980). Marcia (1980) hypothesized that, during the adolescent years, women may not receive the same degree of social support for exploration of identity as do men. A pilot study of high school students provided tentative evidence for that conjecture. High school males in the exploration statuses (Moratoriums and Achievements) tended to be more popular, but females in the committed statuses (Achievements and Foreclosures) tended to be more popular (Matteson, 1978). In short, the pattern of identity statuses for each sex that has occurred on other variables is present here, suggesting that exploration of identity receives social support in males, but stability is sanctioned in females. Because the sample was small ($N = 33$), replication of these results is needed.

The disadvantages of women undergoing the exploration period (higher anxiety, lower self-esteem) appear to be related to the lack of social approval (see Dye, 1975). Studies of achievement motivation provide an interesting test of the hypothesis that lack of social support contributes to the conflicting results for Moratorium women. For both sexes, Moratorium and Identity Achievement youths are higher in achievement motivation (Howard, 1975; Orlofsky, 1978). For men, however, those who do not aspire to achieve (Foreclosures and Diffusions) experience most conflict. For women, those with highest aspirations (Moratoriums and Achievements) have greatest fear of success. It appears that women experience considerable conflict over their achievement striving. Women in the Foreclosure status, having low achievement motivation to begin with, avoid that conflict (Orlofsky, 1978).

Thus, although the search for identity brings women the same benefits it brings men—greater ego development and personality differentiation—

it also brings women the risk of social rejection. The Foreclosure status is functional for women in the way that conformity is functional for the adolescent; it does not bring an authentic sense of selfhood, but it's safe. Fortunately, some evidence suggests that social support is increasing for women engaging in a wider range of roles (Johnson et al., 1979).

Beyond Gender Differences: Gender Roles and Meta-Decisions

Erikson, like most psychologists of his era, assumed the bipolar nature of personality traits, specifically those of masculinity and femininity, and viewed as an important developmental task the achievement of a sex-appropriate gender identity—overcoming "bisexual confusion" through "sexual polarization" (Erikson, 1968, p. 94). This approach assumes that masculinity and femininity are opposites (so that an increase in one necessitates a decrease in the other) and that sexual polarization is the appropriate endpoint of sex-role development.

The recent research literature has challenged the assumption that masculinity and femininity are polar opposites (Hooker, 1965; Constantinople, 1973; Block, 1973; Spence et al., 1973, 1975, 1978; Bem, 1974). Most traits and roles that our culture labels masculine or feminine are independent of each other. Persons high on masculinity may also be high on femininity. Though differences in measurement occur, most recent research involves using separate scales for masculinity and femininity, and comparing research participants high on both ("androgynous"), low on both ("undifferentiated"), gender-typed, and cross-gender typed. The traits and behaviors typically viewed as masculine focus upon "the sense of agency," and feminine-typed traits and behaviors involve "a sense of communion" (Bakan, 1966).

> Agency reflects a sense of self and is manifested in self-assertion, self-protection, and self-expansion. Communion, on the other hand, implies selflessness, a concern with others and a desire to be at one with other organisms. (Spence et al., 1978)

The concept of androgyny, the integration of masculine and feminine traits, has become increasingly popular in social science research on sex-role development. In contrast to Erikson's model, Block (1973) has proposed that androgyny is a higher level of development than gender-role polarity. She suggests a model for gender-role development that parallels Loevinger and Wessler's (1970) model of ego development. According to her model, children move toward increasing role differentiation and the development of stereotypes during late childhood and adolescence, but then begin examining gender vis à vis the cultural gender types they have internalized, and differentiate their own views of masculine and feminine from the cultural stereotypes, leading to an integration of masculine and feminine aspects of themselves. A similar view of development is outlined by Hefner et al. (1975), who described three stages of gender-role development: undifferentiated, polarized, and transcendent. Gender-role transcendence may be a better label than androgyny because it stresses individual differences rather than a "unisex" style.

Consider the identity interview formats in view of this developmental theory: to transcend gender roles, an individual must accept as part of one's repertory both agentic and communal behaviors, and select situation-appropriate rather than gender-appropriate behaviors (see Table 4.1). For the most part, identity status research has assessed exploration among alternatives within a particular domain. For example, we have assumed one's identity will center on one's occupation, and have assessed the search among largely agentic alternatives. The early interview formats, used first with men, mainly had to do with agentic areas: the roles one will play in employment and politics. The formats developed later, and used first with women, have been more communal in content, such as the sexual-ideology interview. It is now clear that both agentic and communal domains are important for both men and women.

Following Block's model, we would expect early life decisions to involve a search among alternatives within an area perceived as "masculine" or "feminine" (e.g., occupational decisions for boys). But if the youth reaches the stage of gender-role transcendence, decisions will need to be made on the relative importance of agentic versus communal functions. For example, the question may shift from "What vocation should I choose?" to "How important is job fulfilment compared to fulfilment in family life?" The interview formats on values, sex roles, and personal life-styles, and the Archer format on family and career decisions (see Chapters 8–10) can be viewed as assessing meta-decisions. The gender-role interview, for example, questions the youth about decisions involving priorities between traditionally "masculine" and "feminine" activities. It seems important to distinguish persons who have weighed alternatives *within* the "masculine" areas (e.g., occupation), or *within* the "feminine" areas (e.g., raising a family) from those who have weighed life-style decisions and considered the full range of possibilities. The evidence suggests that women are more likely than men to undergo meta-decision exploration (Shanken, 1984, Archer, 1985a) as we might suspect from the recent changes in women's roles.

It is a heuristic assumption that sex-role decisions are likely to be "watershed" decisions, because so many of our cultural perceptions have been polarized along gender-role lines. We must recognize that we are imposing a priori the categories of "masculine" and "feminine" activities; these may not be the existential categories around which that individual makes decisions. Only by studying an individual over time could we learn which decisions in her life turned out to be meta-decisions; the content and the categories themselves would be idiographic.

Despite these theoretical problems, it seems important to distinguish persons who have weighed life-style decisions considering the full range of possibilities and consciously decided on their priorities.

Within-Gender Differences and the Life Span

The influence of the women's movement and its effects upon the identity of adult women encouraged researchers to turn their attention beyond the adolescent years in studying female identity. O'Connell (1976) asked middle-aged women to respond to a written, open-ended inventory collecting retrospective data on different periods in their lives. She distinguished "personal" and "reflected" identity.

> Personal identity is an awareness of, and emphasis upon, one's talents, endowments, capabilities, and needs; its focus is on one's unique qualities from which one's self-esteem and feelings of worth are derived. . . . A reflected sense of identity emphasizes the significant others rather than one's own personal characteristics; its focus is external. Self-esteem [is] derived from one's participation in the lives of significant others. It is . . . identity by association. (O'Connell, 1976)

This study is noteworthy in that the data were analyzed using different pathways of development, in terms of the women's work and family history. (See Figure 4.1, which visually portrays her results.) No important differences appeared between women who had interrupted paid employment during childrearing and resumed it afterward (neotraditional), and those who continued as full-time homemakers (traditional), but these groups differed strikingly from mothers who were continuously committed to their careers. The latter group conceived of their identity as stronger, and described identity more personally throughout the life periods. The more traditional groups did not develop a strong personal identity until their children left for school. Strength of identity increased significantly for all three groups of women upon marriage, suggesting that "intimacy apparently contributes to (women's) self-definition." But when that increase is proportionately distributed (according to the ratio of responses) into "personal" and "reflected" identity, only the nontraditional group increases in personal identity through marriage.

It is theoretically possible for personal identity to appear around awareness of one's talents and capabilities within interpersonal relationships. If a person's identity is focused on interpersonal concerns it does not necessarily mean it is a "merged" or "reflected" identity.

Measurements such as the identity statuses, the intimacy statuses, and O'Connell's inventory need to be used together to clarify the issues of the relationship between merged and personal identity and intimacy. Those

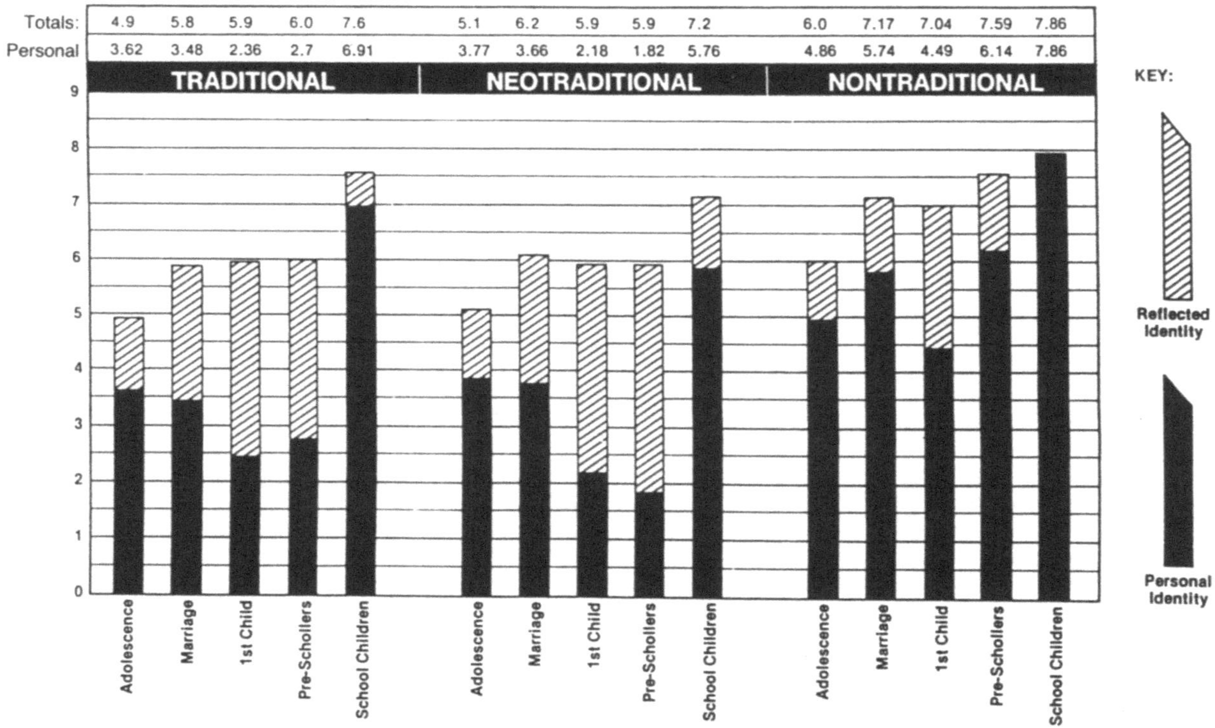

FIGURE 4.1. Personal and Reflected Identity in Women. Based on 'data from retrospective responses of middle-aged women, in Agnes N. O'Connell, "The relationship between life style and identity synthesis and resynthesis in traditional, neotraditional and nontraditional women," *Journal of Personality*, vol. 44, no. 4 (December 1976), pp. 675–688. See Tables I, II. Calculating scores of personal identity from ratio (Table II) applied to strength of identity (Table I) is Matteson's extrapolation.

planning studies in this area are urged to consider three concerns, stated briefly here and elaborated in the last section of this chapter. First, studies should include respondents of both genders drawn from the same population, to allow valid comparisons between the genders. Second, considerable impressionistic research suggests that a reappraisal of masculinity and femininity occurs in midlife for men as well as women;[1] the nature of the mid-life identity process is more likely to be illuminated if we gather and compare data for both genders.[2] Third, though I would not deny the historic value of gathering retrospective data from middle-aged women, our understanding of the identity process is much more likely to be furthered by studies (e.g.) beginning with a comparison of an adolescent and a middle-aged group, and following each group until the adolescents are in middle age. It seems clear that issues of masculinity, femininity, and the life span will best be resolved by studies including both genders and using cohort-sequential (cross-lagged) designs (Schaie & Baltes, 1975).

Comparative Pathways: Studies with Both Genders and Several Domains

Much of the theory on gender differences in identity hinges on whether males and females center their identity in different content areas (the "domains" of the interviews) and whether they mature at the same rate. Thus we turn to studies which have used both male and female subjects, and which rated identity in each of the domains, not just an overall identity status. Studies meeting both of these criteria are arranged according to age of subjects in Table 4.2.

The Sequence of Maturation and the Domains

To clarify my use of terms in this section, let me summarize my conceptualization of the domains used in the various research interviews and their possible connections to masculinity and femininity. Table 4.1 shows

---

[1] Levinson's (1978) interviews suggest that mid-life crisis is common in men across a wide span of vocational and socioeconomic strata. His studies do not use the identity status measures and can't be directly compared to ours. The oldest males reported in a published identity status study are those in Marcia's follow-up (1976), who would be about 28 years of age, compared to a range of 21 to 59 for Miller's women subjects. Only 6 percent of Marcia's men were undergoing "crisis" (Moratoriums) compared to 28 percent of Miller's women. Differences in ages, and in populations, make it uncertain whether or not this is a genuine gender difference.

[2] It will take some creativity to develop a parallel measure of the priorities men set for family life and vocations and various states in their lives. Archer has led the way (see Archer, 1985a, 1985b), using an interview on family versus career on three age groups and on a sample of divorced men and women.

TABLE 4.2. Percentages in mature statuses, by domains[A].

Study	Age of subjects	Occupation		Politics		Religion		Sex ideology		Sex roles		Family roles		Friendship		Dating		Intimacy		Overall Identity	
		M	F	M	F	M	F	M	F	M	F	M	F	M	F	M	F	M	F	M	F
Archer, 1984	x = 12	**25**	13							04	04	0	**13**								
Archer, 1982[B]	11–18	23	**30**	01	03	16	19			06	**14**										
Archer, 1984	x = 16	**38**	29							17	13	13	**33**								
Matteson, 1979[B]	17	**37**	20							25	**30**							31	**50**		
Matteson, 1974[C]	17–18	47	**69**	**53**	47	38	39			38	**51**									55	57
Grotevant & Thorbecke, 1982[B]	17–18	60	**66**	36	36	51	55			26	**49**			48	73	32	**43**			**74**	65
Poppen, 1974[B]	17–21	52	56	**44**	27	42	38	38	**63**											50	**82**
Waterman & Nevid, 1977[B]	17–22	40	41	26	22	36	40	24	**54**												
Heyduk, 1982	16–23	68	**92**			55	57	64	**69**	41	**47**									50	**82**
Adams & Fitch, 1983	17–22	72	72	**32**	14	**51**	31													**57**	47
Hodgson & Fischer, 1979[B]	18–21	**56**	28	**36**	14	**50**	28	40	**50**	30	**58**							50	**72**		
Orlofsky, 1978[B]	19–21	51	54	33	32	40	39	44	43											35	**52**
Schiedel & Marcia (in press)	18–24																	28	**50**	48	**55**
Rothman, 1978[B]	x = 21	80	**87**	**49**	34	49	**57**	**89**	81											60	**70**
Kacerguis & Adams, 1980[B]	19–25	**71**	66	14	**32**	**55**	39											**50**	**52**	55	52
Whitbourne & Tesch (in press)[B,D]	x = 21 (students)	37	**42**	**10**	02	15	19			**13**	08							62	**76**		
Whitbourne & Tesch, 1982[D]	x = 25 (alumni)	**62**	53	34	31	35	**40**			44	**67**							62	**70**	44	**52**
Shanken, 1984	22–29	62	**76**	**62**	41	46	**53**	54	**76**											54	**65**
Shanken, 1984	30–35	60	**69**	**53**	38	**67**	46	60	**85**											**73**	62
Zampich, 1980	33–56	**43**	27	**43**	30	43	43			40	**50**									40	40

Bold type signifies gender with score higher by 5 percent or more.

[A] More mature status for identity are moratorium or achievement: for intimacy are pre-intimate and intimate.

[B] Data received in personal communications with author; not in the published version.

[C] Personal values interview was used because religion interview was inappropriate for Denmark.

[D] The "merged" intimacy category used in this study was deleted in calculating percentages for more accurate comparison with the other studies.

the interview domains on the right, and two levels of categorization or groupings of these in the middle and left columns.

At face value, only occupational identity is clearly related to the "masculine" trait of agency. The feminine or communal area can be tapped in two ways, with one or more of the interpersonal identity interviews, or with the Orlofsky intimacy interview. The ideological area of identity may become important because of either masculine or feminine concerns, or may become an area of meta-decisions because of conflicts among other areas (e.g., between agentic and interpersonal concerns, or between self and other concerns).

The Hodgson study (Hodgson & Fischer, 1979, and personal correspondence) is a useful model because it includes many of the elements needed in identity and intimacy research. Sociocultural (ORP) and communal (SI, SR, and Intimacy) interview areas were used with respondents of both genders from the same population. The gender of interviewers was counterbalanced (a precaution ignored in most studies except Matteson, 1974, 1979). Within-gender differences as well as comparisons between genders were addressed by grouping the subjects by "pathways." Respondents in advanced identity statuses (Moratorium and Achievement) on the ORP but in low statuses (Diffusion and Foreclosure) on the SI and SR were considered to be following the masculine pathway; respondents with the reverse patterns, mature in interpersonal but low in sociocultural domains, were labeled as following the feminine pathway. Respondents in mature statuses in both sociocultural and interpersonal areas were referred to as following an androgynous pathway; those low in both areas were labeled "no pathway."

The comparison of these four pathways parallels work being done in the broader social science literature on gender roles. As would be expected, males tended to be classified as in the masculine pathway (36%), and females the feminine pathway (20%), though a high percentage of these undergraduates were not in mature statuses in either area (38% of males and 58% of females). A higher percentage of males (26%) than females (10%) were androgynous, in contrast to findings using standardized masculinity and femininity measures of androgyny. Twelve percent of females were following the masculine pathway; they were in mature statuses in sociocultural domains, but were in low statuses in the communal areas. No men in this sample followed the feminine pathway; thus no evidence appeared of cultural support for cross-gender-typed identity in men.

Fortunately, the Hodgson study also included some measures of dependent variables as well as comparisons between domains. This combination produced results that help resolve some of the confusion in previous studies on self-esteem. Hodgson found lower self-esteem among women classified as no pathway or masculine pathway, but higher self-esteem if they were in the female or androgynous pathways. This result suggests that identity achievement in traditionally masculine areas (ORP) does not in itself lower women's self-esteem. It appears that women can find support for identity achievement if they do so in a distinctively feminine way (Matteson, 1975). That is, if women do not neglect the communal areas, they may "add on" sociocultural areas of identity struggle as well (just as women can be accepted in the workforce, as long as they also continue all their responsibilities for home and family).

Grotevant and colleagues refined interviews for the interpersonal domains of identity, again including measures of dependent variables: gender roles, achievement motivation, and a vocational identity test (Grotevant, Thorbecke, & Meyer, 1982; Thorbecke & Grotevant, 1982). They also separately rated exploration and commitment as continuous variables, allowing statistical correlations with the dependent measures. Though the communal areas appear important to males as well as females, males seem to approach interpersonal relations as arenas for competition and mastery, and use friendship to facilitate achievement goals (see Josselson et al., 1977). For females, by contrast, commitment to friendships is inversely correlated with competitiveness, fitting Gilligan's theory (1982). Together, the Hodgson and the Grotevant studies show that the communal areas are important to both sexes, but may have different qualitative meanings for males (competitive, achieving) and for females (with the agentic areas being socially accepted only after the communal areas are secure).

The Relationship Between Identity and Intimacy

Erikson's epigenetic theory assumes not only that identity precedes intimacy, but that identity forms a necessary base for the development of intimacy. Clearly the identity and intimacy statuses are related, in that high status on one tends to be associated with high status on the other. However, unpublished data from a study of high school students (Matteson, 1979; see Table 4.2), using interviews in agentic and interpersonal identity and in intimacy (Table 4.1) led me to doubt Erikson's stepwise sequence, at least for women.

Hodgson's data also suggested that intimacy may develop in women before a clear identity has appeared, even in the interpersonal areas. In fact, nearly half the women in the low statuses of identity had reached high levels of intimacy. Sixty-six percent of the women were high in intimacy though only 42 percent were high in identity.

A look at the data compiled in Table 4.2 reveals that Hodgson's results are not unique. The most apparent gender differences in the table affect intimacy. Women equal or exceed men in percentages in the higher intimacy statuses in every study shown. And the percentage of women in high-intimacy statuses is greater than in any other domain in four out of six cases. Throughout the diverse populations sampled, women generally appear to be more advanced in intimacy than in identity. Because no age progression is apparent in the 17- to 25-year-old span, we cannot conclude that intimacy development precedes identity, or vice versa. We can only conclude for this age span that intimacy has priority over identity in women's development.

Even for men the sequence does not seem to be "epigenetic" in the sense that Erikson's theory proposes. Hodgson's male respondents in the masculine and "no" pathways scored much *lower* on intimacy than did androgynous pathway males. (See section on the importance of different domains, below.)

The only longitudinal identity study that also assessed intimacy was the Adams and Fitch study (1981, 1982, 1983), but they did not assess identity in the interpersonal areas. It did show that *for men*, high identity status (ORP) in the first year was significantly related to high intimacy status (Orlofsky) in the second year. The relationship did not hold beyond the second year, possibly because of the attrition in respondents participating in the later data collection. For women there was no evidence that the identity to intimacy sequence held; even the positive relationship between overall identity status and intimacy was problematic.

So far, the data reviewed suggest that identity may precede intimacy for men, but not for women. But if identity is not a necessary condition for intimacy, what is the relationship between these two? The Schiedel and Marcia (1985) study was designed to explore this question further; it included both sociocultural and interpersonal portions of the identity interview, the intimacy interview, and a measure of gender roles (Bem, 1974). As in the Hodgson study, men (with one exception) tended to develop high levels of intimacy only if identity had been achieved. But one-third of the women who were low in identity were nonetheless high in intimacy. This result validated what our review of Table 4.2 suggests, that some women deal successfully with intimacy issues prior to identity issues. And the one exception in the male data, a male who followed the "female pathway," stood as a lonely challenge to Erikson's theory, as if to say "the theory doesn't even work for all men!" Cross-gender pathways of development may be beginning to occur for men, just as they have for women.

A look at Table 4.3 suggests that this man is not alone, if we reanalyze data from other studies assessing both identity and intimacy. Only respondents in the highest two intimacy statuses are presented here, and so the high percentage in the top two identity statuses is no surprise. It is striking, however, that between 9 and 48 percent of the respondents are able to attain high levels of intimacy without having developed mature identities. That is, roughly 30 percent of the participants who achieve mature intimacy do so prior to or independent from achievement of mature identity. Though a higher percentage of females attain intimacy without mature identity (roughly 35 percent), the proportion for males (roughly 27 percent) is far too high to be attributed to mistakes in

TABLE 4.3. Identity status of subjects high in intimacy.

Study	Low identity		High identity	
	Males	Females	Males	Females
Kacerguis & Adams, 1980[A]	44	36	56	64
Orlofsky et al., 1973[B]	10		90	
Prager, 1977		40		60
Schiedel & Marcia, 1983	9	30	91	70
Whitbourne & Tesch, 1982 (alumni)	43	35	57	65
Zampich, 1980[C]	23		77	

High intimacy subjects are those classified as intimate or pre-intimate. Low identity subjects are foreclosures and diffusions; high identity are moratoriums and achievements.
[A] Unpublished data; personal correspondence with G. Adams.
[B] A fifth identity status, alienated achievement, was used in this study. These subjects were deleted in calculating percentages for the sake of comparison with the other studies.
[C] Data were not reported separately for males and females.

assignment to identity or intimacy categories. Regardless of gender, overall identity does not seem to be a prerequisite for intimacy.

A possible revision of the theory would be that identity and intimacy each involve an array of simultaneously developing and interacting personality traits and interpersonal skills. The two (identity and intimacy) interact with and amplify each other, but neither is necessarily first; neither is the "base" on which the other is built. Returning to Bakan's terms, no evidence suggests that agentic traits must precede communal or the reverse. Longitudinal data for women on agentic and communal traits suggest that behavioral development progresses simultaneously in both areas throughout the period of approximately ages 15 to 21 (Sola, 1980).

This view of identity and intimacy as interactive, rather than Erikson's view of identity as primary, fits the Hodgson data in which the interpersonal areas of identity are better predictors than the agentic ones of a man's level of intimacy. Schiedel and Marcia (1985) found that high identity status was related to high masculinity scores (measured independently from femininity), and high intimacy development for males was related to high femininity scores. (This finding did not hold for females, perhaps because almost all females are high enough in femininity to achieve the level necessary for intimacy). (See below for more on the relationship of masculinity and femininity.)

To summarize, though identity may positively correlate with intimacy, it does not appear to be a prerequisite. Further, males appear less well trained in the communal skills, and trail behind women in the development of intimacy. There is weak evidence that in young adulthood men catch up to women in intimacy. Two studies with older samples have shown no gender differences in level of intimacy. The sample in one (Imberman, 1983) was limited to married couples, however, and thus may have excluded those lower on intimacy; the other sample was from a highly educated and sophisticated group and also may not allow generalization (Shanken, 1984).

Is Some Area of Secure Self a Prerequisite for Intimacy?

Once we recognize that overall identity is not necessary for the development of intimacy, we are led to look for some other prerequisite to intimacy. Hodgson reported in his data that *any* of the "pathways" (feminine, masculine, and androgynous) was more likely to lead to intimacy for women than "no pathway." That is, overall identity was not more predictive than identity in just the interpersonal, or just the sociocultural areas; but respondents with any area of mature identity were more likely to achieve intimacy than subjects with no area of mature identity. Prager (1977), Kacerguis and Adams (1980), Imberman (1983), Stolesen (1981) and Shanken (1984) found no relationship between overall identity status and intimacy status in women. Further data analysis by Kacerguis & Adams (1980), however, showed that when identity was rated separately by areas (rather than assigning an overall identity status), women in the committed categories of identity were more likely to be in the higher intimacy statuses. A positive relationship between commitment and intimacy was found for *both* males and females in a later study (Shanken, 1984). In both of the studies just cited the relationship within domains was with commitment, not maturity of identity. In another study (Tesch, 1980), though overall identity status did not relate to intimacy, women who achieved identity in the political domain were more likely to be in the highest intimacy status. Still another study (O'Connell, 1976, see p. 78) has shown that women's personal identity is fostered by having some "life of her own," such as an occupational commitment. Results such as these led me to hypothesize that, though identity may not precede intimacy for women, "some area of secure self (either through achieved identity or through commitment) seems related to intimacy" (Matteson, 1980). Borrowing from the jargon of family-interaction theory (Minuchin, 1974), the issue is one of "personal boundaries." This conceptualization does not assume that mature identity must be developed in some domain. Nor does it assume that personal boundaries must be developed prior to intimacy; intimacy may develop first, but that precipitates the development of personal boundaries, if it is to be mature intimacy rather than dependent or merged intimacy.

Once it was recognized that the traditional feminine style had been to develop interpersonal and intimacy areas first, the issue of "stability" was interpreted in a new light. One must develop a sense of stable self from which to give and receive intimately and still take care of oneself. It is in precisely this area of personal boundaries (susceptibility to outside influence) that female Foreclosures and Achievements look most alike. In instrumental achievement, a highly differentiated personality is most functional. In communal interaction, intrapersonal complexity is less important than boundary issues. With this speculation we can begin to make sense of the evidence (reviewed in Matteson, 1980) that any one area of either personal stability or Identity Achievement is predictive of higher intimacy. Additional support comes from the fact that, for both sexes, self-disclosure with an intimate other is higher for persons in the committed identity statuses (Kinsler, 1972; Zampich, 1980).

Unfortunately, reanalysis of existing data showed the "boundary" hypotheses (that some area of secure self precedes, or at least correlates with identity) fares only slightly better than the original "identity precedes intimacy" hypothesis. It holds for most men (but not all), but it fails to account for a large minority of women.

Despite the greater likelihood of intimacy where there is some area of mature identity, Hodgson's data reveal that 27 percent of his male subjects and 42 percent of his female subjects who were high in intimacy came from the "no pathway" group. To further test whether it is possible to develop mature intimacy before a person has clear boundaries, I examined previous studies to see whether Diffusion subjects achieve intimacy.

Of the six studies with males in the sample, only one reported any Diffusion males in high intimacy statuses (Kacerguis & Adams, 1980, in contrast to Zampich, 1980; Heyduk, 1982; Tesch & Whitbourne, 1982; Adams & Fitch, 1983, and Schiedel & Marcia, 1985). Four of the five studies with Diffusion women in the sample, however, report some Diffusion women in the high intimacy statuses (Prager, 1982; Tesch & Whitbourne, 1982; Schiedel & Marcia, 1985; Kacerguis & Adams, 1980; in contrast to Adams & Fitch, 1983, who found none). One might assume that Diffusion respondents could, at best, achieve a dependent or merged intimacy; yet one study carefully differentiated merged intimacy from mature intimacy, and nonetheless assigned two of the four Diffusion women to the Intimate, and one to the Pre-intimate category (Tesch & Whitbourne, 1982).

Though this reanalysis of data is not an ideal test of the issue, that intimacy without clear boundaries is more frequent in women than men parallels the greater percentage of Intimate women from the "no pathways" group in Hodgson's data. Diffusion and intimacy seem to coexist in some women (though rarely in men), suggesting that, in these women, intimacy precedes development of clear boundaries.

As research outside the identity field suggests (Gilligan, 1982) the masculine path may lead first through separation that defines and empowers the self; the feminine path leads through attachment that creates community, out of which individuation may occur. (See Archer, 1985a,c, for some problems with this view.) It is clear that women generally achieve intimacy earlier than their male cohorts (though women increasingly are also achieving identity) and that intimacy does not depend on the prior formation of identity, or even personal boundaries.

In fact, using a measure related to intimacy, intensity of friendships, identity status has been found to be a far less powerful predictor than is the biological gender of the subject. And feminine and androgynous subjects of both sexes develop more intense friendships than masculine subjects. The connections between identity and intimacy in dyadic systems have only begun to be assessed (Arora & Marcia, unpublished) and are too complex to review here.

The positive relationships that have been found between identity and intimacy, and between personal boundaries and intimacy, cannot be taken to imply a sequential or dependent relationship. Because intimacy does occur with diffusion, the positive relationship cannot be causal. The positive relationship is most likely to be due to a third factor. For example, the women who are more willing to make identity or job commitments may also be higher in intimacy status because of a broader personality trait, such as the *willingness to get involved*, which affects both identity and intimacy.

Summary of the Identity–Intimacy Connection

The data have forced a retreat from:

1. Erikson's original position that identity is the foundation for intimacy, to
2. the hypothesis of some identity researchers that some area of secure self (or boundaries) is a prerequisite to intimacy, to my finally
3. abandoning any belief that agentic development is causally linked to communal development. The levels of positive correlations that do exist seem most likely to result from common factors of learning in both areas of development and to personality characteristics (such as willingness to be involved) that are functional in both agentic and communal areas.

Much more study is needed to unravel the ways in which identity development and interpersonal development interact and support each other, to distinguish between reflected identity and more mature identity, to distinguish between merged intimacy and more mature intimacy, and to clarify sequences over time in the same respondents. Lacking such refined cross-sequential studies, we turn now to the second issue illuminated by studies with separate assessment of the domains, the relative importance of the different domains to male and female identity.

Gender differences in the importance of the interpersonal versus the sociocultural areas have been assessed in several studies. The usual hypotheses predict that occupation, or the whole sociocultural area, will be important for men, and the interpersonal area will be important for women. Many of the studies summarized in Table 4.2, as well as some studies with only male or only female subjects, have addressed the relative importance of the different domains. At least five approaches to assessing "relative importance" have been used, though little attention has been paid to the rationales for these approaches.

1. *Comparative percentages of males, and of females, in the mature statuses of each domain* (summarized in Table 4.2). Restricting ourselves to the identity statuses, females clearly excel males in the interpersonal domains. Only in the political domain do males sometimes excel. Comparing domains within gender, occupation seems the most important domain for both males and females. Longitudinal studies with two grade school and high school populations verify that women are now maturing in identity as early as men, and suggest that women in these age groups are less likely to remain foreclosed (Archer, 1989c).
2. *Relationships of mature identity in a particular domain to mature intimacy* (based on the studies in Table 4.2). Though there is a relationship between overall identity status and intimacy for males, there is no pattern suggesting which domains contribute to that relationship, despite numerous studies.
3. *Self-report*. Four studies have yielded contradictory results (Meilman, 1979, and Rogow et al., 1983 on men; Schiedel & Marcia, 1985, and Kroger, 1987 on both genders).
4. *Correlations between particular domains and overall identity status*. Five studies with women and seven with men show no pattern for women, but suggest that for men the interpersonal and ideological areas are becoming more important. Differences in populations sampled make this generalization highly tentative. (The studies cited in (3) above, plus Schenkel & Marcia, 1972; Heyduk, 1983; Shanken, 1984; Meilman, 1979; Waterman & Nevid, 1977).
5. *Predictive power with dependent variables*. Four studies have used this method for both sexes (Vreeland, 1982; Matteson, 1977a, 1979; and Schuster, 1982). The results are complex, with different domains predicting different variables. It is clear that both the sociocultural and the interpersonal areas are important for both genders.

Summarizing, methods 2, 3, and 5 produce no pattern to suggest that some domains are consistently more important or predictive for one gender than the other. Methods 1 and 4 show women consistently more mature than men in the interpersonal domains; men are more likely to be committed in the political domain.

Methodological Issues in the Study of Femininity, Masculinity, and the Identity Statuses

A review of the voluminous literature on gender differences and sex roles (see Matteson, unpublished earlier version) shows a number of blind alleys that have been explored and abandoned—a history from which identity research can learn.

1. *Distinguishing traits from roles*. The characteristics stereotypically ascribed to each sex are not necessarily those needed to function in the traditional roles. These need to be measured separately. The functions of childrearing, for example, require many agentic traits (Bem, 1975); and in the crucial "feminine area" of social interaction, it is women with high masculinity scores who excel (Wells, 1980). Once the distinction between attributes and behavior is clear, it is not a surprise to find that a woman viewed as "very masculine" can function as a homemaker and mother, and an "effeminate" man may be effective in his role as provider for the family.
2. *Recording within-gender differences*. Sometimes persons with "masculine" interests are more similar in functioning, regardless of biological gender, than are persons of the same gender with different interests (e.g., Norris & Katz, 1970). And frequently the differences between typical and atypical subgroups within each gender parallel the differences between genders (e.g., Norris et al., 1978).
3. *Separate scaling of masculinity and femininity is necessary*. We have already discussed the fallacy of thinking of these traits as bipolar. Two examples of how separate scaling has clarified the empirical relationships must suffice. Bipolar scales led to the mistaken belief that women's higher intuitive (vs. rational) decision-making styles correlated with their higher femininity. Separate scaling has shown that it is not high femininity, but low masculinity, which predicts higher intuitive decision making in women (Moreland et al., 1979). There is no evidence that high scores in "masculine" traits militate against high scores in feminine traits, or vice versa, as thoroughly demonstrated in a review of the relationship of individualism to such traits as social interdependence (Archer & Waterman, 1988).
4. *Test for possible "sleeper effects."* Clear interpretations of the effects of masculinity and femininity require analysis of scores over several years of development. The relationship between low masculinity and intuitive style just reported does not appear during the early high school years. It first becomes significant when subjects reach their senior year in high school (Sola, 1976) and continues through the college years (Moreland et al., 1979). As mentioned earlier, the adolescent years appear to involve a simultaneous increase in both masculine and feminine characteristics (Sola, 1976). During these years the increase in masculine scores appears to be more marked than the increase in feminine scores, at least for women (Phye & Sola, 1984). We can speculate that this increase happens to an even greater extent for men. Subjects who do not undergo sufficient increase in masculinity continue to make intuitive rather than rational decisions; thus the effect appears only after masculine scores have increased for the group.

A less complex illustration of the need for follow-up studies for clear interpretation comes from an early longitudinal study. Results during the high school years suggested that boys who were most masculine had all the advantages over their less masculine peers (Mussen & Jones, 1957). These same males, however, when the follow-up data were gathered during the middle years, were not so unambiguously well off. Some of the feminine traits that had made their peers unpopular during adolescence turned out to be functional and positive later in life (Jones, 1957, 1965; Mussen, 1962). In masculinity and femininity, it appears to be particularly risky to judge consequences based on data from only one stage of development. Again, cohort-sequential studies of both sexes seem most valuable.

Femininity, Masculinity, and the Identity Process

Returning to identity status research, the two variables that have defined the process of identity formation are (a) exploration of alternatives, and (b) commitment. Exploration of alternatives, as it is actually measured in the interviews, seems to be highly related to "expressiveness." Moratorium subjects (presently involved in exploration) seem more expressive and tend to take longer on the identity status interviews than respondents in the other statuses.[3] In a study by Munro and Adams (1977), separate measures of expressiveness and instrumentality (based on the conceptions of Parsons & Bales, 1955) were used to predict identity achievement. Contrary to prediction, no difference between statuses occurred on the instrumental scale. It was the expressive scale that revealed significant differences. Moratoriums were found to be most expressive, with Achievements next. The differences between Moratoriums and the less mature statuses (Diffusion and Foreclosure) were significant, a pattern that held for both genders and for both college and working-class youths in the sample.[4]

These results seem congruent with the direct observations of Moratorium family triad interactions. These families had the highest interaction rate, and expressed more positive and negative emotions than did the triads from the less mature statuses (Matteson, 1974). The Foreclosure families tended to be the most task-oriented (instrumental) and were most likely to complete the assigned task.

---

[3] The difference in interview length was sufficient to raise concern about possibly confounding length of interview with assessment of exploration. In one study (Matteson, 1979) this variable was controlled by restricting the time for each section of the interview.

[4] For both genders, scales of exploration and commitment (rather than the identity status categories) show exploration to be the more salient variable in correlations with other personality variables as well (Grotevant & Cooper, 1985; Matteson, 1977a).

More recent studies have used scales of masculinity and femininity, and followed Bem's procedure of comparing groups high on only one scale ("masculine" and "feminine" groups) to those high on both scales ("androgynous") and on neither ("undifferentiated"). Despite differences in the measures, the three additional studies using identity statuses (Orlofsky, 1977; Prager, 1982; Waterman & Whitbourne, 1982) found a pattern similar to that just reported. Foreclosures, regardless of sex, were overwhelmingly in sex-typed categories (males were masculine, females feminine). Feminine characteristics seemed necessary during exploration of alternatives, but masculine traits seemed necessary to reach Identity Achievement.[5] Using scales to assess the interviews, instead of the identity statuses, Grotevant & Thorbecke (1982) confirmed this finding. The outcome of Identity Achievement seems to require a moderately high level of masculine traits, though these traits can coexist with feminine traits, and need not deflate or discount the femininity of a female Identity Achievement. This interpretation parallels the longitudinal data on decision-making styles for women: high masculinity is a necessary condition, though high femininity does not suppress the emergence of a rational decision-making style (Sola, 1976; Phye & Sola, 1984).

Schiedel and Marcia (1985) reversed Grotevant's methods, using the rating scales (rather than sex-role categories) of masculinity and femininity, and added intimacy interviews as well as identity. They confirmed the pattern of higher masculinity scores for Identity Achievements. For males, they found higher femininity scores were needed to achieve high intimacy statuses. (Females appear to score high enough on femininity, and so higher levels are not needed to achieve intimacy). Valdez's (1984) finding for women suggest the reverse of the pattern just reported for men—higher levels of masculinity needed for identity, but not for intimacy. This relationship fits the view that in women, intimacy develops earlier, and identity requires further maturation and integration. For men the reverse is true, with identity developing earlier and intimacy developing only in those who reach more advanced levels. These findings make sense in the light of Block's model of gender-role development described earlier.

---

[5] Schenkel's (1975) early study used a bipolar scale of masculinity-femininity, and can't be interpreted by types. The results fit the developmental pattern (F D M A) in the direction of increasing masculinity, and do not conflict with the findings reported. Grotevant & Thorbecke (1982) found a similar though not identical distribution using occupational identity. The major difference is a higher proportion of Identity Achievements among the feminine subjects. Using the Objective Measure of Ego Identity Status with high school subjects, Behar (1983) found androgynous youths most likely to be Identity Achievements. Androgynous subjects also scored highest on Constantinople's identity measure (Della Selva & Dusek, 1984).

Healthy Functioning

Parallel to the interest in determining which identity statuses are most functional, interest has been considerable in determining the relationships between the gender-role styles and healthy functioning. In both Orlofsky's and Prager's studies, high self-esteem was closely related to masculinity or androgyny; undifferentiated subjects had the lowest self-esteem.

The relationship between gender-role styles and measures of mental health is a complex one however.[6] At first, the concept of androgyny was presented as uniformly positive, stressing the advantages of being flexible and capable of both agentic and communal behaviors. However, a careful piece of research with multiple measures of mental health led Jones et al. (1978) to conclude that measures of mental health and well-being have tended to be more positively related to masculinity than to femininity. The measures Jones used, and for that matter most measures of mental health, are loaded on the instrumental side; instrumental behaviors are more valued in the work world regardless of gender. But communal behaviors are valued in men, as well as women, in the family. Children express the wish for more nurturant qualities, particularly in relation to their fathers (Lifshitz, 1978). When femininity is measured by positive communal items such as interpersonal awareness, it correlates positively with self-esteem. It is the items on emotional vulnerability that result in low self-esteem scores for highly feminine subjects (Spence & Helmreich, 1978).

In a response to Jones, Wells (1980) has argued that "the effect of gender-role identity on psychological adjustment is complex and is dependent upon both the sex of the respondent and the index of adjustment." Androgyny, as usually measured, does not necessarily provide an advantage over traditional identity in sex-typed situations; in situations involving behaviors that have been stereotyped as appropriate for the other gender, a cross-gender-role identity is advantageous.

Androgyny does allow greater flexibility (as Jones et al., 1978, admit despite their critical review of Bem's work) and does not seem to be associated with poorer adjustment of high school boys even in instrumental areas (Wells, 1980). The only setting in which it can be argued that masculine sex typing is more advantageous than androgyny is in highly competitive college environments (Jones et al., 1978). This advantage is probably attributable to the low rewards given to communal behaviors in this setting.

---

[6] I have used the phrase gender-role style rather than sex-role orientation to avoid confusion with sexual orientation. Our popular culture frequently confuses sexual orientation (homosexuality, bisexuality, heterosexuality), gender identity (one's concept of oneself as a man, or as a woman), and gender-role style (masculine, feminine, androgynous). These are discrete concepts, and may or may not be correlated.

Conclusions on Femininity and Masculinity

The two variables that underlie the identity statuses (exploration and commitment) seem highly related to the variables involved in sex typing (see Table 4.4). A positive relationship appears to connect exploration and expressive/feminine traits, and to connect commitment and instrumental/masculine traits. This relationship is not easily attributable to methods of assessment; it has been demonstrated using very different forms of measurement.

The integration of masculine and feminine behaviors (androgyny, or sex-role transcendence) and the achievement of commitment after exploration (Identity Achievement status) appear to be generally related to positive mental health for both sexes. This conclusion must be drawn with the caution that most measures of mental health are situation-specific. It is more meaningful to talk about the specific situations in which agentic behaviors or communal behaviors are functional—and likewise, the specific settings in which, for example, Foreclosure women (or masculine men) function as well as do Achievement women (or androgynous men).

Summary, Hypotheses, and Theoretical Directions

The Decision-Making Model

The identity status investigations began as an attempt to understand the process of identity formation, or, as I prefer to call it, the process of making life decisions. A sequence of operations can be seen as prototypic: a recognition that a particular area of concern warrants some decision; an assessment of one's own needs and desires in relation to the alternatives available; an exploration through some form of tentative but direct involvement when possible; and a gradually growing sense of "this is me," with a commitment that provides some direction and continuity for that individual. Some sequence of movement through exploration to commitment, and with it greater autonomy, is implied in the conceptualization of the developmental progression of identity statuses (see Matteson, 1975, Ch. 15). This prototype gains support from most of the data on men's identity formation, particularly in occupational identity. It also parallels the optimal strategies for decision making as analyzed in general research on decision making (Janis & Mann, 1977).

With this decision-making model as background, let us remind ourselves of the areas in which identity status research has produced similar data for both males and females. Foreclosures show low anxiety; they have not been faced with a need for a change in their direction, but move smoothly to affirm what has been expected of them. New decisions are unnecessary, and the lack of crisis means lack of anxiety. By contrast, youths in the midst of decision making experience the highest anxiety, as shown by

Table 4.4. Identity and sex-role variables.

Identity status	Levels of variables					
	Exploration[A]	Expressiveness[B]	Femininity[C]	Commitment[A]	Instrumentalness[D]	Masculinity[C]
Achievement	high	high	mixed: androgynous or masculine types	high	unknown	high
Moratorium	high	high	high	low	low	mixed: androgynous and feminine types
Diffusion	low	low	mixed: feminine or undifferentiated types	low	low	low
Foreclosure	low	low	sex typed	high	high	sex typed

Data are based on:
[A] By definition. Supported by separate scaling of these variables (Matteson, 1977, 1978; Grotevant et al., 1982).
[B] Munro & Adams, 1977; using a written instrument. Matteson, 1974, using direct observations.
[C] Orlofsky, 1977; Prager, 1986; Schiedel & Marcia, 1985; Thorbecke & Grotevant, 1982.
[D] Matteson, 1974, using direct observations; no achievements in the sample. Munro & Adams (1977) found no significant differences on their scale of instrumentalness.

the scores of Moratoriums of both sexes. Once a decision is reached (Achievement), anxiety is reduced, unless the decision is at variance with cultural sex-role stereotypes. Cross-sex identity achievement occurs mainly in women and produces anxiety if same-sex-typed achievement has not already provided security. The decision-making process (Moratorium) appears to be related to greater personality differentiation, to increased cognitive and moral complexity. These decision-making characteristics are present in Achievements of both sexes, even though the moratorium is over and the anxiety has subsided. The most ambiguous findings have to do with susceptibility to outside influence; further investigation is needed for both sexes on a variety of measures. Overall, in spite of the issues of anxiety and inadequate cultural support, the evidence says that exploration is an important variable in women's identity as well as man's, and that identity achievement in masculine areas is functional for women if it is not at the expense of achievement in feminine areas.

It seems reasonable to summarize that the data on development in agentic areas, for both sexes, fits the decision-making model fairly well. That is, increased individuation, masculinity, and optimal decision making seem closely related.

Where the Model Fails

The decision-making model of identity development as presently operationalized is inadequate in dealing with some important findings from women's identity studies. The first is that Foreclosure status appears to be adaptive for women, at least on some variables, and does not appear to have the rigid defensive character that it has for men. The second is that intimacy appears to develop earlier and to higher levels in women than does identity. It seems hard to interpret the data in *any* other way than to conclude that for women intimacy precedes identity.

The emerging data on women's identity development may challenge the adequacy of the decision-making model for describing the relationship between identity and intimacy.

Rethinking the Developmental Sequence

Both a critical review of identity-intimacy studies (Matteson, unpublished) and the data from scales of agentic and communal traits (especially Sola, 1976) suggest the concurrent development of these two aspects of personality for both genders. Women tend to develop earlier than men in the communal areas; men's development may have exceeded women's in the agentic areas in the past, though it no longer appears to do so.

It might be useful to look at how the "decision" gets made to pursue identity in the agentic areas, or in the communal areas. It is most likely that this meta-decision is not a conscious one for most adolescents and has its roots in sex typing that occurs earlier in life. At least as early as fourth grade, girls appear more concerned with relationships than boys, but girls are also just as concerned with industry issues as boys are (Cooke, Apolloni, & Cooke, 1977). By sixth grade the self-worth of boys and girls is associated with different areas, with interpersonal issues being more salient for girls and agentic areas for boys (Bukowski & Newcomb, 1983).

Because it appears that intimacy frequently precedes identity, what sort of "self" is brought to the intimate relationship? Though some boundaries, some area of firm or committed self, correlates with intimacy, we have been forced to reject the hypothesis that some area of secure self is a prerequisite for intimacy. It is quite clear that high intimacy is possible even when an individual's boundaries are very diffuse (see discussion of Table 4.3 above). O'Connell's (1976) distinction between personal and reflected identity may be helpful, but there is a danger that reflected identity will be assumed an inferior style before there has been sufficient study of the communal area. There may be some "cost" to developing an early intimacy: the development of agentic areas and the differentiation of personality may be delayed. There may also be a "cost" to highly individuated identity if it takes a competitive and achievement-oriented direction that interferes with development of communal areas. At this early stage of knowledge, it is necessary to discipline ourselves to avoid self-before-others assumptions. Just as Marcia (1980) asked "What is the effect (for women) . . . on the identity process of being encouraged to always look outside one's self?"; we need to ask "What is the effect for men on the communal or intimacy process of being encouraged to always look to oneself, rather than others?"

Both genders appear to have in common a concurrent increase in both agentic and communal areas, suggesting that usually one area complements rather than interferes with the other. Perhaps it is this concurrent rise that accounts for positive correlations between identity and intimacy. It is not at all clear that a masculine style (with agentic areas developing ahead of communal) or a feminine style (with communal areas exceeding agentic) or even an androgynous style is best.[7]

The studies assessing masculine, feminine, undifferentiated and androgynous types among the four identity statuses suggest a developmental sequence paralleling Block's theory of sex-role maturation. Though feminine (expressive) characteristics are important to the moratorium period for both sexes, the move out of Moratorium to Identity Achievement seems to require masculine characteristics. Masculine and androgynous types are most common in the Identity Achievement category. When scores, rather than types, are used, the masculinity score of Identity

---

[7] It is preferable to speak of "masculine style" or "feminine style," recognizing within-sex differences; speaking of "male" or "female" styles ignores the reality that some men follow the feminine style, some women the masculine style.

Achievers is significantly higher than the other identity statuses for both males and females (Schiedel & Marcia, 1985). Because the hypothesized direction of sex-role development is from undifferentiated, through sex typed, to androgynous, the move from Moratorium to Achievement for males can parallel the move from undifferentiated to either masculine or androgynous types. For men, then, Identity Achievement can occur as part of the gradual movement from undifferentiated to either masculine or androgynous sex-role identity. For women, however, Identity Achievement necessitates a move away from sex-typed identity. Because Identity Achievement requires personality characteristics that our culture associates with masculinity, the move from undifferentiated to sex-typed roles in women results in Foreclosure rather than achievement of identity. To achieve identity, a woman must accept either an androgynous or a cross-sex-typed style. Thus the pattern of sex-role development favors identity achievement for stereotypically "masculine" men over traditionally feminine women.

It seems a likely hypothesis that the identity process as measured by the identity statuses, the decision-making process itself, and masculinity are highly related, positively correlated, developmental processes. Given the "feminine" personality characteristics associated with communal development, however, it may not be appropriate to attempt to assess communal development with a measurement of identity based on the optimal decision-making model. We shall return later to conceptual issues in communal development, and appropriate measurements.

Hypotheses about Identity/Intimacy Development of Women

A number of hypotheses take shape from this review to form the skeleton of a theory of typical female development. The evidence for most of them has already been presented and is not repeated or referenced.

1. Femininity is defined in our culture as communal skills and interests (Spence & Helmreich, 1978).
2. Identity development in women generally receives social support only if femininity is already well secured.
3. The development of intimacy leads to the need for some personal boundaries, a stable self (though this step may follow, rather than proceed, intimacy). A high level of individuation and personality differentiation are not necessary for intimacy.
4. As a woman moves through late adolescence, she experiences increased pressure to develop in communal and intimacy areas. Some settings may support prolonged identity struggle in men and accept a deferral of intimacy issues; the deferral of intimacy issues in women is not generally supported.

5. The early identity studies with women suggested that if a woman had not reached an achieved identity early enough, there was social pressure to divert her energy from identity search to development of intimacy. Sustained intimacy requires personal boundaries, so that the consequence of this shift was foreclosed identity.
6. It is now clear that most college women continue to progress in identity issues simultaneously with giving attention to intimacy. Whether young working women (noncollege women) are able to do so, or whether they must defer identity development to comply with society's demand for intimacy development, deserves further study.

The so-called lack of support for female identity is, more accurately, lack of support for cross-sexed identity; that is, highly individualized identity without communal concerns. In the past the development of communal concerns may have had the effect of "foreclosing" some areas of identity development, or at least foreclosing the development of "personal identity" because of the immediate need for personal boundaries. In other words, energy went into boundary issues and relationships, rather than intrapsychic issues and differentiation.

The studies of masculinity and femininity in the identity statuses suggest a move away from sex-role polarities during the college years. Possibly there is some support for sex-role transcendence in the university community. But as the student prepares to leave that community, she or he must begin to face the strong cultural pressure for fitting into traditional sex roles. For the male, this requirement means pressure toward masculinity, which may aid the final step toward achieving identity.

But the move toward gender polarization may inhibit development of intimacy in the male. For example, a man may achieve occupational identity in a highly masculine trade or profession, and undergo neither a search for identity in ideological areas nor development of communal areas. Such men, though high on identity, would score low on intimacy. The description fits males following the masculine pathway in the Hodgson & Fischer study (1979), and a similar group of men in an earlier study (Orlofsky et al., 1973). These lead to the following hypotheses about development for both men and women:

7. Certain "feminine" characteristics provide a necessary foundation for developing intimacy.
8. Certain "masculine" characteristics provide a necessary foundation for developing identity.

Masculine and feminine characteristics mostly being additive rather than oppositional, persons possessing high levels of both can be expected to succeed at both intimacy and identity issues. But because the culture continues to view these traits as polarities, cultural support will be contingent on achieving in the "sex-appropriate" area first. It is not so much that our culture undermines identity in women; rather, it considers intimacy a high priority for women. The reverse is also true; it considers identity the high priority for men, with the unintended effect of retarding development of intimacy among men not sufficiently high in masculine and feminine characteristics. Just as women of previous generations, having different identity differentiation in adolescence, may catch up with men in identity in midlife, after their feminine (intimacy) areas are secure (Marcia and Miller, 1980), men may do the reverse; they may catch up to women in the communal area in midlife (Zampich, 1980).

How Do Communal Areas Develop?

At this stage in the history of identity and intimacy research, we cannot begin to answer this question. My intent here is to encourage researchers to reexamine past research and to attempt some new theorizing (lest research, like history, be forced to repeat itself).

The unfolding of a life-style that focuses upon relationships may be rather different from the process of life decision making in sociocultural areas such as occupation. The model that underlies the identity statuses, the model for optimal decision making of Janis & Mann (1977)—that is, a careful survey and assessment of options leading to a decision—may not be as appropriate to the unfolding of the communal areas; deep interpersonal relationships are not necessarily characterized by goal-oriented decisions. As the literature on decision making attests, most decisions in life are not made in the optimal style. We muddle through, using the approach that Janis and Mann (1977) call "satisficing." We accept a course of action that will suffice, a good-enough approach (Simon, 1976). Further, we do not use the same strategy in making every decision. If I am purchasing a new car or a major appliance, I may systematically explore alternatives, but if I am buying only one item of clothing, the satisficing approach works fine. Research is needed to explore new categories based on decision-making styles other than the optimal style, and relate these to the various identity areas.

The identity statuses at first were used to describe the process and style an individual adopted to achieve an overall identity. The concept of an overall identity status reflected the dream of discovering a clear model showing how the process between childhood and adulthood is negotiated to culminate in a particular life-style.[8] The method of assessing an overall identity status served us well as a beginning approximation in exploratory research. We now need to move away from the overall status model toward more specification (paralleling the move in mainstream personality theory from general personality traits to situation-specific traits). Identity

---

[8] I use the word life-style here, rather than identity, to emphasize that both identity and intimacy issues may be incorporated.

researchers have begun to move in that direction by separately assessing the different content areas. The next step may be to determine the strategy of decision making used in each content area (and to assess which strategies are most appropriate to particular areas).[9]

For example, instead of describing Sue as a Moratorium it might be more useful to say that she is using an optimal strategy for making occupational life decisions, but is developing her communal style by satisficing. The emergence of a life-style is most likely to involve a number of life decisions, which may not all be made using the same strategy.

Perhaps data from future research will lead to dropping the decision-making model entirely for the communal area. Possibly communal development is better described as an additive learning process, with several important perceptual shifts, rather than a decision-making process. One strength of the Orlofsky intimacy categories is that they do not assume a particular process of development;[10] using these in addition to the identity status categories has already been encouraged.

Research in the communal areas is still in a beginning stage. We have rated girls' earlier investment in interpersonal concerns. These areas continue to be more important to college women; for instance, they invest more in trying to understand their parents' perspectives than do men (White et al., 1986). Some depth studies of individuals over this period of years, using exploratory interviews to probe beneath the statuses to the sequence of decisions and perceptions involved in the emergence of a life-style, could be fruitful. Structured interviews based on alternative hypotheses about how decisions are made and priorities are set seem more valuable than clinical interviews and unfocused exploratory research (Valdez, 1984 is a good model of research using contrasting hypotheses on the relationship of identity and intimacy). Using these more intensive case studies from a subsample of respondents who are part of a larger longitudinal identity status study has many advantages.[11]

---

[9] Grotevant and his collaborators have taken a step in that direction by examining more carefully particular content areas; e.g., Thorbecke & Grotevant, 1982, p. 488.

[10] Orlofsky's intimacy statuses, though they may not be the final word, at least were developed by looking at the interpersonal domain afresh, and attempting to see which categories appeared, rather than trying to force interpersonal development into categories formulated for more goal-oriented areas of decision making.

[11] It would be preferable to collect these more intensive data on a randomized subsample of respondents who are part of a larger sample also being studied at two or more times in their development. This technique would allow a comparison of the main and subsample of standard measures at the last data-collection point, in order to assess the effects of the experimenter's frequent interventions for the subsample. (A series of interviews on decision making might precipitate a change in decision-making style, or a movement to meta-decision making).

The study of sex differences in identity development has drawn attention to the optimal decision-making model implicit in the identity status approach. It has led us to question the appropriateness of that model for describing development in the communal area. Suggestions for future studies will be developed in more technical detail in the next section of this chapter. (If you do not plan an empirical study, skip to the last section of this chapter, "A fear and a hope.")

Suggestions for Future Studies

Throughout this chapter a number of methodological problems have been mentioned. Many difficulties in interpretation that have been encountered could have been avoided by better research designs. Table 4.5 lists de-

TABLE 4.5. Desirable elements in identity/intimacy research.

Design
Cohort-sequential design, combining longitudinal and cross-sectional developmental designs, using cross-lag statistics.
* At minimum, arrangements are made with subjects for possible follow-up.
* Hypothesis-testing, rather than exploratory.
Subjects
* Both males and females from the same population.
Two or more populations or social groups are compared.
Variables; Assessment of at least
* An agentic area (e.g., occupational identity).
* A communal area (e.g., sex-role identity, or intimacy).
* Communal area assessed as an aspect of both identity (Marcia's categories) and intimacy (Orlofsky's categories).
* A measurement of masculinity and femininity on separate but comparable scale.
* Identity status categories and scales of exploration and commitment.
* Dependent variable(s) measured blind from interviews.
Procedures
* Sex of interviewers counterbalanced.
* Interview areas presented in systematically varied order (separate, blind ratings of each interview area).
Analysis of results
* Test of differences among statuses.
* Test of differences between mature and immature statuses (AM/DF).
* Test of differences between stable and unstable statuses (AF/MD).
Data analyzed: for differences
* Between high and low identity statuses (AM/DF).
* Between stable and unstable identity statuses (AF/MD).
* Between sexes.
* Within sexes, for masculinity/femininity subgroups (e.g., sex-typed, androgynous, cross-sex-typed, and undifferentiated).

* Denotes desirable and possible even in very limited studies.

sirable elements that can aid researchers in planning their projects. Most of the items are marked with an asterisk, indicating that it is possible to include the elements in the design of studies of limited scope (such as dissertations). As the review of research throughout this chapter indicates, however, many of the unmarked items are well worth the added effort they entail because of the clarity they will add to the results.

Next I give my rationale for the suggestions in Table 4.5.

Design

The concept of identity statuses implies a developmental progression. The statuses need to be studied using the best research designs for assessing development over time. The risks of biasing results because of sample errors are great when using cross-sectional designs to compare different age groups. For example, when a group of college students includes a larger proportion of Identity Achievements than does a group of high school students, one does not know if this difference is due to age or to the likelihood that a higher proportion of Achieved students than of Diffusion students go on to college. On the other hand, when one group of respondents is followed over a period of time, it is not clear whether the changes are due to age or to general cultural-historic changes. If a group of sixteen-year-olds sampled in 1964 were reassessed on attitudes toward authority in 1974 (at age twenty-six) and were found to have become more critical of authority, the change could be due to development, but it also might result from changes in public attitudes precipitated by such historic events as the Vietnam war and the Watergate scandal. A design that combines both cross-sectional and longitudinal methods helps to control for the limits of each method (See Bayley, 1974; Ausubel & Sullivan, 1970; Schaie & Baltes, 1975). This design, referred to as either cross-lagged or cohort-sequential design, entails considerable time and effort. For the researcher planning a less extensive project, I suggest beginning with a cross-sectional design (gathering data from two age groups) but informing the participants that you may be contacting them for a follow-up (e.g., gaining permission to obtain addresses through the school), you may later be able to complete a cross-lagged design. This minimal investment may bring substantial returns in the future.

Enough research has been done using the identity status approach to leave little justification for further "exploratory" studies. It should be possible, after carefully reviewing identity status literature, to clarify the questions one wishes to address and then to develop some general hypotheses. It is important to take two further steps in literature review: (1) review the instruments that have been used to assess the dependent variables to be studied, and (2) review the empirical research in that area outside identity status research. For example, researchers on gender differences need to be cognizant of the discussions and debates occurring in the study of gender differences as a whole, and to avoid planning research that leads up an alley that has already been mapped as a dead end.

Participants

Earlier in this chapter reasons are given for including in future research on gender differences both males and females from the same sample. The avalanche of women's studies included many with all-female samples, in which phenomena were observed and presented as if they were unique to women, only later to discover the same phenomena occurring in male development. (The fear-of-success motive is an example. See Horner, 1972; Tresemer, 1977; Romer, 1977; Hoffman, 1974). The error above is in danger of being repeated in the area of mid-life crisis. The evidence of a mid-life crisis is equally strong for men (Levinson, 1978) and for women. Though Marcia and Miller's (1980) and O'Connell's (1976) retrospective studies of women's identity need replication, further investigations should involve both sexes, as in Archer (1989).

A second concern about the populations sampled in our studies is that most of our knowledge comes from respondents with a college education. It is possible that mid-life crisis is a phenomenon of the educated middle class (though Levinson's impressionistic data on men suggest otherwise). We need studies of rather different samples across the same age groups—studies involving participants from other subcultures, ethnic groups, levels of educational attainment, and socioeconomic statuses. Data must be collected at the same time from several groups and compared. The studies of Waterman et al. (1971, 1974, 1976) comparing liberal arts and engineering students are an example. Much needs to be learned about the milieux that support exploration and commitment in each of the identity domains.

Variables and Instruments

The argument for including an assessment of both a "masculine" (sociocultural) and a "feminine" (communal) area for both sexes has already been made, and the need to look for within-sex differences (particularly in masculine, feminine, and androgynous styles) has been presented. Because it is not now clear how to best conceptualize the development of the communal process, it seems advantageous to assess the communal areas using more than one measure, such as an identity status interview in the interpersonal area and the intimacy interview.

The choice of instruments for measuring the dependent variables deserves critical thoughtfulness. The experimenter should not only formulate general hypotheses about the relationship between statuses and the dependent variables, but should try to anticipate how participants in each of the statuses might respond to each instrument. Let's illustrate: because the Foreclosure status appears to have different consequences for each sex, or at least for the sex-typed members of each sex, it is of specific interest. There is reason to believe, however, that Foreclosures, more than those in other statuses, may be prone to give socially desirable responses on paper-and-pencil tests. Despite the glowing self-descriptions of Foreclosure families, when absorbed in a task situation they had the highest ratio of negative emotional expression (Matteson, 1974). Thus, further studies of the Foreclosure status are more likely to yield useful information if they do not rely solely on paper-and-pencil tests, but make use of direct observations of behavior.

Categories and the Analysis of Data

Category systems (the statuses of identity, or intimacy) are appealing because of their simplicity. Some ways of analyzing the data from categories can increase the information yielded. For example, the importance of stability in women's identity, and the conflicting results with different dependent variables, are discussed above. The relative importance of "maturity" vs. "stability" for each sex can be determined without adding further instrumentation to the study.[12] In addition to testing for differences between the statuses on the dependent variables (F/D/M/A), tests for differences should be run between the mature and immature statuses (AM/FD) and between stable and unstable statuses (FA/DM).

A caution in combining categories comes from the observation that, in older populations, the intimate and pre-intimate groups are very different on some variables. Certainly the researcher needs to "eyeball" (and publish) the means and standard deviations of the variables for each group before combining them.

Adding Scales to the Categories

Methods

Elsewhere I have urged use of separate scales of exploration and commitment in addition to the identity status categories (Matteson, 1977a). Using such scales, the variables of exploration (which approximates "maturity") and commitment (which approximates "stability") can be

[12] When comparing the relative importance of stability or maturity, it is not valid simply to state, for instance, that more variables reached significance for the stability groupings than for the maturity groupings, because the numbers and degrees of freedom are not likely to be the same. One must check to see if the same means for the two maturity groups would have been significant if the numbers in the groups had been the same as in the two stability groups.

measured on a continuum rather than in either/or categories, which increases precision and allows the use of certain higher-powered statistics. This procedure need not require much additional time. Rather than using separate raters to assign subjects to identity status categories, one can construct the categories directly from the scores on exploration and commitment by using the median-split method.[13]

Conceptual Issues

My interest in scaling exploration and commitment rests not just in its statistical power but in a more basic conceptual issue. We need to clarify

---

[13] I'll briefly explain the median-split method as used in research on sex-role types. When data on masculinity and femininity scales are obtained on a sample, the median score for each scale is computed. Then subjects are assigned to categories according to their position above or below that median on each scale: high feminine, low masculine = feminine type; high masculine, low feminine = masculine type; high on both scales = androgynous; low on both scales = undifferentiated.

Some problems with the median-split method are minimized by a compromise method proposed by Orlofsky et al. (1977), and used by Spence & Helmreich (1978) and Tesch (1984). Categories similar to the identity statuses could be constructed from the exploration and commitment scales in the same manner: high commitment, low exploration = Foreclosure; low commitment, high exploration = Moratorium; low on both scales = Diffusion; high on both scales = Achievement. Grotevant et al. (1982) have described and used such an approach with good results. The method has obvious advantages: the two crucial variables can be independently rated and the categories are objectively derived from these variables.

There are also some disadvantages. First, the clinical judgments of the categories may actually be closer to the "data" and more valid than such a purely numerical manipulation. Second, use of the median-split method in studying gender roles has opened controversy yet to be resolved. Its use in identity status research would lead to the same problem: if each sample is split on its own median, the result is shifting definitions of the categories. A respondent might be assigned to one category as part of one sample, but if a respondent with the same scores were taken from a sample with higher medians, that respondent might be assigned to a completely different category. Further, because in every sample approximately equal numbers of respondents are assigned to each category, it becomes impossible to study the changes in percentages of persons in specific categories. Moratorium or Foreclosure become labels that are relative to a particular group.

One may argue that interpretations of the identity status categories as presently used may also be relative. (See Chapter 7.) I suspect that those of us who have studied mostly high-school-age samples may set our subjective criterion for "Achievement" a bit lower than experimenters who have studied only college populations, for example. But there are advantages in not having relativity rigidly built into the system. If the same experimenters rate the participants throughout a longitudinal study, constancy in use of categories is probably sufficient to measure the shift in percentages in a status over time. This possible measurement of developmental change would be lost if the median-split method were used (unless, of course, the median for the first period of testing were used as the standard for the follow-up data).

what we are actually assessing when we use the identity status method. The interviews were initially designed to assess the process of identity; that is, of how life decisions are being made. It is that inquiry which interests me. As the four statuses become reified, there is a risk they will be used as one more set of "personality types" (as I believe has been done in attempting to assign them post hoc to earlier personality studies; see Mallory, 1989). Given the history of typologies in personality theory, I think this is a mistaken direction.

The scales, if used in clearly conceptualized hypothesis testing, may be one tool for teasing out the processes in decision making. A decision can be assessed sequentially on the degree of exploration and the degree of commitment that followed. Again, it would be a mistake to reify exploration and commitment as stable "personality traits"; the question is when and where these processes are being used.

Procedures

The earlier discussion of the Hodgson & Fischer study (about pathways of identity—masculine, feminine, and androgynous) pointed out the importance of using double blinds and counterbalancing to prevent contaminating data and confounding variables (Meyers & Grossen, 1974; Anderson & Borkowski, 1972). It may have been defensible in the early stages of identity research to ignore these methodological refinements; it is no longer wise to do so. The procedures for double blinds and counterbalancing are relatively simple and do not usually involve added cost if planned in the research design from the beginning.

Cautions in Interpretation

Until recently, much more research was being done on abnormal or troubled adolescents than on normal adolescents. This emphasis has important implications for validating many of the measures we use in research on adolescence.

Imagine a continuum of adjustment extending from dysfunctional through normal to gifted adolescents. I assume that, on many variables, scores plotted along that axis might show a linear relationship. If adjustment scores were plotted in relation to socioeconomic status, for example, a linear relationship would be likely to appear, with low status and low adjustment at one end and high status and high adjustment at the other; the highest ratio of gifted individuals would probably be in the upper socioeconomic classes. I suspect that on other variables, however, the relationships would be curvilinear. For example, on measures of creativity, frequencies of uncommon (unique, individualistic, bizarre) responses would be likely to occur at each end of the continuum of adjustment; participants with bizarre cognitive patterns at the dysfunctional end, and highly creative subjects at the fully functional end of the continuum, would score high on uncommon responses.

Though the hypothetical examples just given are purposely oversimplified, the concept is important. We must be both cautious and contextual in interpreting results from instruments that have been validated mostly at one end of the continuum of adjustment.

An example from my research with adolescents' families will illustrate. Previous family interaction studies had been limited to clinical populations, usually schizophrenics' families. One commonly used measure was a count of the frequency of interruptions and simultaneous talking (hereafter, "interruptions" for short). Interruptions occurred much more frequently in "schizophrenogenic families" than in the normal families used as controls, and were interpreted as an indication of pathological communication. In my study of Danish family interactions, we found interruptions were much more frequent in Moratorium youths' families. Had I used a linear interpretation of this measure, I would have been forced to conclude that Moratorium families were pathological. However, a later study using a similar measure with married couples found that couples with exceptionally good communication patterns interrupted each other more often than the more normal couples. This discovery suggested that frequency of interruptions, if plotted across the full span of families from pathological to superior-functioning, might show a U-shaped curve; both highly expressive successful communicators and pathological family systems may be characterized by these behaviors. Thus it seemed more parsimonious to interpret simultaneous talking and interruptions as part of the high excitement and expressive communication pattern of Moratoriums. (See also Gottman, 1980, for further evidence of this interpretation.)

This realization leads to a second caution. When using category systems, the personal bias of the researcher may contaminate interpretation of the data. Because I happen to enjoy Moratoriums, it is easy for me to interpret their behavior positively. And because the theory has treated Moratoriums and Achievements as the more mature statuses, there is a risk that the data may be distorted and only the good traits of these youths may be emphasized. In reality, foreclosed identity may function in superior ways on some tasks, which may be true of males as well as females. It could be predicted, for example, that tasks which require carefully following directions and do not reward creativity or questioning will be better performed by Foreclosures than Moratoriums. We need to remind ourselves (lest value-laden perceptions foreclose our looking at this issue) that many of the tasks which need doing in life are of precisely this mundane type. Once again the literature on androgyny is instructive. At first the androgynous type was described glowing words. It is now clear that on some measures masculine types do better, on other measures, feminine types (Wells, 1980). We must become situation-specific in deciding which type is "functional" or preferable.

I suspect that part of the appeal of identity status research is our personal identification with one of the statuses. If so, it behooves us to be all the more cautious to avoid imposing our values upon the data, and upon persons with whom we do not so readily identify.

A Fear and a Hope

In closing, I express a fear and a hope. I have some anxiety that this book, by moving toward increased standardization of identity status research, will foreclose improvement of the instruments and rating systems. We must not keep reinventing new formats but must begin refining and purifying the present formats for each content area. But it would be a serious mistake, particularly from the viewpoint of gender difference and feminine identity development, to assume that the instruments are now in final form.

Perhaps this chapter and this book will nudge identity research beyond some of its present characteristics. Too many theses and published studies still repeat the methodological mistakes of our early studies. And far too many of these repeat the theoretically sloppy conclusion that "overall, the results provide support for Erikson's epigenetic theory."

Several of us who do identity research share a sense that much of Erikson's theory is challenged by the results of studies on female identity (Matteson, 1975, 1979; Hodgson & Fischer, 1979; Marcia, 1980; Rowe & Marcia, 1980).

We began this exploration with a theory of male identity development assuming that identity was focused on intrapersonal concerns, that the identity process had characteristics of exploration and commitment similar to those in optimal decision making, that the process culminated in late adolescence, with resolution of identity preceding development of intimacy. Now, none of these characteristics can be assumed for female development, and most of them can be challenged as overgeneralized for male development as well.

There is a humanistic vision in Erikson's writings that goes deeper than his epigenetic schema and his formulation of male and female development. It is a vision of a society shaped and pervaded by communal values:

> Mankind needs a guiding vision. And fate usually makes it only too clear what the next vision must be: today, it must be a world order which would permit all children chosen to be born to develop to an adulthood that may learn to humanize its inventions—experientially as well as technologically. I cannot see how such an adulthood could evolve except through an equal involvement of women and of their special modes of experience in the over-all planning and governing so far monopolized by men. (Erikson, 1975, p. 247)

Perhaps identity and intimacy research, which began as an attempt to operationalize Erikson's system, must abandon the system in order to come of age. If more mature research provides information that will help us actualize Erikson's vision, it will be a far greater tribute to his generative powers. This is my hope.

5
Intimacy Status: Theory and Research

Jacob L. Orlofsky

Whereas Eriksonian theory identifies identity formation as the primary developmental issue in adolescence, it views development of intimacy and establishment of an intimate mode of interpersonal relationships as paramount in young adulthood. Successful resolution of the tasks in this period is reflected in individuals forming an intimate orientation, evidenced in their capacity to commit themselves to enduring intimate relationships (such as marriage and close friendships) and in the high degree of communication and closeness that characterizes these relationships. Failure in the task is reflected in inability to establish and maintain close relationships, in withdrawal, and in isolation.

The Concept of Intimacy

Intimacy is the quality of interaction between individuals, but—from an Eriksonian perspective—it may also be considered a *capacity* of the individual. According to Erikson, the individual with a capacity for intimacy is able "to commit himself to concrete affiliations and partnerships and to develop the ethical strength to abide by such commitments even though they may call for significant sacrifices and compromises" (1963, p. 263). Intimacy involves openness and sharing, a mutual trust. It also involves self-abandon and openness to experiences of interpersonal "fusion" without fear of ego loss: in mutual play, sexual excitement, and orgasm, "in the solidarity of close affiliations . . . in experiences of inspiration by teachers and of intuition from the recesses of the self" (1963, p. 264).

Other theorists emphasize communication and growth-promoting aspects of intimacy but share Erikson's view that individuals differ in their capacity for intimacy. Rogers (1972), for example, stressed communication, commitment, breaking down of expectations, and continued development of each partner as an individual as elements differentiating intimate from less intimate relationships. Fromm (1956) described genuine intimacy as requiring responsibility, mutual respect, care, and knowledge, and distinguished it from immature love, or "pseudointimacy." Maslow (1954) made similar distinctions between the "being" love of self-actualizing persons and immature forms of love based on "deficiency" needs.

Discussions of intimacy often focus on marital relationships, but intimacy may color any relationship involving emotional commitments between adults, not only those institutionalized through marriage. As Whitbourne and Weinstock (1979) point out, "numerous types of relationships may be intimate: close friendships between persons of the same or opposite sex, relationships between older and younger adults, homosexual and heterosexual relationships between adults that have not been legally sanctioned, and the various encounters a person may have with others throughout the adult years" (p. 152). Thus, intimacy is of concern throughout life and may characterize many types of relationships of varying duration and involvement. In this sense, intimacy is a continually evolving capacity involving openness and sharing, care, and mutual trust. These developments meet a major test, however, during young adulthood, when individuals are faced with the task of choosing long-term, perhaps lifelong, partners and establishing bonds of mutual love and respect that will serve as a continuing foundation for cooperatively dealing with household tasks, family income, recreation and leisure pursuits, sexuality, raising children, and relating to other social systems such as relatives, friends, and the community. These challenges and the compromises and sacrifices they require demand a stability and responsibility that may hardly be expected prior to adulthood. Hence, intimacy is particularly at issue in early adulthood and may be considered the phase-specific task of this period.

Measurement of Intimacy

Erikson described the developmental stage in terms of the two polar outcomes, intimacy and isolation. Early efforts to assess intimacy focused on these two poles. One measure, developed by Yufit (1956), consisted of two self-report scales. One was composed of items judged to be characteristic of an "intimate" individual, the other, of items representing "isolation." Individuals scoring high on one scale and low on the other are considered to be intimate or isolated, respectively. A similar measure is the intimacy-isolation subscale of Constantinople's (1969) Inventory of Psychosocial Development. Some validating evidence has been obtained for both Yufit's and Constantinople's measures, so that intimates and isolates as defined by the scales have been found to differ on personality variables (such as warmth, impulse expression and inhibition) in expected directions. These scales, however, have a number of drawbacks. First, they assess only general characteristics (e.g., sociability, warmth) rather than the individual's behavior in relationships or the quality of his or her interaction. A second limitation is their susceptibility to social desirability responding (Orlofsky, 1978; Waterman, Beubel, & Waterman, 1970). Finally, studies utilizing these scales (e.g., Yufit, 1956) have focused only on individuals who score at the extremes of the continuum, so that the majority with less extreme "resolutions" have been ignored. The scales need not be used in this manner, but the bipolar concepts employed encourage this kind of use. To be sure, this bias is consistent with Erikson's description of the stage in terms of the two polar outcomes. Certainly, however, people rarely are completely intimate or completely isolated. Nor is anyone likely to arise from the crisis with either total capacity for intimacy or total resignation to isolation. In fact, the range of possible outcomes, or ways of resolving the intimacy "crisis," is broad.

This type of thinking guided the intimacy status approach which my colleagues and I developed (Orlofsky, Marcia, & Lesser, 1973; Orlofsky, 1974) and which is the subject of this chapter. Conceptualizing the intimacy-isolation crisis as a developmental task for which more than just two polar outcomes are possible and modeling our approach upon the identity status typology developed by Marcia (1966), we generated theoretical descriptions of several alternative types of resolution, each with elements of both "intimacy" and "isolation."

Before we discuss these intimacy statuses, realize that they were developed initially to describe the interpersonal styles or orientations of college men, and specifically those with heterosexual orientation.[1] The statuses have been adapted for use with women and with noncollege populations, and with homosexual individuals as well. Because most of the research has been with college men, however, the criteria and theoretical descriptions that follow are likely to be most applicable to this group.

Three general criteria are used to determine an individual's intimacy status: (1) the extent of the individual's involvement with male and female friends, (2) whether he is involved or has been involved recently in an enduring—committed—love relationship, as with a dating partner or spouse, or some other such "primary" relationship, and (3) the depth and quality of the individual's friendships and dating or love relationship(s). This third criterion is connected generally with the intimacy orientedness

---

[1] Most of my intimacy research with college students has used juniors and seniors (avoiding freshmen and sophomores), so that most subjects are at least twenty years of age. Even this group, however, may be slightly younger than those Erikson had in mind in writing about the intimacy crisis of young adulthood. Few of the college students studied have been married. Except for Isolate subjects, however, most have had at least some dating and sexual experiences, and a good number have been either engaged or involved in exclusive relationships. Thus, these upper-division college students have seemed to me to be quite appropriate as subjects for research on intimacy development.

TABLE 5.1. Criteria for assessing intimacy status.

	Depth of Relationships		
	None	Shallow	Deep
	Isolate		
Uncommitted		Stereotyped	Pre-intimate
Committed		Pseudo-intimate	Intimate

of the individual's interpersonal attitudes and behavior. It includes the degree of communication between partners, mutual care and respect, capacity to accept and resolve differences equitably, and maturity of sexual attitudes and behavior.

These criteria combine to define five intimacy statuses, as represented in Table 5.1. Brief descriptions of the intimacy statuses follow.[2]

The *Intimate* individual forms deep relationships with male and female friends and is involved in an enduring, committed relationship with a girlfriend or wife. The peer relationships of the *Pre-intimate* resemble those of the Intimate except that the Pre-intimate has not entered into an enduring heterosexual love relationship. He may be ambivalent about commitment and may attempt to develop "pure" love relationships free of possessiveness and obligations. The *Pseudo-intimate* has entered into a somewhat permanent heterosexual relationship, but this, like his other relationships, lacks closeness and depth (e.g., there is little sharing of feelings; his view of girlfriend tends to be limited and superficial). The *Stereotyped Relationships* individual maintains some friendships and dating relationships. These relationships tend to be superficial and conventional, however, with a low degree of personal communication and closeness. The *Isolate* withdraws from social situations, and, except for a few casual acquaintances with whom he occasionally interacts, lacks personal relationships with peers.

As you can see from the foregoing descriptions and from Table 5.1, the five statuses were not intended to represent a simple linear measurement of intimacy. For example, the Pre-intimate is seen as more intimacy-oriented than the Pseudo-intimate individual in his interpersonal attitudes and in his self-disclosing style of relating with others. In some respects, though, the Pseudo-intimate is more "intimate" than the Pre-intimate; the former appears less conflicted in the area of commitment, having established a somewhat stable, enduring dating or love relationship. Thus the intimacy statuses were conceptualized not as a linear measure of intimacy but as differing styles of coping with close interpersonal relation-

[2] With the application of the intimacy status approach to women in more recent work, the statuses have been expanded to include additional categories, which are described in a later section.

ships, each, except for the two polar statuses, with elements of both intimacy and isolation.

Assessment of Intimacy Status

To rate individuals for intimacy status, we need detailed information on their interpersonal attitudes and behavior. In many cases (e.g., for rating the person's communication with friends), it is not enough to rely on the person's self-report. Rather, some objective perspective is needed that can compare the person's behavior and self-report with that of other individuals. For this reason a semistructured interview was chosen for examining individuals' interpersonal attitudes and behaviors and rating their capacity for intimacy. The interview is sufficiently structured to ensure a standardized method but permits enough flexibility to accommodate individual lines of questioning.

The interview consists of two sections. The first part inquires about the individual's closest friendships, particularly with same-sex friends. Topics include shared activities, types of things discussed or not discussed, feelings toward friends, and values in relationships. The second part, dealing with dating and love relationships, focuses on the extent of the individual's dating experience and whether he is dating one partner steadily or exclusively. Questions about the specific relationships concentrate on the feelings toward partner(s), degree of commitment, sexual activity, openness of communication, how differences or problems are resolved, and so on. A rating manual including illustrative sketches of characters fitting each category is used for making ratings.[3]

Individuals are assigned two part-ratings, one for friendships using the "depth"-of-relationship criterion (Intimate, Stereotyped, or Isolate) and the other for dating relationships using both the depth and commitment criteria (one of the five statuses). These two part-ratings are then combined into an overall intimacy status rating (one of the five statuses). If the two part-ratings differ (e.g., Stereotyped in friendships, Isolate in dating relationships), the general "tone" of the interview is used, or the second part-rating is weighted more heavily in determining the overall status.

Most research employing the intimacy statuses has used at least two or three interviewers and raters. Because subjective judgment enters into rating decisions, it is necessary to determine whether independent raters agree in their classification of subjects.

Table 5.2 lists inter-rater reliability for a number of studies. As the table shows, in five studies assessing inter-rater reliability between two independent judges, the average agreement has been 81 percent (ranging

[3] The interview and rating manual are found in the Appendix.

TABLE 5.2. Inter-rater reliability for intimacy status ratings.

Investigation	N interviews in reliability check	N judges	Criterion	% agreement
Orlofsky, Marcia, & Lesser, 1973	32	2	unanimous	81
Orlofsky, 1976	20	3	two-thirds	95
Hodgson & Fischer, 1979	100	2	unanimous	79
Kacerguis & Adams, 1980	15	2	unanimous	82
Orlofsky & Ginsberg, 1981	20	4	three-fourths	95
Tesch & Whitbourne, 1982	92	2	unanimous	82
Levitz-Jones & Orlofsky, 1985	20	3	two-thirds	95
Schiedel & Marcia, 1985	20	2	unanimous	80
Prager, 1986	50	3	two-thirds	89

from 79 to 82 percent) (Hodgson & Fischer, 1979; Kacerguis & Adams, 1980; Orlofsky, Marcia, & Lesser, 1973; Schiedel & Marcia, 1985; Tesch & Whitbourne, 1982). In three studies assessing inter-rater reliability among three or four judges, 95 percent agreement was attained in each case with a criterion of majority (i.e., two-thirds or three-fourths) agreement (Levitz-Jones & Orlofsky, 1985; Orlofsky, 1976; Orlofsky & Ginsburg, 1981). A fourth study (Prager, 1986) found two-thirds agreement in 89 percent of the cases. These figures are comparable to those obtained for identity status ratings (Marcia, 1980) and represent adequate inter-rater reliability for this type of assessment.

Validity of Intimacy Status Ratings

Once we have determined that intimacy status can be reliably measured, the next question is whether the statuses provide a valid discrimination of capacity for intimacy. One way of determining whether the statuses represent differing levels of this capacity is to compare them with other measures of intimacy. Orlofsky et al. (1973) used Yufit's (1956) Intimacy-Isolation scale for this purpose. It was expected that Intimates and Preintimates—those who establish "deep" relationships with others—would score higher on this self-report measure of intimacy than Pseudo-intimate and Stereotyped individuals, and that these "superficial"-relationship statuses would score higher than Isolates. These expectations were confirmed (Orlofsky et al., 1973; Orlofsky, 1974). A similar pattern of status differences was obtained with Constantinople's (1969) Inventory of Psychosocial Development intimacy-isolation subscale in a later study (Orlofsky, 1978). Both sets of findings lend construct validity to the intimacy statuses. Furthermore, they suggest that the "depth"-of-relationships criterion may reflect a more basic dimension of intimacy capacity in college men than the commitment criterion and that the five statuses can be combined into three "major" statuses (Intimate plus Pre-intimate, Stereotyped plus Pseudo-intimate, Isolate) representing a continuum of high, medium, and low intimacy.

Still, data from self-report questionnaires are not sufficient indicators of validity for the statuses, which are themselves determined by subjects' self-report in an interview situation. To properly assess and extend the validity of the intimacy status constructs, they must be used to predict behavior outside the realm of self-report questionnaire responses. This was the objective of the next study.

Orlofsky (1976) examined the validity of the statuses by investigating their relationship to a measure of "partner perception." Here is the rationale for this measure as a criterion for intimacy: Part of being intimate with another person involves being able to perceive and respond to the other's needs, even when they are not clearly expressed. This capacity presupposes knowledge of the other on many levels, knowledge gained by sharing feelings and experiences with the other over time. Thus, the more intimate the relationship and the more sensitive each partner is to the needs and feelings of the other, the more knowledge each should have of the other, his or her self-concept, feelings, and attitudes. Subjects participated in this study in dyads with one of their closest male or female friends. Degree of mutual knowledge and understanding was measured by subjects' and partners' ability to accurately predict each other's responses to a personality and attitude inventory. As expected, subjects rated high in intimacy status by virtue of the depth of their communication with partners (Intimate and Pre-intimate) were more accurate in their predictions of their partners' responses than those who maintained active but more superficial relationships (Pseudo-intimate and Stereotyped), and these medium-level intimacy subjects were more accurate than Isolate subjects and their partners. These findings are consistent with the expectation that "high" intimacy subjects are more sensitive to and communicate at a deeper level with their partners than "medium" and "low" (Isolate) intimacy subjects.

Further support for the statuses has been found in studies of self-disclosure and communication. Using Jourard's (1971) self-disclosure questionnaire with a sample of adult men and women (ages 33–56), Zampich (1981) found that men and women rated Intimate reported greater self-disclosure than stereotyped individuals. This pattern held regardless of whether subjects were rating their disclosure to a spouse, a same-sex friend, or an opposite-sex friend. Using a similar method, Prager (1986) also found that Intimate men and women disclosed more private information over a broader range of topics to their romantic partners than non-Intimate subjects. However, when the target person was one's closest friend (as opposed to romantic partner), Intimate and non-Intimate subjects did not differ in their rated self-disclosure.

Prager (1986) also examined whether individuals in the intimacy statuses differed in their self-disclosure when they were disclosing to a "significant other" or to a casual acquaintance. High intimacy subjects did not differ from non-Intimate status subjects in the extent of their self-disclosure to casual acquaintances, but they did disclose more when the target person was a significant other. Furthermore, they were more selective in their disclosure, disclosing more to the significant other than to the casual acquaintance. Prager interpreted this selectivity of Intimate individuals as their being attuned to the situational appropriateness of self-disclosure and able to modulate their disclosure levels to those with whom they are communicating.

In another study with more direct assessments of subjects' communication, Prager (1989) observed conversations of married couples and rated the intimacy level of the statements each partner made as they discussed various topics. Consistent with predictions, dyads with two Intimate status spouses discussed more private and personal material than dyads with two non-Intimate status partners, and mixed-status dyads with an Intimate and a non-Intimate partner gave intermediate scores. High intimacy couples also reported greater marital satisfaction than couples with non-Intimate status partners.

Personality Differences among the Intimacy Statuses

The research discussed thus far shows Intimates and Pre-intimates as forming deep friendships and love relationships characterized by a high degree of personal communication and mutual understanding. Isolates present an opposite picture of interpersonal anxiety and withdrawal. Between these two extremes is the active but shallow interpersonal style of the Pseudo-intimate and Stereotyped statuses. What accounts for these interstatus differences in closeness and communication? One suggestion is that they stem from how comfortable individuals are with aspects of their emotional experience (Orlofsky & Ginsburg, 1981). Because close relationships may stimulate intense feelings of affection, dependency, anger, jealousy, and so on, individuals who are open to and not threatened by their feelings are able to establish and sustain closeness. They are aware of their feelings, have insight into their reactions, and are able to conceptualize their feelings. As a result they can articulate their feelings and communicate them to their partners in ways that enhance rather than disrupt their relationships. The close relationships they are thus able to establish provide further opportunities for new feelings that also require conceptualization. Thus a healthy, growthful process occurs in which insight into one's feelings and needs is furthered by relating with others, and the capacity to relate is facilitated in turn by growing insight. This is the pattern that might be expected to characterize Intimate and Pre-intimate individuals.

By the same token, discomfort with one's feelings may lead to a defensive repudiation of them, or to explosive discharge of feelings. Neither alternative is likely to foster further closeness or increased insight. Thus, defensiveness toward one's feelings can lead to a superficial, shallow style of relating, in which interpersonal issues and conflicts are avoided (Pseudo-intimate and Stereotyped orientations), or, for greater threat and discomfort, to the extreme avoidance found in Isolate individuals.

Summarizing this line of reasoning, interpersonal closeness and communication are closely related to cognitive and emotional development, and the two facilitate each other. This idea was tested by Orlofsky and Ginsburg (1981), who compared the statuses' performance on a measure designed to assess subjects' ability to conceptualize and articulate their emotional experience. This "affect cognition" measure, developed by Rachman (1965), rates respondents' Thematic Apperception Test (Murray, 1943) stories for their degree of conceptual elaboration of affect. Rachman's procedure rates stories along a four-point scale ranging from little or no conceptual elaboration of affect (e.g., "this picture seems like a happy one"); through "attributed" affect and "defined" (i.e., increasingly elaborated) affect; to the most highly differentiated affective reaction, where the affect expressed is clearly connected with the context and/or with ensuing behavior (e.g., "He got so angry at her for embarrassing him that he stormed out of the house"). The writing of such higher-level stories requires the subject to create characters who experience and conceptualize their emotional experience. Thus, the level of affect attributed to the respondent's story characters is viewed as reflecting his own characteristic level of affective experience and conceptualization.

Consistent with the rationale described above, Intimate and Pre-intimate men scored higher in affect cognition than men in the other statuses. Isolates attained moderate scores, and Pseudo-intimate and Stereotyped men were lowest in affect cognition. This ordering of the statuses is interesting in that it parallels findings in other research on affect cognition and activity orientation in adolescents. Gerber (1968) found that youths scoring high in affect cognition engaged in both interoceptive and exteroceptive activities with high frequency. Those with moderate scores engaged in predominantly interoceptive activities, and those with low scores were exteroceptive in orientation. Thus, individuals high in affect cognition are open to and able to develop meanings for their feelings and then "move on." They are introspective but also able to "complete" their internal exploration and go on to other inner or outer stimuli. Individuals low in affect cognition occupy themselves with external stimuli and activities and are relatively insensitive to inner stimuli. Those with moderate affect cognition scores can partially develop and elaborate the meanings of their inner experience. But they seem "caught" in their internal experience, unable or unwilling to come out of it and involve themselves in external stimuli and activities (Gerber, 1968).

In parallel fashion, Intimates' and Pre-intimates' high affect cognition scores suggest individuals who are open to and able to develop meanings for and express their feelings. Their close relationships with others might be characterized as integrating intero- and exteroceptive modes. Isolates withdraw from contact with others. Interpersonally they live in the interoceptive mode, preoccupied with themselves, unable or unwilling to go beyond their fantasies of relationships. Like Gerber's interoceptive youngsters they experience and develop their emotions only in part, so that they remain caught in their inner frame of reference. They do so because they cannot fully develop, act on, and resolve their feelings in an interpersonal vacuum. Furthermore, it is likely that the anxiety attached to their unresolved feelings reinforces their withdrawal. There is a different kind of isolation in the active but shallow (exteroceptive) interpersonal style of Pseudo-intimate and Stereotyped individuals. Because they are unable or unwilling to explore and communicate their feelings, their relationships remain shallow and stagnant.

Developmental Factors

The research on college men reviewed thus far suggests some basic differences among the statuses in interpersonal style and personality. Furthermore, all the studies but one have found no age differences among the statuses.[4] Thus, though it is possible and perhaps probable that developmental shifts from less mature to more mature statuses occur during adolescence and early adulthood, it appears that differences in capacity for intimacy among the statuses are a function not merely of age but of some basic differences in personality. What do these differences stem from? What antecedent conditions have individuals in the statuses experienced that may have influenced their interpersonal development?

One way of approaching these questions is suggested by Eriksonian theory. According to Erikson, successful resolution of each developmental crisis depends on favorably resolving the preceding stages. Thus, the young adult's capacity for intimacy is partially a function of his or her success in coping with prior developmental issues. The individual who has emerged from previous crises with a dominant sense of basic trust,

[4] One study (Orlofsky & Ginsburg, 1981) did find a younger mean age for the Stereotyped status than for the other statuses. Because this study also obtained a larger Stereotyped group (one-third of the sample) than has been found in other studies, perhaps some of these individuals were "developmental" stereotypes (i.e., younger individuals who with additional experience would develop into a more mature position), and others were "characterologically" stereotyped.

autonomy, initiative, industry, and identity should theoretically be better able to establish intimate relationships than an individual with a residual sense of mistrust, self-doubt, guilt, inferiority, and role confusion. A recent study lends support to this hypothesis and provides suggestions for which prior developmental issues may be particularly significant for development of intimacy. Orlofsky (1978) examined college men's scores on Constantinople's (1969) Inventory of Psychosocial Development (IPD), a self-report measure with subscales representing the first six Eriksonian stages (trust, autonomy, initiative, industry, identity, and intimacy). Strong relationships were found between intimacy status and most of the IPD subscales, supporting Erikson's contention that positive resolution of earlier developmental issues is a partial prerequisite for intimacy development in young adults. Of particular interest were findings on the Trust subscale, on which Isolates scored lower than the other groups, and on the Autonomy subscale, on which Intimates and Pre-intimates were highest, followed by Pseudo-intimate and Stereotyped individuals, with Isolates lowest. These findings suggest that the interpersonal problems of Isolate individuals may be traced to difficulties encountered at the earliest developmental stage, when the establishment of a basic sense of trust in self and others is at stake. Eriksonian theory posits that unsuccessful resolutions tend to accumulate from one stage to another. Hence, Isolates' unresolved conflicts over trust would be likely to hinder them in dealing, not only with intimacy issues, but with most subsequent developmental crises (e.g., autonomy, initiative, identity). In fact, Isolates did score lowest of the groups on all the other scales—exhibiting difficulties at all the stages but one (industry). Their high industry scores may reflect defensive preoccupation with work and achievement as an attempt to avoid anxiety associated with interpersonal relationships, or work may be an area in which Isolates can gain some gratification and self-esteem.

Pseudo-intimate and Stereotyped individuals appear to have a basic foundation of trust. Their lower scores on the autonomy scale suggest that their difficulties may begin at this next stage, where establishment of a sense of separateness and self-control are at stake. Unfavorable resolution of these issues might interfere with later development of intimacy in Stereotyped and Pseudo-intimate individuals by contributing to their avoidance of closeness and sharing. Experiences of closeness and vulnerability may be threatening to individuals who are uncertain of their autonomy and separateness and wary of others' potential influence over them. Lack of autonomy may contribute to intimacy difficulties in another way, through excessive dependency and need for security. Thus, the Pseudo-intimate individual's tendency to seek a permanent partner may be motivated more by fear of being alone than by interest in the partner. This picture of the Pseudo-intimate as motivated by need for security and fear of independence is consistent with the impression these individuals often give of treating their girlfriends or wives as extensions of themselves rather than as separate autonomous beings. The Pseudo-intimate often appears controlling of his girlfriend, intolerant of any sign of individuality on her part. His frequent choice of a dependent, insecure, malleable partner is consistent with this inclination.[5] Intimates and Pre-intimates, in contrast, seem to have well-established autonomy, and their relationships appear to be motivated more by mutual stimulation and fulfilment than by striving for security. Intimates also were found to score highest in industry and in identity, both findings suggesting that part of the Intimate college man's capacity for intimacy and readiness for long-term commitments may derive from his clarity of self-definition and self-efficacy.

The latter finding is particularly interesting because of its consistency with a series of studies investigating the role of identity achievement as an antecedent and partial prerequisite for intimacy. As already discussed, Eriksonian theory posits that successful resolution of each developmental crisis depends on favorable resolution of prior crises. Nowhere is Erikson more explicit about this tendency than for identity and intimacy. "'True engagement' with others is the result and the test of firm self-delineation" (Erikson, 1959, p. 95). Only when identity formation is well under way can true intimacy, which is "a counter-pointing as well as a fusing of identities," take place (1968, p. 135).

The first study to test this relationship between identity status and intimacy status (Orlofsky et al., 1973) found that Intimate men were almost invariably identity achievers, Pre-intimates were most frequently in the moratorium status, and Stereotyped and Pseudo-intimate men tended to be foreclosed or diffuse in identity. Only a few men in that college sample were Isolates. Most of these men, however, were diffuse in identity. Thus, consistent with Eriksonian theory, men in the higher intimacy statuses tended to be drawn from the higher or more developmentally mature identity positions, and those in the low intimacy statuses tended to be drawn from the lower or less mature identity positions.

The association between the Pre-intimate status and identity moratorium is a special example of the relationship between identity development and intimacy, and it suggests an explanation for the Pre-intimate's apparent ambivalence about commitment alongside his striving for an open, disclosing style of communication. Perhaps Pre-intimates avoid long-term interpersonal commitments because of their unfinished identity concerns. Uncertain about the outcome of their identity search, they shy away from

[5] In the partner perception study (Orlofsky, 1976) described above, in which subjects brought close male or female friends to participate with them as their partners, it was found from individual interviews administered to the partners that four of the seven female partners accompanying Pseudo-intimate subjects fitted this description of being insecure, malleable, and dependent. Two others not fitting this description expressed serious dissatisfaction with their relationship.

"permanent" relationships in which some stability and consistency are expected of them. On the other hand, the Pre-intimate's active identity search may exert a positive influence on his intimacy development, underlying his strivings for intense communication with friends. Relationships with others appear to serve an identity-clarifying function, in part, for the Pre-intimate. His "deep" discussions with others (about personal values and attitudes, feelings toward each other, and so on) provide him with a useful source of identity-establishing feedback, helping him to discover himself at the same time as he "discovers" others. In this sense, strivings for identity and intimacy appear to facilitate each other.

The study with college men just described is not the only research that has investigated the relationship between identity resolution and intimacy status. A number of other studies have been conducted using women as well as men and noncollege as well as college populations. One study (Prager, 1977) failed to find any relationship between the two stages in college women. All other studies reported, however, have made findings similar to those of Orlofsky et al. (1973). Fitch and Adams (1983), Hodgson and Fischer (1979), Kacerguis and Adams (1980), and Schiedel and Marcia (1985) all found a relationship between identity status and intimacy status for college men and women, so that individuals high in intimacy status tended to be more advanced in identity development than those low in intimacy status. Findings have been similar for men in their late twenties (Marcia, 1976) and for men and women in their middle adult years (Tesch & Whitbourne, 1982; Zampich, 1981).[6] Although the cross-sectional design of these studies does not allow firm conclusions that identity precedes intimacy, as Erikson theorizes, the studies do demonstrate at least a clear association between capacity for intimacy and development of identity.

It is noteworthy that five of the six studies examining both male and female subjects have found a stronger identity and intimacy relationship for men than for women (Fitch & Adams, 1983; Hodgson & Fischer, 1979; Schiedel & Marcia, 1985; Tesch & Whitbourne, 1982; Zampich, 1981). It has been suggested that young women may be further developed

[6] One difference between the studies using college students and those employing adults is that the latter have suggested somewhat fewer positive implications for the Pre-intimate status. By virtue of the depth of communication characterizing Pre-intimates' relationships, Pre-intimacy has been viewed as one of the more advanced intimacy statuses for college students. Tesch and Whitbourne (1982) found, however, that Pre-intimates in their adult sample were frequently diffuse in identity (Zampich, 1981, did not include a Pre-intimate category in her research with an adult sample). Tesch and Whitbourne concluded that adults in their late twenties or early thirties who have not yet committed themselves to a long-term relationship may be quite different (e.g., less mature) from those who have made such commitments, and they advise against combining Pre-intimates with Intimate subjects for data-analysis when working with adult samples.

in their intimacy capacity than men, given the greater emphasis on expressive social skills in women and instrumental skills in men (Bem, 1975; Parsons & Bales, 1955), and development of intimacy may even precede development of identity in women (Douvan & Adelson, 1966). This difference could explain why capacity for intimacy appeared less related to identity development for women than for men in these studies. Support for this idea that women may be more advanced than men in their development of intimacy was found by Hodgson and Fischer (1979) and Schiedel and Marcia (1985), who found that a substantially larger proportion of women than men in their college samples rated high (Intimate and Pre-intimate) in intimacy status. However, another study examining college students of both sexes (Kacerguis & Adams, 1980) did not find a difference in the proportion of men and women rated high or low in intimacy, and neither did the studies examining adults.[7] Thus, it is still unclear whether men and women differ in their development of intimacy or if the relationship between identity and intimacy development differs for the sexes. More detailed consideration of these issues may be found in Matteson (1980). Other issues relating to differences in intimacy between men and women are discussed in a later section of this chapter.

One final antecedent of intimacy status has been examined. Orlofsky (1978) studied college men's reports of their peer relationships during childhood and adolescence and found that Isolates had less interpersonal involvement and success throughout childhood than men in the other statuses. Isolates reported having fewer friends and experiencing less popularity among school mates from grade school on. They reported participating in fewer extracurricular activities during junior high, high school, and the first two years of college than the other statuses. Finally, together with stereotyped men, they were slowest in establishing heterosexual relationships; their first dating experience occurred, on the average, two or more years later than that of men in the other statuses. These findings suggest that the social isolation of these young men was lasting and did not begin during college. They suggest further that lowered involvement with peers during childhood may interfere with the individual's developing social skills and ease in relating to others and may therefore predispose him toward a continued marginal social adjustment into adulthood. Orlofsky (1978) found little evidence of differences among the other statuses in prior peer relationships. The only difference was the late-beginning dating age of Stereotyped men, a factor that may account for the superficial, immature quality of their current heterosocial relationships.

[7] Information about the frequencies of men and women in the high and low intimacy statuses is not available in the Fitch and Adams (1983) study that utilized a college sample.

Developmental Pathways

The typical Stereotyped individual tends to have only superficial, immature relationships with others, but at least he maintains—and enjoys—relationships. But the typical Isolate has little to do with male or female peers, having few if any friends. Furthermore, his isolation from his peer group generally extends, as we have seen, far back into childhood. This finding, along with the findings of poor psychosocial development for the Isolate group, suggests profound personality differences between Isolates and the other statuses.

The differences among the non-Isolate statuses seem to be stylistic and differentiated at a somewhat later age, perhaps during adolescence because of varying types of social exposure and experience. Or they may reflect different developmental levels or stages of interpersonal concerns through which most individuals normally pass, some more slowly than others, during their teens and twenties. If so, these are the most likely developmental sequences (at least for men). Most individuals would start from a somewhat stereotyped position.

Following a significant interpersonal experience, like a close chum relationship (e.g., Sullivan, 1953), the young person might begin to perceive possibilities for greater closeness in relationships and develop communication skills for establishing intimate relationships (Pre-intimate). After taking greater risks in sexual relationships and/or resolving identity concerns, he might begin to establish an intimate, committed sexual relationship. On the other hand, the Stereotyped individual, because of painful or unrewarding interpersonal experiences, might fail to develop "intimate" attitudes. This individual might remain in a somewhat distant stereotyped position, or he might seek a security-motivated commitment (Pseudo-intimacy). One or two unsatisfactory relationships later, he might, with encouragement from girlfriend or wife—or marriage counselor—begin to take greater risks in his relationships and become more intimate in his interpersonal attitudes and behavior.

Whether these developmental sequences are normative is a question for future research. At present, we do not even know how stable intimacy status is. Research results discussed in earlier sections of this chapter suggest some basic personality differences among individuals of varying intimacy status. These variations do not, however, rule out the possibility of developmental shifts, at least for some individuals, during adolescence and early adulthood. Follow-up studies, say at yearly intervals, may be helpful in clarifying how much change occurs as well as providing data on the sequence of changes in status.

The most likely developmental changes would be from Pre-intimate to Intimate and from Stereotyped to Pseudo-intimate. More interesting would be major changes in status, such as Stereotyped to Pre-intimate or Intimate, or Pseudo-intimate to Intimate. Do developmental shifts such as these occur, and if so, are they the norm, or do they require major corrective experiences such as psychotherapy? It is easy to imagine many of the "middle" intimacy status individuals benefiting from corrective experiences. For example, many Stereotyped individuals might become Pre-intimate if they were exposed to individuals with more intimacy-oriented attitudes and life-styles. Perhaps sensitivity training would introduce this type of individual to alternative attitudes and more effective styles of relating to others. Similarly, the Pseudo-intimate might benefit from couples therapy or marriage counseling. The Isolate, on the other hand, seems most thoroughly stuck. His difficulties in trusting others, his flimsy identity, and his lasting pattern of isolation argue against easy change. He would seem to require at least long-term relationship-oriented psychotherapy before he could develop enough confidence in himself and trust in others to lay the foundations for satisfying interpersonal relationships.

Intimacy Status in Women

The intimacy statuses were originally formulated to describe basic interpersonal styles exhibited by young men. The basic criteria of depth of communication and affectional bonds and progress toward commitment to an enduring love relationship seemed particularly appropriate for assessing the intimacy behaviors of this population. Evidence that the statuses differ predictably in personality and interpersonal behavior suggests that these criteria do discriminate well young men's maturity of intimacy.

There is some question, however, about whether these criteria—particularly the depth-of-relationships criterion, which is most discriminating for men—provide adequate discrimination of individual differences in women's capacity for intimacy. It is generally well established that women tend to be more self-disclosing than men (Himelstein & Lubin, 1965; Hood & Black, 1971; Jourard & Landsman, 1960; Jourard & Lasakow, 1958; Jourard & Richman, 1963; Pederson & Breglio, 1968; Pederson & Higbee, 1969) and that they are, on the average, more relationship-oriented and expressive of feelings than men (Bem, Martyna, & Watson, 1976; Douvan & Adelson, 1966; Orlofsky & Windle, 1978). Differences such as these suggest that women may be more advanced in the "depth" aspects of their intimacy development than men, and therefore that many, perhaps most, young women might be rated in the "deep" (Intimate and Pre-intimate) intimacy statuses. Though support for this anticipation has been mixed (Hodgson & Fischer, 1979; Kacerguis & Adams, 1980; Schiedel & Marcia, 1985), as discussed above, it is possible that "depth" of relationships may not be as discriminating a criterion for women's capacity for intimacy as it is for men's and that other criteria may be more discriminating. In part because of their socialization and the roles traditionally occupied by women in American society, dependency issues may be particularly significant for women. Mature intimacy can occur only between two autonomous individuals who are psychically independent. Thus, unresolved dependency issues that dispose the woman to "merge" with her partner and subordinate herself to him can limit her capacity for intimacy. Observations I made (Orlofsky, 1976) from a series of pilot interviews I conducted with college-age women suggested that this may be a frequent dynamic in women's approach to intimate relationships. Accordingly I proposed adding a Dependency status to the five-status classification system to describe women who are motivated largely by needs for security and who give up their own self-determination to their partners. It was not assumed that dependency strivings were characteristic only of women or that they are not primary in the personality dynamics of many men as well. In fact, I have suggested elsewhere that dependency issues may play a central role in the dynamics of many Pseudo-intimate men (Orlofsky, 1978).[8] The primary difference between these Pseudo-intimate men and Dependent women is that Dependent women express more directly their dependency and security needs and Pseudo-intimate men cover their needs with a show of self-sufficiency and noninvolvement because of these ego-threatening, unmasculine feelings. Thus, Pseudo-intimacy in men and Dependency in women may be dynamically related and represent basically similar orientations.

These speculations have not yet been tested. However, there have been some more formal efforts to describe and validate a dependency type of intimacy status. Two types of dependency statuses have been proposed. Whitbourne and Weinstock (1979) have proposed what they call a Merger position as a sixth intimacy status. Merger ratings are applied to individuals whose relationships are characterized by unequal power, so that one partner's wishes generally get subordinated to the other's.

My colleagues and I have proposed a similar addition of a Merger status, although our conceptualization differs. In our version, the Merger status refers not only to unequal power and self-subordination but also to difficulty in accepting the partner as a person separate from oneself, a high degree of possessiveness and jealousy, and a perception of oneself as unable to get along or find any happiness without the partner. We believe this interpersonal style can apply to individuals whether or not they are involved in an enduring (committed) relationship. Thus we proposed "committed" and "uncommitted" versions of the status, one to describe a dependent individual involved in a long-term, committed relationship,

---

[8] In this 1978 paper, discussed in an earlier section of this chapter, I remarked that Pseudo-intimate men tend to treat their girlfirends or wives largely as extensions of themselves rather than as separate, autonomous people, and that they tend to discourage the partner's independent activities.

TABLE 5.3. Expansion of the intimacy statuses to include Dependency and Merger statuses.

	Depth of Relationships			
	None	Shallow	Dependent	Deep
	Isolate			
Uncommitted		Stereotyped	Dependent	Preintimate
Committed		Pseudointimate	Merger	Intimate

and the other to describe insecure individuals who tend to seek out dependency relationships but have not yet established a long-term one. An advantage of this conceptualization is its parallel with the current practice of distinguishing between committed and uncommitted statuses while being able to combine them for "major" status comparisons. The classification scheme resulting from addition of the Merger statuses appears in Table 5.3.

Ellen Levitz-Jones and I revised the intimacy interview and rating manual to include the Merger statuses.[9] Though formulated specifically for women, the expanded intimacy status scheme may be applicable to men as well. Recently a single version of the intimacy interview was written along with a revised rating manual for use with either sex. The interview and rating manual are included in the Appendix.

Only a handful of studies have examined the validity of a merger status. Tesch and Whitbourne (1982), using their version of the merger status, found that only a few of the adult men and women (ages 21–35) in their sample received Merger ratings (8 of 48 men and 5 of 44 women). Their data suggest that Merger individuals may be less likely to have achieved an identity than Intimates, a finding that would support the validity of this status. However, no formal comparisons were reported by the authors to substantiate this difference.

In a study I conducted in collaboration with Ellen Levitz-Jones, we examined the profiles Merger status and other college women attained on a projective test assessing separation-individuation and attachment style, the Separation Anxiety Test (SAT) (Hansburg, 1980). Consistent with expectations that Merger individuals are burdened by inadequate separation-individuation and insecure attachments to love objects, women rated as committed or uncommitted Merger attained more pathological profiles on the SAT than women in the high intimacy statuses (Intimate and Pre-intimate). They displayed a lower capacity for individuation and self-reliance, even in relatively mild separation situations, a higher need to defend against the reality or impact of separation, and a greater

[9] Bellew-Smith and Korn (1986), working independently, developed a very similar conceptualization of committed and uncommitted Merger statuses and a similar interview and rating procedure.

tendency toward self-blame and depression in the face of separation from attachment figures. Somewhat contrary to expectations, women with a superficial, distancing relationship style (Pseudo-intimate and Stereotyped statuses) did not exhibit an avoidant pattern of excessive detachment and self-sufficiency in their SAT responses. Rather, their pattern of scores closely resembled that attained by Merger women, including the same anxious, insecure reactions, low self-reliance, maladaptive defensive reactions, and intropunitive tendencies (Levitz-Jones & Orlofsky, 1985). These findings suggest that Stereotyped and Pseudo-intimate women have much the same underlying anxious-insecure base that Merger women have. They just tend to deal with the problem in different ways. Merger individuals try to deal with their underlying insecurity by clinging to others and attempting to fuse with them, whereas Stereotyped and Pseudo-intimate women attempt to cope by remaining standoffish or only superficially involved with others.

One other study examining the Merger status has been published. Bellew-Smith and Korn (1986) found that committed and uncommitted Merger women scored lower on a self-report measure of ego identity than women in the other intimacy statuses, as well as higher in needs for succorrance.

These studies provide some support for the Merger construct, but additional work is necessary to round out information about individuals who adopt this style. Still other questions concern the applicability of the Merger construct for men. Do men and women differ on the average in their maturity of intimacy? For men and women who have not achieved a high level of such maturity, is one relationship style more typical of one sex than the other, such as a Pseudo-intimate or Stereotyped position for men and Merger for women? Research in progress should begin to provide answers to some of these questions.

Merger or dependency is not the only additional status that has been suggested by researchers studying intimacy in women. Prager (1977) suggested a Constricted Intimate status. Some of the women in her college sample were not readily classifiable according to the original five-status classification system. Some women expressed a desire to become more open to others and to learn to express themselves more genuinely, but found this change difficult to carry out. They experienced a discrepancy between the level of closeness they wished to achieve and the level they were able to achieve. These women were not Intimate, but they did not match the shallowness and superficiality of Stereotyped women. Thus Prager felt that an additional category was necessary to classify these individuals, hence the label Constricted Intimate. This status referred to women who "(1) are exploring more intimate ways of relating yet continue to hold back in significant ways, or (2) have achieved a fair degree of intimacy with women compared to highly limited relationships with men, or (3) claim a great deal of intimacy with others, yet do not or cannot articulate this relationship precisely or give examples. All these women have a discrepancy of some kind between their ideals and their behavior" (Prager, 1977, pp. 47–48).

Although a fair number of women in her college sample were rated Constricted Intimate (11 of 87, or 13 percent, with six statuses rated) no differences were found between this and the other statuses on measures of identity, sex role, or self-esteem. More recent research with adult men and women did, however, provide support for the Constricted Intimate status. Using three major statuses (Intimate, Constricted Intimate, and Stereotyped), Zampich (1981) found that many (30, or half) of her adult subjects were rated Constricted Intimate. As would be expected, these subjects scored in the middle range (between Intimate and Stereotyped subjects) on a measure of self-disclosure. Furthermore, they tended to be overrepresented in the foreclosure identity status (Intimates tended to be identity achievers and Stereotyped subjects tended to be either diffuse or foreclosed in identity). These findings provide support for this status for an adult sample (ages 33–56, mean age 45), although its utility for a younger (college) population is yet to be demonstrated.

I see the Constricted Intimate status as representing a midpoint between the Intimate/Pre-intimate and Pseudo-intimate/Stereotyped statuses along the depth dimension rather than as a qualitatively different status. These individuals strive for deeper communication than those in the latter groups but are not functioning at a level attained by the former statuses. Thus, although adding this status may contribute greater precision to the rating process, the gain appears more quantitative than qualitative.

Evaluation

The foregoing discussion points up probably the greatest difficulty with the intimacy status constructs—the use of discrete categories to measure continuous variables. Though ideal types serve a valuable function in concretizing concepts for theoretical discussion, typologies are rather crude as assessment devices. Individuals rarely fit neatly into one category in the sense of exhibiting all the criteria for that category perfectly. Few individuals are totally committed or totally lacking in commitment; few are completely self-disclosing or completely closed in their relationships. Rather, there are degrees of commitment and degrees of communication. This limitation does not mean that we cannot successfully superimpose discrete categories upon these continuous dimensions, but that cutoff points for distinguishing between categories may be rather arbitrary. Research has demonstrated that intimacy status can be reliably classified. Independent raters in each study, blind to each other's ratings, have shown generally good agreement. I wonder, however, if reliability is adequate *across* studies or from one group of researchers to another. The studies cited have varied somewhat in the proportions of individuals rated in each intimacy status. On occasion, findings in one study have not been replicated in another conducted with a different subject population by another research group. These varying proportions and results may reflect actual differences among the populations studied. They may also, however, have resulted from subtle differences in the way the research groups interpret the rating criteria.

If such differences are actually occurring in the interviewing or rating procedures utilized by different researchers, what can we do to correct this inequity? I have two suggestions. First, we need to test inter-rater reliability across different research groups working at different institutions. This test could be accomplished by having research groups exchange samples of tape-recorded interviews for rating. Second, we need to go beyond the less exacting typological assessments and develop rating scales to measure the intimacy criteria. Given the reality that there are degrees of commitment and depth of relationships, greater precision in measuring these criteria can be achieved with rating scales than with the typology. Care must be taken in constructing these rating scales so that clear behavioral referents are specified for each dimension. It would be desirable to have at least five- and perhaps seven-point scales for each dimension.[10] Rating scales might be generated not just for each of the general criteria (depth, commitment, autonomy, and so on) but for facets of each of these criteria. For example, the depth criterion might be divided into rating scales for depth of communication of personal concerns and problems (intrapersonal disclosure), depth of communication of feelings and reactions toward partner (interpersonal disclosure), depth of caring and affection experienced toward partner(s), and so on. Rating scales such as these need not completely supplant the typology. Rather, they can be used to supplement the categories and even to bring greater objectivity to the classification. For example, points 1 and 2 on a 7-point depth-rating dimension can be used to justify a status rating of Isolate; points 3, 4, and 5 can refer to the middle-level statuses (Pseudo-intimate and Stereotyped); and points 6 and 7 can refer to the higher-level statuses (Intimate and Pre-intimate). Thus the intimacy status constructs can be retained for their heuristic value and to facilitate theoretical discussion, and greater objectivity can be brought to classification by the rating scales. In addition,

[10]The original five-status classification system might be described as embodying three-point rating scales for the depth-of-relationships and commitment dimensions, with Isolate, Stereotyped plus Pseudo-intimate, and Intimate plus Pre-intimate statuses representing the three depth-of-relationship points, and Isolate, Stereotyped plus Pre-intimate, and Intimate plus Pseudo-intimate statuses representing the three extent-of-commitment points.

these scales can be used to supplement the intimacy status categories with continuous data for statistical analysis.[11]

Conclusion

Despite the lack of more precise rating scales thus far, evidence is growing that the intimacy statuses represent a scientifically valid and useful approach to the study for intimacy. Research has yielded theoretically consistent findings, and a number of suggestions promise greater understanding of individual differences in capacity for intimacy. Much work remains, however, to corroborate and enlarge the understandings already gained. The work on dependency or merger relationships is only beginning. This effort represents a promising and substantial addition to the original conceptualization of intimacy orientations, but it is too early to evaluate the merits of this addition or even to determine the specific form it should take. The results of several current projects should shed some light on the relative merits of various dependency constructs. Questions also remain about developmental issues confronting males and females and whether different constructions are needed to account for men's and women's intimacy orientations. More research is needed to examine the range of correlates, antecedents, and social-skills components of intimacy and to study growth-enhancing experiences that can lead to positive changes in individuals' intimacy behavior throughout adulthood. Finally, our studies should begin to focus more on couples and not just on individuals.

The intimacy status approach is based on the assumption that individuals themselves possess a level and style of maturity of intimacy that they bring to each of their relationships. It assumes further that their intimacy status can be assessed apart from their particular relationships. For the researcher grounded in personality study these seem like reasonable assumptions. In certain respects, however, they are open to question, because intimacy, after all, is not something that occurs in isolation: it occurs between people. This reminder leads to questions about how far we can separate an individual's maturity of intimacy from the context of his or her relationships. Obviously, individuals are not equally intimate

[11] Actually, some very promising work developing continuous scales to rate maturity of intimacy has been done recently by Kathleen White and her associates at Boston University. White et al. (1986) adapted the intimacy interview for use with couples and developed scales to rate their subjects on a number of separate but related intimacy components. These include communication, caring, orientation (or perspective taking), commitment, and sexuality. Each component is rated along a continuum rooted in a Kohlberg (1973) or Loevinger (1976) type of stage conceptualization, with six stages representing three basic levels: self-focused, role-focused, and individuated-connected.

with all their acquaintances. Or consider an individual involved with a partner who has generally pseudo-intimate, distancing style. This person might appear less mature (perhaps dependent and insecure or perhaps distancing as well) than if he or she were involved with a different partner more capable of mature relatedness.

These considerations suggest that perhaps we should turn our energy to assessing and studying relationships rather than individuals. Or perhaps we can combine the two foci and study *individuals-in-relationships*. We might then investigate whether people tend to select partners who are similar to themselves in maturity of intimacy or style. What types of relationships do similar and different status partners fashion with each other? Does one partner's style tend to win out over the other's so that the one socializes the other, in effect, to his or her style? Prager's (1989) study of intimacy status and couple communication is a good start toward studying individuals-in-relationships (and the relationship they develop together). Other issues that might be investigated include conflict-resolution strategies, length of relationship, and relationship satisfaction in various relationship pairings. Information from this type of research can provide some balance to the emphasis thus far placed on the individual, and it may prove quite useful in designing effective interventions and treatments for various types of relationship problems seen by clinicians.

Part II
The Determination of Ego Identity Status

6
Interviewers and Interviewing

DAVID R. MATTESON

Throughout science, the accuracy of our understanding rests fundamentally upon the quality of the data we collect. The limits of the identity-interview approach should be recognized before embarking on a study; they are well summarized by Bourne (1978b, pp. 375–382). He correctly points out that probably no instrument can incorporate all components of Erikson's broad concept of identity, but concludes that the identity interviews strike an optimal balance between the opposing demands of interpretive depth versus empirical rigor and generalizability.

The main problems with the interview method are addressed briefly here. More detailed critiques of the advantages and disadvantages of the interview method in research can be found in Selltiz et al. (1976, pp. 294ff.), Cannell & Kahn (1953), Richardson et al. (1965), and Douglas (1985, pp. 67ff.).

The first problem is social desirability in self-report data. It is important in evaluating this problem to distinguish between the social desirability of particular responses in the interview and the social desirability of a particular identity status. The former is partially mitigated by the skill of the interviewer. For example, it is common for respondents, when asked about their parents' influence on their choice of occupation, to report that their parents left the decision entirely up to them ("as long as you're happy"). An experienced interviewer continues in a way that probes beyond this socially desirable response; for example: "Do you think your parents may have had a preference for one field over another, even if they never would have tried to pressure you about it?" About a third of the respondents, once they've established their parents' positive intentions, will respond to this probe by revealing the parents' preferences (Waterman, personal communication).

Second, we should recognize that the final ratings assigned are not "self-reports," although they are based on information that the respondent presented. Even when the research objectives call for information that the individual is unable to provide directly, the interview is often an effective means of obtaining the desired data, as in the studies of prejudice and ethnocentrism by Adorno et al. (1950). The use of interviews and raters is especially appropriate when the respondent is not qualified to make a direct judgment of certain characteristics in himself, but is able to provide personal information from which a trained rater can make such a judgment (Cannell & Kahn, 1953, p. 331). The identity interview is not a self-report instrument, in that the respondents do not know the categories being used. It is possible that responses to some questions will be affected by social desirability, but it seems unlikely that the cumulative effect of socially desirable responses to particular items would result in a interviewee's being categorized incorrectly. In contrast, unidimensional ego identity scales might be affected by social-desirability responses, because of the face validity of the items and the obvious social desirability of scoring in the "mature" direction. (For the advantages of an objective measure, see Adams, Benion, & Huh, 1989.)

A second common objection to the semistructured interview is that the stimuli presented are not uniform. However, the uniformity of a questionnaire, with its standardized order and wording of questions, "may be more apparent than real" (Selltiz et al., 1976) because the same words may have diverse meanings for different people, or may be misunderstood (Richardson et al., 1965). In an interview, a question that has been misunderstood can be reworded, an unclear response can be followed up, and questions can build on the previous responses of the respondent. "The interviewer varies the questions so as to obtain *uniformity of meaning* for each respondent" (Richardson et al., 1965, p. 151; italics mine). Additional advantages of the interview include the likelihood that interviewees will take the questions more seriously and are less prone to giving random or careless answers and that, despite the less anonymous situation, respondents will tend to share more intimate and more negative self-disclosures in face-to-face interviews than they do in less personally supportive situations (Henson et al., 1977).

Of course, the success of the interview technique is highly dependent upon the interviewer's ability to build rapport with the respondent. Differences between interviewers pose a final problem, which can be minimized by: (1) systematic assignment of interviewers, and (2) careful training of interviewers.

Much evidence in social psychology research shows that research participants respond differently to interviewers of different sexes, different races, and so on (Benny et al., 1956). In one study, significantly more of the respondents interviewed by females (compared to those interviewed by males) were judged to be Diffusions (Archer, 1982). This possible confounding can be avoided by counterbalancing gender of the interviewers in the research design; that is, using both male and female interviewers and varying gender of interviewer and gender of participant so that half the male respondents interviewed are seen by male interviewers, half by female interviewers (Matteson, 1974, 1978; Hodgson & Fischer, 1979). It might also be wise to use interviewers of different ages, especially in research with high school age research participants where interviewers similar in age to the interviewees' parents might be responded to differently. Even in the smallest project, two or more interviewers can be systematically assigned and checks can be made to ensure that interviewer differences do not affect the tests of hypotheses. Characteristics of the interviewers can be treated as variables in the research design, and potentially salient characteristics (sex, race, age) can be randomly or systematically varied.

Much can be done to ensure greater accuracy and reliability of the data through careful selection and training of both interviewers and raters.

Selecting the Interviewers

The art of conducting an interview involves at least these skills:

1. Creating a friendly atmosphere (developing rapport).
2. Asking the questions properly and intelligibly.
3. Spontaneously clarifying misunderstood questions.
4. Electing expansion and elaboration of incomplete or insufficient responses.
5. Clarifying apparently conflicting or incompatible responses. (Richardson et al., 1965)

These skills are generally taught in elementary courses on counseling. It saves considerable training time to choose interviewers from among students who have already succeeded in courses on basic counseling skills. More advanced counseling students may, however, tend to encourage movement into deeper emotional responses, and need reminders that a research interview has a different purpose than a counseling interview and that too much encouragement of feelings is inappropriate.

Obviously the interviewer must be able to develop a relaxed and friendly atmosphere to gain the respondent's participation and optimize cooperation. She must grasp the concepts being assessed (e.g., exploration and commitment) and be able to spontaneously reword questions and formulate new ones to ensure that the respondent provides sufficient information from which to assess identity or intimacy.[1]

Because it is standard practice to audio-record the identity status interview and have the raters make assessments directly from the recordings, it is not important that our interviewers be proficient in written recording skills. This is a great advantage because it permits using interviewers of lower socioeconomic background. My impression is that many persons

[1] To avoid the clumsiness of "his/her" and similar combinations, I have referred to the interviewer and researcher as *her* and the respondent as *him* throughout this chapter.

(e.g., in the mental health programs of community colleges) do not have highly developed writing skills, but are perfectly adequate in the oral skills necessary for semistructured interviews. Identity studies in noncollege populations are sorely needed, and research designs that systematically assign interviewers according to socioeconomic background appear practical and are recommended.

Finally, as part of the selection process I suggest conducting an identity status interview with the potential interviewers and raters. I hypothesize that individuals who have reached the Achievement status in at least one area will make better interviewers and raters than those in other statuses. My rationale is that it is difficult for raters to recognize and assess processes that do not resonate with one's personal experience. Similarly, interviewers may overlook areas that need further inquiry, if key processes (such as exploration, or commitment) are not part of their life experience. In addition, there is evidence that Identity Achievements are better at facilitative listening skills (Genthner & Neuber, 1975).

Having research carried out by an "elite" group has interesting implications, but is not unique to this area. We frequently have those who rate high on a variable do the assessment—whether it is I.Q., moral development, or a concrete skill (e.g., piloting a plane).

Training the Interviewers

The performance of interviewers before training has been shown to be a poor indicator of potential skill; the relationship between assessment of interview skills before and after training is very low (Richardson et al. 1965). This condition suggests that good interviewing depends upon good training, yet very little research has been done to determine exactly what skills are involved in a good research interview, and we have even fewer data on the characteristics of a good training program.

Much of the literature consists of rules of thumb, essentially nonsystematic compilations, the "folklore" of interviewing based on experience. Few scientific studies test these common-sense injunctions. It probably is accurate to characterize interviewer training as the passing on of this folklore. Social science research has documented that incredibly subtle interpersonal influences can affect all our research (Orne, 1962; Rosenthal & Jacobson, 1966). Thus some humility is appropriate regardless of the methods used to collect data.

Trainers of counselors and of research interviewers have increasingly moved to a step-by-step model of training. This model involves isolating specific observable behaviors that are believed to constitute effective interviewing, having trainees observe models of these behaviors, and then having them practice the behaviors in a sequence of settings with supervision and feedback until they are ready to perform interviews in the field alone (Egan, 1990; Ivey et al., 1968; Zimmer & Park, 1967). The following learning experiences are typically included in such a training program:

—Explaining the nature and purpose of the interviews to be conducted.
—Reading the manual and discussing any questions raised by it.
—Role-playing sample interviews to become familiar with the content to be discussed.
—Listening to a recorded model interview.
—Practicing interviews in the training setting (with other trainees).
—Practicing interviews at home (with friends or acquaintances).
—Practicing interviews in the field.
—Getting feedback on recorded interviews from the field.

These elements usually occur in the order listed, allowing a progression toward increased independence for the trainees. For variety, other elements may be introduced, when further experiences are needed, such as the trainer demonstrating an interview with a trainee as respondent, and use of videotapes in interviews between trainees.

The specific skills that need to be taught depend, of course, upon the trainees' past training and present skill. I present here some of the broader skills in the order in which I usually teach them, but with the warning that the training involves constant feedback and informal evaluation, which frequently determines the next step in training. I do not structure each training period in advance from start to finish.

Beginning the Interview

Though the first priority in the actual interview is to develop rapport, I do not start my training with this focus. Doing so puts too much stress on the interpersonal relationship at a time when both the interview materials and the other trainees are "strangers." I focus instead on the content of the semistructured interview and have trainees practice the opening remarks. Prior to the interviews I will have spoken to classrooms of students; thus the respondents they see have already had a chance to ask some questions about the purpose of the study. They have already been told that individual information will not be available to teachers or administrators in the school system (or college), but is confidential; they have already decided to volunteer. I explain this procedure to the interviewers, and suggest that they begin the interview with as few details about the research as possible, to avoid raising unnecessary questions or biasing the responses. A typical interview begins as follows:[2]

[2] Dialogues between I and R in this chapter are quoted from recordings of interviews with high school students, changed only as necessary to disguise identity and with minor omissions for brevity, with the one exception mentioned in footnote 4.

Interviewer (I): Hi, I'm Arlene. [Introductions.] I know you're in Mr. Bank's class, but I don't know how old you are and what year of school you're in.

Respondent (R): I'm seventeen, and I'm a Junior.

I: Fine. There are two parts of the interview that I'm going to do with you this period. In the first part, I want to ask you some questions about friendship. I want to remind you that the interview is confidential—no one who hears it will know your name. But if I ask you something that you think is too personal, just tell me to go on to the next question. Okay?

R: Yes.

I: Any questions?

R: Not that I can think of.

I: Then let's begin. If some questions come up as we go along, feel free to ask.

This beginning is fairly typical of our interviews with high school students. By being friendly but moving quickly into the interview itself, any anxiety the respondent may feel is soon alleviated and questions that may bias the response are usually avoided. When questions are asked, interviewers should answer them honestly, but avoid describing the specific variables being assessed (exploration and commitment). After the trainees have practiced beginning interviews with each other, I model answering some of the questions that might occur. This is an example from another of our high school interviews:

I: Any questions?

R: Uhm, who listens to the tapes?

I: The cassettes are gonna be listened to by the other university students who are involved in the research, and the professor probably will be listening to some, too. They're going to help us put information into the computer. No one will know your full name, and no one except the people doing the research will hear the tape.[3]

R: Okay. What's the subject? Is it a certain subject?

I: Well, it has three areas. One has to do with occupations, one with friendships, and one with gender roles—roles of men and women.

R: Okay.

I: The ones that I'm going to be talking with you about have to do with friendships and occupations.

R: Okay. Why aren't you going to go into the gender roles?

I: Well, it's set up ahead of time. We have time in one period to cover only two areas, and so we take turns on the ones we do.

---

[3] See the section below, "Common Problems in Interviewing," for an additional illustration of how the interviewer explains confidentiality to the high school respondents.

The example helps the trainees to realize that inquisitive youths may ask questions simply out of curiosity, and that a lot of explanation probably would not answer the specific questions this youth raised. By responding to the individual questions, better rapport is established without providing information that may contaminate the study and may be irrelevant to the respondent. I do provide interviewers with a basic description of the research that I have used in the classrooms, which shows them how to describe the purpose of the investigations without being specific about variables.

Developing Rapport

Facilitating open and honest sharing of information demands sensitivity to the respondent's needs without losing sight of the function of the interview—gathering information. Generally the respondent enters the interview with three needs: (1) he needs to feel that the interview will be enjoyable; (2) he needs to confirm that he is capable of giving the kinds of responses that the interviewer is looking for; and (3) he needs to see that his participation in the research is worthwhile (Cannell & Kahn, 1953; ISR, 1969). Because most people enjoy talking about themselves, it is usually easy to develop rapport during the identity or intimacy interviews. In most of the formats, the questions begin with items that are fairly general and easy to answer. If the interviewer shows the respondent that she is listening and following his line of thought, rapport and motivation seem to develop naturally. Very often our respondents state at the end of the interview that they liked being listened to and that they have not previously had the chance to think things out aloud. The students typically find that the questions evoke sufficient personal interest to keep them motivated, and yet are not threatening.

The basic interviewer responses necessary are minimal encouragers (nods, "uh-huhs"), reflections of content, and the other responses frequently referred to as "active listening" (Gordon, 1970) or "attending skills" (Carkhuff, 1972). These can be found in most introductory texts on counseling (e.g., Egan, 1990). The usefulness of such minimal encouragers as "and then . . . ?"; "yes, go on . . . ," "Anything else?"; "Can you say more about that?"; or "Can you be more specific?" is pointed out to trainees. Also emphasized is the effective use of short periods of silence. It is important to help the trainees to distinguish a response that encourages but does not evaluate ("uh hum"), from one that passes judgment ("that's right"). A minimal encourager commonly used in social conversation, "good," or "that's good," has been shown to bias respondents' ensuing responses, but "uh-hum" does not (Hildum & Brown, 1956).

Reflections of content are particularly useful in helping the respondent to feel understood. They can also be used to summarize several statements, to be certain the interviewer has captured the meaning of the respondent's answers, and to help the subject collect his thoughts, providing direction for the next response. It is valuable to distinguish reflection of content from reflection of feeling. Limited responsiveness to feelings is often helpful in developing and maintaining rapport, but it is not appropriate in a research interview to encourage opening up deeper feelings. The accurate reflection of content is helpful in reassuring respondents who begin to move into feelings and become uncomfortable. As with any other technique, it is possible to overuse reflection of content so that it becomes a ridiculous echo, but this slip is easily caught when tapes are supervised and feedback is provided.

Once the skills for encouraging elaboration have been learned, it is useful to practice the interviews from the start, pointing out that encouragements work best when used from the very beginning of an interview (Richardson et al., 1965).

Once the skill is mastered, one caution about encouragements is needed. Direct requests to "tell me more" may backfire if used with a hostile or highly suspicious respondent (Richardson et al., 1965). In such cases it is safer to stick to the less obtrusive minimal encouragers.

Perhaps the most potent encourager of all is simply waiting. A brief pause, rather than rushing on to the next question, often results in further elaboration. Of course long silences that lead the respondent to feel anxious are not appropriate. Generally a pause of about three seconds is effective; silences of ten seconds or longer may produce anxiety and lead to the respondent's producing shorter responses (Gordon, 1954; Saslow et al., 1957).

Once the interviewers have become comfortable with using encouragers and reflections, they can practice linking; that is, connecting the next question to something that the respondent has already said. When the interviewer can spontaneously relate the questions to the respondent's own context, the questions not only make more sense, they convey that the interviewer is genuinely interested in that respondent. This signal enhances the respondent's feeling of active participation and increases the validity and depth of the responses (Richardson et al., 1965).

At the beginning of an intimacy interview, which followed an identity interview, the interviewer makes a statement (I4) illustrating the value of linking:

> I1: I'd like to ask you if there's anybody you're particularly close to here at Eisenhower High?
>
> R: A close relationship . . . do you mean like a friend? [I nods.] I don't have a close one.
>
> I2: You don't have one who particularly stands out. Can you tell me a little about your relationships with your associates?

R: My associates, ah . . . at school you mean? [I: Uh, huh.] It's shallow. It's more or less—we all hang around together. . . .
I3: Is there any one person you see frequently, more frequently than the others, in or out of school?
R: No.
I4: I think you mentioned in the other part of the interview that you had some friends who didn't go to school here. How about those guys?
R: Yeah, ah, I'm staying at this one place, right now, with these two other guys, and ah, one guy went to school in Manchester, England, and ah, one guy went to school at Illinois State, and, you know, they tell me a lot of things.
I5: How close are you to either of them?
R: Pretty close. I mean, if I have a problem or something like that, I can go to them and talk about it.
I6: Can you describe any close experiences you've had?
R: [Gives a long description of having problems with a girlfriend and discussing it with one of his apartment mates.]

In this instance, the first questions the interviewer asked (I1 and I2) were poorly worded and too circumscribed. By the time the interviewer recognized this flaw (I3), a low response set was already developing. The linkage with the previous, more free-flowing interview (I4) was successful in breaking that set.

It is important for interviewers to realize that once a respondent has begun to feel comfortable and to give more personal and subjective answers that a switch by the interviewer to an objective and impersonal question will break the flow and be experienced as "highly disturbing" by the respondent (Richardson et al., 1965). Of course, the interviewer must move on to other questions and keep the respondent discussing what is relevant to the research. When the interviewer can do so by linking the question to what has just been said, it directs the respondent without producing an abrupt break in the personal sharing.

Effective Inquiry

By this stage in the training, the interviewers have begun to move away from reading the questions to spontaneously posing their own questions. If the trainees are novices, they may have the tendency to use closed or restricted questions when more open questions are preferable.

I: Do you think, for example, that boys should open the doors for girls?

This question is closed, in that it requires only a yes or no answer. Further, it puts words in the respondent's mouth by choosing a specific instance. Early in the sex-role interview, a more open question is preferable, such as:

> I: Are there specific things that you think guys should do that you wouldn't expect of girls?

It is common for beginning interviewers to offer multiple-choice questions (as in I2 below), which make assumptions about the possible options:

> I1: Have you discussed your choice of occupation with your parents?
> R: Yes.
> I2: Did they agree, or disagree?

A better response would have been:

> I2: How did they respond?

Open questions frequently begin with "what" (to elicit facts), "how" (generally more people oriented), "could you," "can you," "would you" (providing great flexibility of response) (Evans et al., 1979).

Providing trainees with these beginning words frequently helps them formulate open questions.

There is increasing agreement that the question "why?" is not usually a productive probe (Passons, 1975; Perls, 1951; Smith, J.M., 1972); therefore I discourage its use. Usually, asking a respondent "how" something came about will elicit the content aimed at with a "why" question.

Closed or restricted questions also have their place in an interview, and it is important that the trainees not develop rigid avoidance of them. Closed questions generally involve an assumption. When that assumption is warranted, a closed question may facilitate rapport. If the respondent has given you good reason to expect a particular answer, a question embodying that expectation demonstrates that you have been following accurately (Richardson et al., 1965).

> I: And, when a boy opens the door, would you feel special and feminine?

The question functions almost as a reflection of previous content, clarifying whether the present understanding is correct. Closed questions are also helpful in focusing a respondent on a point.

> I: I'm still not clear. Do you think your father is opposed to your choice, or just not interested?

The training task is not to eliminate the option of closed questions, but to be sure the interviewer has at her disposal the ability to compose open questions, and thus can decide which is appropriate to the situation.

An additional aspect of effective inquiry is the intonation of questions. Some trainees, when reading questions, tend to lower their voices (falling tone) at the end of an item, instead of raising their voice (rising tone) as in spontaneously asking a question. The rising tone communicates an expectation that the respondent may have something to report. The falling tone unwittingly communicates boredom and lack of expectation or interest in a response, and research shows that it decreases not only the amount of response elicited, but the motivation and interest of the respondent (Barath & Cannell, 1977). The risk of receiving distorted and incomplete information from such questions is high (Richardson et al., 1965).

It is essential to effective inquiry that the interviewers understand the intent of the questions and not reword them in ways that fail to provide the information needed. For example, one of the interviewers in a study with high school students failed to remember that the purpose of the "friendship" (intimacy) interview was to assess relationships between peers, and accepted the respondent's choice of a teacher as her closest friend, and thus completed this whole section of the interview without obtaining any information on the degree of intimacy the respondent could develop with peers. Unfortunately, this misperception of the purpose of the interview had not surfaced during the training program.

Self-Disclosures

Even the most cooperative respondents may find a conversation uncomfortable when the flow of information is in only one direction. It is important that the interviewer not offer personal information that can bias the interview and not permit the interview to degenerate into a social conversation. If the interviewer is very responsive, in using the minimal encouragers mentioned above, in feeding back information offered, and in nonverbal signs of interest, this flow of responses makes up for the lack of information offered, and the problem seldom appears. It is also possible to increase the mutuality of the give-and-take by teaching less naturally responsive trainees types of self-disclosure that do not reveal opinions that would bias the responses elicited. For example, if a female respondent discussing occupational possibilities comments:

> R: My grandmother, and even my Dad, think I'm weird to consider being a truckdriver, but . . .
>
> I: Sometimes it's hard for adults to recognize how much job areas are opening up to either sex. If it interests you, you might explore it.[4]

The interviewer's statement is very general and factual, following the respondent's line of thinking, yet makes the exchange more mutual.

[4] This is a hypothetical dialogue, not a quotation.

Similar effects can be achieved by providing factual information about oneself, such as acknowledging common interests, places in which the interviewer has lived or visited when these places are first mentioned by the respondent, and similar tactics used in small talk. But it is best to delay such disclosures until the respondent has assimilated some sense of his role in the interview, so that he doesn't misunderstand these disclosures to suggest that a social chat is all that is expected of him (Richardson et al., 1965).

When the interviewer is asked by the respondent for personal opinions or values, however, the request can be politely deferred: "Could we discuss that after we've finished the interview?" (Smith, 1972); or humorously deflected, "My job is to get the opinions, not to have them!"—spoken in a warm and humorous tone.[5] This tactic makes it clear that the interviewer is willing to share, but prevents such sharing from biasing the information sought in the research. Of course, when the interviewer prefers not to share information, her personal prerogative should be courteously expressed.

Clarifying Responses

The interviewers are instructed to improve the quality of responses that lack specificity or clarity by asking further questions (Richardson et al., 1965). To do so intelligently, they must be clear on the purposes of the interviews and how they will be rated. When I am conducting an interview, I may covertly ask myself: "Am I sure this youth is Diffused, or might he be in Moratorium?"; and "What do I need to know to be sure?" Of course, an interviewer cannot do this shifting until she has had experience with the rating process. Thus it is helpful during the training to have the interviewers act as raters, perhaps rating each other's practice tapes. The commonest problem is that the interviewer has accepted a vague, uncertain answer and not tested it. Of course if an "I don't know" response seems clear and nondefensive, it should be accepted at face value as a genuine lack of opinion, and no further probe should be used. Sometimes, when the respondent says "I don't know," accompanied by a puzzled look, it is an indication that he hasn't understood the question. The interviewer may rephrase it and succeed in getting a response. In other cases, the respondent needs to sense real interest from the interviewer before he will volunteer a fuller response. Here is example from a high school girl, several exchanges into the occupational interview:

> I1: Do you have, just generally, some ideas about what areas you're most interested in?

---

[5] Ann McLaughlin, "Interviewing techniques." Unpublished, personal correspondence.

R: Ummm. [Pause.] Not really. [Pause.] But I know that I wouldn't want to be behind a desk all my life. [I: Uh huhm.] Like a secretary; I don't think I could handle that.
I2: So it's clear that that's out.
R: Yeah.
I3: What are some of the possibilities that are in?
R: Um. Dealing with people, but I don't know how, I mean, a lot of people talk about physical therapy or speech therapy, but I don't really know much about those.
I4: From what you do know, are those possibilities?
R: They could be, but I haven't really gone into any of . . . like I've just been taking general courses all four years. And so I haven't. . . .
I5: The only thing you're really clear on is that it's going to deal with people.
R: Yes, but not too serious, 'cause I'm not a real . . . like I'm not unstable, but I'm very sensitive and emotional, so if I was like a psychologist or something like that I don't know if I could handle all the problems. I'd probably make them my own problems. . . .

This information gathering could have stopped at "Not really," if the interviewer had not paused and waited for more, and after that, reflected the student's meaning (I2), and rephrased the question in the context of what she had said (I3). This move brings a positive response, followed by a disclaimer (which again could have ended the exploration). The interviewer picks up the ball again (I4), encouraging expansion. After another disclaiming response, the interviewer reflects the positive piece of information (I5) and finally gets a more thorough response. Obviously (from that response) the youth has evaluated work with people in the light of her sense of her own limitations, but is reluctant to reveal her tentative thoughts until prompted and encouraged. The interviewer must learn to come back assuredly with clarifying probes: "How do you mean . . . ?"; "In what ways?"; "Can you explain more fully what you meant by . . . ?" It is reassuring to trainees to know that pausing to think of such a probe is okay, and that the silence may actually be facilitative.

Frequently, when a question receives an evasive response, simply rewording it results in clarification.

I: Do you ever talk about it with other students?
R: Not really, I just say I have no idea what I'm gonna do. That's about as far as I go.
I: You don't have any friends you've discussed the possibility with . . . ?
R: Um. [Pause.] A friend of the family. [Proceeds to tell of his trust and sharing with this friend.]

Rephrasing broadened the scope of the question from "students" to "friends" and brought a response.

Two other variations of the "I don't know" response deserve mention. Sometimes the interviewer observes facial expression or gesture accompanying the noncomittal statement suggesting that the respondent is afraid to speak his mind. This reticence can frequently be overcome by reassurance: "Well, I just want your opinion on it," or "There really aren't any 'right' or 'wrong' answers to these questions."

Often the interviewer may notice eye movements suggesting that the respondent is trying to organize his thoughts or that an "I don't know" is a stall for time. In both cases, allow for a pause, then use a probe such as, "Well, lots of people have never thought about this before, but I'd like to hear your ideas about it, just the way it seems to you."

Techniques other than probes and rephrasing of questions may be taught to help interviewers deal with ambiguous or vague responses.

Sometimes the respondent may infer something and not clearly and directly state it. Picking up on the inference may result in clarification: "I take it you didn't agree with him; did I understand you rightly?" If the client seems shy or fearful, a gentler wording may be more successful: "I'm not sure I fully understood you. Did you mean . . . ?"

Inconsistencies should be challenged in a way that doesn't put the respondent on the defensive. One format is to accept responsibility for the confusion: "I'm sorry, apparently I misunderstood you. I thought you said earlier. . . ." This technique gets the inconsistency up front, but without blaming the respondent, which usually results in the respondent's either resolving the confusion or admitting that the inconsistency lies in his own thinking. The following illustration, which occurred midway through the sex-role interview with a high school girl, is an example of confrontation and nonjudgmental acceptance:

I1: Can you picture a situation where you'd continue working and he [future husband] would quit?
R: Well, if I were making more money! [Laughs heartily.]
I2: Really?! [Mild surprise because of contrast to previous statements.] If you were making more, then you'd keep working.
R: Yeah [Softly, sounding doubtful.]
I3: Are you sure about that?
R: [More firmly.] I would think so. Because if I . . . [Pause.], but I can't really imagine him earning less money.
I4: So you think it's unlikely?
R: I can't picture any man doing that.
I5: [Surprised.] You can't picture a guy wanting to do that? [Pushing her to try to imagine it.]
R: Not any guy I would marry!
I6: Can you say what your picture is of a guy who might do that?
R: It just seems like he's . . . he's just living off me. I don't like that. [She then recognizes that the reverse might be true of the traditional woman, and discusses this possibility.]

I7: You seem to be saying—I'm not sure—are you saying it's better for the wife than for the husband to stay home, but that it might not be good for either one?
R: [More clearly.] Yeah.
I8: But you are saying it's better for the wife than for the husband—is that right?
R: Yeah [Sheepishly, sensing the conflict with her own egalitarian statements.] I think so. [Stressing that the personal value isn't absolute.]
I9: That's fine. I just wanted to be clear. [Accepting her present position.]

The interviewer uses humor and challenge to bring out the inconsistencies, but provides acceptance of the respondent's present state of incongruity and makes no attempt to reach a resolution. The intent is to get a clear picture of the respondent's present status, not to produce consistency that does not presently exist. The humor used in this instance (I5) is a bit like the closed questions we ask children, knowing that the opposite is true: "But you don't like ice cream cones, do you?" This type of closed question can be useful when a response is unclear. The slant of the question is so obvious that the respondent can clearly rebut it, yet it pushes the respondent to picture the scene and express her deeper response to it.

Acceptance of differences can be shown by prefacing a question. For example, in the intimacy interviews, when the early questions suggest that the respondent is an "isolate," the interviewer could make it easier for him to state that (or rebut it) by asking:

I: Some adolescents feel that the dating games and other social events of your age group aren't really right for them. Do you ever have this feeling?

The lead "some adolescents feel . . ." makes it easier to admit a socially undesirable behavior or feeling.

Providing Structure and Limits

With some respondents the problem is not to get them to open up, but to limit the responses and to direct the discussion toward relevant issues and away from anecdotes. Typically, this shift can be accomplished by a subtle interruption, which has been called a "guggle."[6] Most people use

[6]The word "guggles" was first used in Richardson et al. (1965, p. 205) to denote these mild interruptions. "Because we had seen no previous mention of this behavior as we have defined it and knew of no word to describe it, we borrowed from Ko-Ko in Gilbert and Sullivan's *Mikado*: 'As he squirmed and struggled and gurgled and guggled, I drew my snickersnee!' "

this soft clearing of the throat as an unconscious habit when they want to say something; and the normal social response is for the speaker to complete his sentence and pause, allowing the interviewer to move on to the next question.

Another means for reducing garrulity is to interrupt and summarize when the respondent pauses for breath. As soon as the summary is affirmed, a new question is posed. The only skill necessary is to spontaneously produce a succinct summary. If rambling occurs frequently, the interviewer can be more directive by explicitly bringing the respondent back to the subject: "We were talking about . . ."; "Now I need to ask you about. . . ."[7]

Occasionally in the intimacy interviews, a topic may trigger a respondent's emotions, and he may handle this feeling by talking too much. If the interviewer summarizes and changes the topic, it prevents the respondent's feelings from gaining momentum. This portion of an interview with a high school girl illustrates:

I: I want to ask you a bunch of questions about friendship. First, do you have any friends you think of yourself as really close to?
R: [Very cautiously.] I used to.
I: You used to have. [Pause.] But they left the area? [Respondent shakes head "no."] Ah, [Pause.] something's happened to the friendship . . . ?
R: [Softly.] Yeah.
I: [Gently.] Okay. Can you describe a little bit what the relationship was like?
R: Well, we had a lot of fun, and we both had the same sense of humor, and she felt the same way I did. [Begins to talk freely, and describes the situation that preceded their ending the friendship.] That kind of thing aggravates me beyond belief. [Nervous laugh.]
I: Yes, it sounds like—it would hurt your feelings.
R: It does. And so it's not worth it. [Pause.]
I: About how long has it been since you've been good friends?
R: [Answers and describes a number of things they used to do together.]
I: So you talked about boyfriends, and things that were funny, ah, were there any things you couldn't talk about?
R: [Casually.] No.
I: [Mildly challenging.] You could have shared about anything?
R: [Thoughtfully.] Yeah. [Begins to show sadness.]
I: [Gently.] I don't mean to get you back into that, but it sounds . . .

[7] Harold D. Grotevant & Catherine R. Cooper, "Probes for Problem Interviewees" in the unpublished Identity Manual used in their research on "Identity formation and role-taking skill in adolescence."

R: [Interrupting.] Oh, it's nothing. But at the time it was. Yes, when it first happened, I didn't even want to come out of the house. . . .

I: How about her? [Moving on with the interview.] Could she share things like that with you?

The interviewer has shown sensitivity to feelings and thus developed rapport, but then returns to the business of conducting the information-gathering. From here on, the interviewer can remain objective and ask more about the relationship, and the respondent can talk about it with a little more distance, and yet can trust the interviewer with the information.

A final means of structuring the interview, when a respondent is overly talkative or rambles and needs focus, has to do with the style of questions posed. Instead of asking broad, open questions, the interviewer may switch to narrower questions, reducing the scope of what is requested. Because the garrulous respondent tends to overelaborate, chances are good that the narrower questions will elicit sufficient information for assessing identity or intimacy. And of course, if the response is incomplete, the interviewer can ask a broader question.

With such a respondent, it may be useful to provide feedback on the quality of his performance. When the respondent gives a lucid and succinct answer, the interviewer may state: "That was a very helpful answer." Studies have shown that the most frequent interviewer behavior, besides asking questions, is giving positive feedback—but unskilled interviewers tend to do so indiscriminately (Marquis & Cannell, 1969). An interviewer who habitually provides active listening responses may continue to do so with a respondent who needs no encouragement, thus providing reinforcement for long and rambling answers. Most respondents are motivated to try to provide useful information: they also need honest feedback, both positive and negative, to recognize the kind of information that is useful to the interviewer. One study of interviews about health information demonstrated that negative as well as positive feedback increased the quality of information the respondents provided; no adverse effects of negative feedback were found, either on motivation or on reaction to the interviewer (Vinokur et al., 1977). Obviously, the negative feedback is stated inoffensively:

I: That's only one alternative. Can you think of any others?

or I: Perhaps if I ask the question again you might think of something. [Repeats question.]

or I: You answered that quickly. We are interested in all kinds of [information]. . . . [Rewords question.] (Vinokur et al., 1977)

The examples of negative feedback in the report of this experiment have to do primarily with inadequate responses. But a statement such as: "I want you to focus your answer specifically on whom you've discussed this with," would provide the respondent with information that his response is too wide-ranging, and would clarify for the respondent a more useful response.

It is pertinent to reemphasize that the criteria for a good interview must be made explicit to trainees. They need to understand not only their task of developing good rapport, but the kind of information needed, so that they can correct the interview as it progresses (Richardson et al., 1965).

Common Problems in Interviewing

Conducting research interviews demands that the interviewer develop closeness through understanding and acceptance, and yet attain the "detachment or objectivity which we associate with a professional–client relationship" (Cannell & Kahn, 1953). When the trainees have learned the separate skills required, some practice in doing total interviews is necessary so that the skills may become integrated and properly sequenced. Typically, open-ended questions and the skills of establishing strong rapport are needed at the initial phase of the interview. The interviewer must learn, once rapport is established, to "retreat" personally and guide the respondent through the interview, spontaneously formulating questions that link to the respondent's previous answers, while listening attentively and observing clues in the respondent's behavior to maintain his motivation to respond fully (Smith, 1972).

This sequence does not hold for all respondents, however. Interviewers must learn not to drop the rapport-building techniques too early with respondents who need encouragement far into the interview. Occasionally, a respondent will become constricted in his replies when the interview becomes more personal (for example, when the interview on occupational identity is followed by the intimacy interview), and all that is needed is reassurance about the anonymity of the interview tapes. A few students may believe that the school administration has some way of checking up on the research data; an explanation of the researcher's independence from the school administration and of the methods of data analysis may be enough to reestablish rapport. The interviewer may reiterate: "All the information given by you is completely confidential. Your name never goes with it. Your answers end up rating scales as numbers that are processed by a computer, and come out as percentages" (Smith, 1972).

The more frequent problem in the identity and intimacy interviews is the reverse, in which rapport leads to deeper trust than intended. Sensitive and responsive interviewers develop good rapport, and the youths are so responsive to being heard and accepted as individuals that they open up more feelings than are appropriate to the research relationship. As suggested by the excerpt about a friendship that had broken up (last section), it is fairly easy to move away from deeper emotions, even if they come out, without leaving the respondent feeling abandoned or not understood.

Where the student is already talking freely, it may be preferable to avoid moving into the emotions at all, as illustrated in this interview on occupational identity:

I: What do your parents think about it?

R: Well, [Pause.] I don't think my parents think a whole lot. . . . [Discouraged and exasperated.] I don't think they really care about exactly what I do. I could tell them, but it would just go in one ear and out the other. . . .

I: [Interviewer lets him talk, but makes no comment. She doesn't cut him off, yet she gives him no encouragers. After about six sentences, the interviewer makes a guggle and interrupts at the next breath stop.]

I: And so there are pains about discussing occupations. I want to ask you. . . .

Thus, the interviewer gets him back to the topic of the interview, and moves on. After this excerpt, each time the interviewer gets sufficient information, she moves objectively to the next question:

R: My Mom doesn't really understand.

I: Are there any other adults who have influenced you?

Even though this sort of response seems to cut off the respondent, she continued to participate and stay motivated, and in fact, the interviewer ran out of time and couldn't complete this section. Such needy respondents are relatively rare, but in each interview setting, I do ferret out faculty and counselors who are good listeners, to whom we may refer students. I instruct interviewers to ask the respondent, at the end of such an interview, whether he has discussed this issue with someone.

I: You've shared with me that this relationship with your parents bothers you, but as you know I will only be seeing you for this one interview. Would this be something you'd like to discuss with Mr. Luoma, for example?

This final example illustrates the value of having the researcher and trainer know the setting in which the interviews will be conducted. Most of the problems that trainees imagine occurring will not, in fact, occur. But the surest way to relieve their anxiety is for the trainer to have conducted interviews in the specific setting and become familiar and comfortable in it.

The enthusiasm and appreciation that so many of the respondents have for being interviewed makes the interviewing rewarding in itself. If the trainer has experienced that, her confidence and positive outlook will be communicated to the trainees.

7
Overview of the Identity Status Scoring Criteria

ALAN S. WATERMAN

The Ego Identity Interview

There is no standard form for the identity status interview, and the material in this book is not intended to define a standard format. Different investigators have chosen from among a variety of domains in which to assess identity and have varied the number and level of complexity of the questions. The principal determinants used in creating the interview have been the research hypotheses under investigation, the age and sex of the participant samples studied, and the academic background and experience of the people employed as interviewers.

The original interview created by Marcia (1964) involved a semi-structured format. A limited number of standard opening questions and follow-up probes were specified in his training manual. The responsibility was placed on the interviewer to create additional follow-up questions, as appropriate, to draw out a participant's pattern for handling identity concerns. Because Marcia and close associates conducted all the interviews in the original study and knew what information was needed for the research, no more precise specification of the interview questions was required. Since then, investigators have employed graduate and undergraduate student interviewers less fully cognizant of the intricacies of identity formation. This change has led to the preparation of more detailed interview schedules spelling out the variety of follow-up probes called for under different circumstances. In the identity interview schedules presented in the Appendix, these more detailed schedules are provided.

The interview first employed by Marcia (1964) covered three domains: occupation, religion, and politics. The initial research was conducted with male college students. When Marcia undertook to work with females he tried two additional domains: family and career conflicts (Marcia & Friedman, 1970) and attitudes toward premarital intercourse (Schenkel & Marcia, 1972), of which only the latter was maintained in his subsequent studies with women. Other investigators have considered other topics important to a person's self-definition and have added corresponding sections to the interview.

Based on the patterns of usage of the various topics in the interview, a division can be made between core domains that are now employed in a large percentage of studies and supplemental domains that, as yet, have been used just occasionally. Because the interview schedules for the supplemental domains are newly developed, it is possible that some will eventually become core topics, at least with particular age groups.

At present the core domains are:

1. vocational choice (Marcia, 1964)
2. religious beliefs (Marcia, 1964)
3. political ideology (Marcia, 1964)
4. gender-role attitudes (Matteson, 1974)
5. beliefs about sexual expression (Schenkel & Marcia, 1972)

The supplemental domains are:

1. avocational interests (Meilman, 1979)
2. relationships with friends (Grotevant & Cooper, 1985)
3. relationships with dates (Grotevant & Cooper, 1985)
4. role of spouse (Archer, 1981)
5. role of parent (Archer, 1981)
6. priorities assigned to family and career goals (Marcia & Friedman, 1970; Waterman, 1980)

In the following section, the identity-related issues for the core and supplemental domains are briefly summarized. Several of the domains are examined in greater detail in subsequent chapters, focusing on how they apply to early and middle adolescents, late adolescents, and adults.

The Identity Interview Domains

Core Domains

Vocational Choice

The central question in this area is decisions about one's life work. Viewed in this way, vocation is *not* equivalent to paid employment. Rather it includes activities performed for pay, homemaker and parenting responsibilities, and volunteer or other activities on which a person spends a substantial proportion of time but without monetary gain, as in artistic pursuits and amateur athletics. Specific identity-related issues include:

1. Should one pursue a paid career or take on full-time homemaker and/or parenting responsibilities?
2. What specific career choice would be best?

3. What relative importance should be attached to intrinsic and extrinsic rewards?
4. What relative importance should be attached to taking risks for possible career advancement versus maintaining stability and economic security?
5. What can be done in anticipation of, or in response to, career burnout?

Religious Beliefs

This domain deals with the extent to which the person has worked out his or her views of subjects generally considered religious. Where the person is not religious in a conventional sense, a personal philosophy of life, particularly about ethics and social responsibility, is appropriately considered under this heading. Specific identity-related issues include these:

1. Should one believe in God or not?
2. What form and frequency of religious observances, including attendance at religious services, should be maintained?
3. Should involvement with an organized religion be maintained, or does one need to develop a highly personal religious orientation, perhaps without group involvement?
4. What positions should be taken on any of various doctrinal issues?
5. Under what circumstances should one change one's religion?
6. If one is not religious, on what basis can ethical judgments be made?
7. How should one feel about interfaith marriage?
8. What type of religious training should be offered to one's children?

Political Ideology

The domain of political ideology, broadly considered, covers the relationship between the individual and the society in which he or she lives. This domain includes, but is not limited to, matters of political parties and partisan issues. Matters of political philosophy are equally relevant. Specific identity-related issues include:

1. Should a political party affiliation be made, and what form of support should be offered to the party selected?
2. Where does one view oneself on a continuum ranging from liberal, through moderate, to conservative?
3. What positions should be taken on any of a variety of political and social issues such as big versus small government; defense, war, and peace; economic policy; foreign policy; environmental protection; and race relations and social justice?

Gender-Role Attitudes

The main question about gender-role attitudes is determining what it means to the respondent to be male or female. Specific identity-related issues include:

1. To what extent does one want to adopt a gender-role pattern that can be characterized as masculine, feminine, or androgynous?
2. How should one feel about sex-typical and/or sex-atypical interests?
3. How should gender-role considerations influence friendship choices?
4. What attitudes should be held on social and political issues associated with women's (or men's) liberation (e.g., the Equal Rights Amendment)?

Beliefs about Sexual Expression

At the center of this topic as a matter of identity concern is the role that sexual activity should play in an individual's life. Specific identity-related issues include:

1. How important is sexual expression in defining oneself?
2. What sexual orientation (heterosexual, homosexual, bisexual) is personally expressive?
3. What relationship should exist between love and sexual activity?
4. How does one feel about personal involvement in premarital sexual activity?
5. How does one feel about personal involvement in extramarital sexual activity?
6. What should one believe about contraceptive use?

Supplemental Domains

Avocational Interests

As a subject of identity concern, the questions in this area focus on the extent to which people define themselves in terms of leisure-time activities (e.g., sports, hobbies, extracurricular activities). Specific identity-related issues include:

1. How important a role should leisure-time activities play in one's life?
2. What avocational interests are most personally rewarding?

Relationships with Friends

As a topic involving relationships, friendships may be thought to have more to do with intimacy than it does with identity. From the perspective of identity, the central question is how one tries to define oneself through relationships with friends. In contrast, intimacy involves considering the ways in which a person actually relates with others (See Chapter 5). Specific identity-related issues include:

1. What does one have to offer to or share with friends?
2. What can a person reasonably expect of his or her friends?

3. What should one's friends reasonably expect in return?
4. On what basis should an individual choose his or her friends?

Relationships with Dates

Again, identity and intimacy issues overlap. The concerns here parallel those for friendships but specifically refer to relationships with a potential or actual romantic component. In some instances this topic will generate content relevant to beliefs about sexual expression. Specific identity-related issues include:

1. What does one have to offer or share with a dating partner?
2. What can a person reasonably expect from a dating partner?
3. What should a dating partner be reasonably able to expect in return?
4. On what basis should an individual choose a dating partner?

Role of Spouse

As with both of the preceding topics, the role of spouse involves both identity and intimacy. The primary identity-related question here refers to whether people choose to define themselves in terms of a relationship with a marital partner. Specific identity-related issues include:

1. Why does a person want to marry or not marry?
2. What does it mean to be a husband or wife?
3. Does one want to be partially defined by another through a marital relationship?
4. What does one want to offer a partner in the role of spouse?
5. What can one reasonably expect from one's partner in a marital relationship?
6. Under what circumstances should a marriage terminate in divorce?

Role of Parent

This domain involves concerns relevant to two of Erikson's stage components, identity and generativity. The core identity-related question here is whether an individual chooses to define himself or herself in terms of parenting activities and responsibilities. Specific identity-related issues include:

1. Why does a person want to be a parent, or why not?
2. What does one want to offer to a child in the role of parent?
3. How does one want to be a parent, that is, what parenting style is most personally expressive?
4. What can one reasonably expect to receive from one's child?

Priorities Assigned to Family and Career Goals

As a topic of identity concern, the subject of family and career priorities refers to the relative weight to be placed on family-related and vocational areas of life. (If this topic is not used, the identity questions listed here can be merged into the two preceding supplemental topics.) Specific identity-related issues include:

1. How should one divide one's time between career and family responsibilities?
2. When conflicts arise between career interests and one's role as spouse, in what way should such conflicts be resolved?
3. When conflicts arise between career interests and one's role as parent, in what way should such conflicts be resolved?

It is evident that an interview respondent will not necessarily show concern with all the identity-related issues listed under any one topic. In assessing an individual's identity status with regard to a specific domain, we must consider the number of issues raised, their subjective importance to the respondent, and their importance relative to the issues that were not a focus of concern.

Keep in mind too that there are no particular answers to the various identity issues that are, in themselves, indicative of a specific identity status. The identity statuses are defined in terms of process, not content, variables. What is needed to arrive at a decision on the assignment of a status is an understanding of how the individual went about handling the task of developing whatever content may be discussed in the interview. The criteria for analyzing the formation of identity elements are presented in the following section.

Operational Definitions of Exploration (Crisis) and Commitment

As described in Chapter 1, the four ego identity statuses are defined by their position along two conceptual dimensions: exploration (crisis) and commitment. These positions are shown in Figure 1.2 (Chapter 1).

To establish an appropriate degree of consistency among interviewers and scorers involved in identity research, it is essential to arrive at operational definitions for each dimension and therefore for the identity statuses themselves. These operational definitions must specify what to listen for in the statements of a respondent so as to identify where that respondent stands on each dimension. There are five such defining criteria for exploration and six for commitment.

Exploration (Crisis)

Exploration (crisis) refers to a period of struggling or active questioning in arriving at decisions about goals, values, and beliefs. The positions on the exploration dimension are: (1) past crisis, (2) in crisis, and (3) absence of crisis. To say that a person is past crisis means that there was a period of exploration when active consideration was given to a variety of potential identity elements, but that period is now over. The person may have successfully resolved the crisis and emerged with a firm sense of direction for the future, or the task may have been abandoned without reaching any meaningful conclusion. Being in crisis implies that one is currently trying to work through identity questions and is striving to make important life decisions. Absence of a crisis means that the individual has never found it necessary to explore competing identity alternatives about personal goals, values, or beliefs. The following are the defining criteria for exploration.

Knowledgeability

The respondent should exhibit awareness of the content and the implications of any alternative that has been or is being seriously considered. It should be evident that the person's knowledge extends beyond a casual or superficial familiarity, such as could be acquired from the mass media. Although it is important that the information conveyed be generally accurate, absolute accuracy is not required for considering the respondent to be knowledgeable. The offering of personal interpretations of material can be taken as added evidence that an alternative has been seriously considered.

Activity Directed Toward the Gathering of Information

An individual in an identity crisis, actively exploring alternatives, should be seeking to acquire information useful in resolving that crisis. Activities directed toward learning more about alternatives under consideration may include reading, taking courses, and discussions with friends, parents, teachers, or others knowledgeable about the material of interest. Although experimentation with several potential identity elements provides the strongest evidence of exploration, behavioral experimentation is not an essential feature of an identity crisis.

Evidence of Considering Alternative Potential Identity Elements

There are two distinct patterns from which the consideration of identity alternatives can be inferred. The first is the simultaneous presence of two or more distinct alternatives. This pattern involves a symbolic fork in the road for which each alternative can be clearly identified. The respondent is keenly aware of the various possibilities and can describe the advantages and disadvantages of each in considerable detail. The situation is one of a multiple approach-avoidance conflict, and there may be extensive wavering back and forth between the alternatives. The second pattern involves the existence of successive changes in goals, values, or beliefs over time. A person who has successively explored alternatives has a history of commitments to a number of choices, each of which has been rejected for some reason. Where the exploration of simultaneously available alternanatives represents a choice of A or B, the successive exploration of alternatives involves a branching program of the type: A or not A; if not A, then B or not B; and so on.

Emotional Tone

During the early stages of identity exploration there is often a feeling of exhilaration, anticipation, and curiosity. It is as if the whole world is open to investigation and one is eager to expand one's horizons by tasting new experiences and possibilities. Later, this feeling may give way to subjective discomfort. To find that exploration, per se, does not provide clear-cut answers can be disheartening. The knowledge that one's goals, values, and beliefs are still indefinite often produces feelings of anxiety, frustration, and/or a sense of urgency. Continued active consideration of alternatives may lead to a state of heightened ambivalence as the person tries to cope with a multiple approach-avoidance conflict situation. The intensity of these emotions will vary widely among individuals as a reflection of their temperaments. In some instances, an identity crisis may seemingly involve considering alternatives on a strictly intellectual level without notable emotional involvement.

A Desire to Make an Early Decision

Because of the subjective discomfort associated with an identity crisis, a respondent will usually want to resolve the indecision as early as realistically possible. An expressed willingness to live indefinitely with uncertainty suggests that the alternatives discussed are not really under active or serious consideration.

The distinction between present exploration (indicative of the Moratorium status) and past exploration (found for the Identity Achievement status and some individuals in the Identity Diffusion status) can usually be made on the basis of whether the respondent phrases the discussion in the present or the past tense. Problems in scoring will exist, however, when a person is just entering or exiting an identity crisis. Where exploration is just beginning, the extent of current activity to gather information may be considered the pivotal criterion. Where an identity crisis is partially but not full resolved, the scoring will depend to a large extent on whether the person believes that answers to the most important questions in the area have been formulated. Often the emotional tone of the interview, whether of increasing confidence or subjective discomfort, will be the determining sign on which to base a conclusion that the phase of exploration has largely passed or is still current. Where a person is on the margin between statuses in a section of the interview, moving from one status to another, the status not chosen as the primary scoring should be included in the scoring as a secondary element. Such secondary scores may contribute to arriving at a global or overall identity status scoring for an individual.

Commitment

Commitment involves making a relatively firm choice about identity elements and engaging in significant activity directed toward implementation of that choice. Commitments can be described as either present or absent. To say that commitments are present means that the individual's identity elements are serving as meaningful guides to action and that thought is not being given to making any major changes in those elements. The absence of commitment implies that the person's ideas are weakly held and that behavior is changeable. There is no strongly felt sense of direction. There may or may not be concern with forming personal commitments at the time. The following are the operational defining criteria for commitment.

Knowledgeability

As with the criteria for exploration, if a person has a genuine commitment to a goal, value, or belief, there should be evidence of reasonably detailed and accurate knowledge of its content and ramifications.

Activity Directed Toward Implementing the Chosen Identity Element

Where exploration entails information-gathering activity, the activity resulting from identity commitments is directed toward expression or realization of the identity choices that have been made. Such activities may involve preparation for future life roles consistent with one's identity elements or may represent their current implementation. A verbalized commitment in the absence of corresponding activity must be considered suspect. Although the extent of the activity indicative of commitment may vary widely among individuals, there should be a sense that the respondent's self-definition is guiding his or her life on a day-to-day or at least month-to-month basis.

Emotional Tone

The presence of identity commitments will usually be expressed in ways that reflect confidence, stability, and optimism about the future. Although there is often awareness of the difficulties that could arise in implementing an identity element, this does not lessen the determination to pursue the chosen course. In general, persons with identity commitments will show stress reactions appropriate to a situation, but do not become easily rattled or show emotional overreactions. In some instances, particularly of the Foreclosure status, commitments may be expressed in a rigid, formalized way suggesting intolerance for other possible values or beliefs. In contrast to the buoyancy of persons with a clear sense of identity, those who lack identity commitments and who are not trying to form them often show a marked lack of enthusiasm. Among the emotions that may characterize such interviews are pessimism, apathy, boredom, unfocused anger, alienation, anxiety, personal confusion, and/or feelings of helplessness and hopelessness. Occasionally a person without commitments may evidence a sense of omnipotentiality (i.e., the feeling that one can become anything one chooses to be) accompanied by a desire never to be permanently pinned down to a specific goal or course of action. This position entails a paradoxical commitment never to become committed.

Identification with Significant Others

In many instances identity commitments originate in identification with parents, other relatives, teachers, or persons learned of through school or the mass media. Such a process is most typical of the Foreclosure status and accounts for the formation of many early commitments, particularly those consistent with the parents' aspirations for their children. It sometimes happens that contrasting goals will be acquired early in life by identification, each goal associated with a different model figure. Except where an *intense* conflict is experienced over the alternatives, a scoring of Foreclosure generally continues to be appropriate. Persons in the Identity Achievement status may also develop their commitments through identification but in these instances the identification usually develops at a later age after a variety of other possible courses of action have been explored.

Projection of One's Personal Future

Identity commitments provide a mechanism for integrating the past with the present and the present with the future. This aspect of identity will be reflected in ability on the part of those with identity commitments to project themselves into the future and describe the type of activities in which they would like to be engaging five to ten years hence. This ability does not mean they expect that the content of identity elements will remain unchanged. Rather, a sense of continuity should be evident between where one is now and where one wishes to be in the future.

Resistance to Being Swayed

In the ego identity interview, questions may be asked to test the strength of an identity commitment by attempting to divert the respondent from the content being described (e.g., How willing would you be to change your plans if something better came along?). Where commitments are present, the respondent should be relatively resistant to deliberate or inadvertent attempts by the interviewer to induce contradictory statements.

As with the dimension of exploration, some individuals will be on a borderline, here between commitment and noncommitment. In these instances, whatever relevant status is not indicated as the primary scoring may be included under the heading of secondary elements.

Distinguishing Identity Crises from Emotional Crises

There is a need to distinguish between those life crises which do and do not have identity implications. Three types of crises can be identified.

1. Primary identity crises—those involving selection of core identity goals, values, and beliefs from among an array of alternatives or the serious and intensive reevaluation of identity elements previously established.
2. Secondary identity crises—those involving consideration of alternative paths toward the expression and implementation of particular identity elements but that do not themselves call into question core commitments.
3. Emotional crises—those which represent the person's emotional reaction to some stressful situation (e.g., loss of a job, death of a loved one).

Emotional crises may or may not give rise to questions in either of the other categories.

The principal concern for identity research is with crises in the first category. To score a respondent as having, or having had, a primary identity crisis requires consideration of distinctly different core goals, values, and beliefs. The person's life must be seen as potentially taking clearly divergent forms or directions depending on the outcome of the decision-making process. Usually the respondent is aware of these implications and it is this awareness that leads to the sense of urgency experienced over the crisis.

In contrast, secondary identity crises are limited to issues of implementation. They may arise from a personally motivated search for the best course of action to put into effect a particular identity element. Alternatively, such crises may result from the situational frustration of some previously chosen path. A secondary crisis is indicated when the response to that frustration is the search for the next best path to the original goal. It is also possible that finding a pathway blocked may initiate reevaluation of the underlying core identity element, in which case a primary identity crisis would be said to exist. On the scoring forms, the existence of a secondary crisis may be appropriately indicated under the heading of secondary elements.

Unlike primary and secondary identity crises, purely emotional crises should play no role in identity status scoring. These crises will be observed most frequently when there is strong family conflict, a personal loss, or when one is thwarted in efforts to reach a personally important objective. Although an emotional crisis may be triggered by circumstances related to a person's sense of identity, such a crisis does not in itself involve any consideration or reevaluation of identity-related goals, values, and beliefs, or of their implementation. Because an emotional crisis can give rise to either a primary or secondary identity crisis, it is necessary to listen carefully for evidence on whether or not an interview respondent is actually trying to define or redefine identity commitments.

Identity Across the Life Span

Erikson discusses the formation of a sense of personal identity as the pivotal issue in the psychological development of adolescents. Confronting and responding to identity issues may be thought to begin even before the high school years and does not stop with entrance into adulthood. It is readily apparent from a life-span perspective that the meaning of identity is very different for a person aged 15 than it is for someone aged 25, or for someone aged 45 (Waterman & Archer, 1990). In identity research, these differences appear both in the identity status interview itself and in the interpretation of the defining criteria for the identity statuses, exploration and commitment. It is therefore necessary to consider our definition of the identity statuses relative to the age of the individual under study.

It is because the identity interview and the defining criteria for the statuses vary over the life span that the succeeding chapters of this book cover three age groups: (1) early and middle adolescents (junior and senior high school students), (2) late adolescents (particularly college students), and (3) adults. The interviews and scoring criteria for each age group are discussed in depth in the respective chapters, but we will briefly describe here some of the age differences.

Differences among the age groups are immediately evident in the time it takes to complete an interview. A typical interview with a high school student covering four content areas will take approximately 20 to 30 minutes. The same four content areas given to a college student usually take 45 minutes to an hour. And with an adult respondent it usually takes one-and-one-half to two hours to cover the same ground. The increasing complexity of thinking and range of relevant experiences are principally responsible for the expanded length of the interview.

The age of the respondent also affects the time devoted to exploring the person's development as opposed to anticipations about the future. As would be expected, a far greater proportion of the interview with adolescents and youths is conducted in the future tense than with adults. Correspondingly, the past tense occupies more time in interviews with adults.

A third difference in the interview among the various age groups is the content of the questioning itself. The lead questions in any content area are essentially the same at each age level, but the follow-up or probe questions are not. The identity issues likely to be raised by adolescents, youths, and adults in response to lead questions are themselves age-related. As a consequence, interviewers must adapt their questioning to the concerns considered most salient by their respondents in the different age groups.

Not only does the age-appropriate content of identity crises and identity commitments vary with the stage of development, the operational definitions of the criteria themselves shift with age. The same statements made by a high school student and an adult could be interpreted quite differently as a function of their life histories and the social expectations held for each. A view that may seem relatively sophisticated when offered by the former could be considered naive if expressed by the latter.

Such shifts in the meaning of the criteria are most apparent for knowledgeability and activity. Within an age level, it is usually not difficult to distinguish persons who are relatively knowledgeable or active from those who are not. But we expect both greater knowledge and activity with increasing age. A statement pertinent to either criterion may be judged quite differently based on the age of the respondent. Age-related shifts also exist for other aspects of our operational definitions, including the desire to make an early decision, projecting one's personal future, and resistance to being swayed.

In adolescence a person first becomes self-consciously aware of the main identity question, "Who am I?" and of the vast array of answers that can be given to it. For any one aspect of identity, an adolescent is likely to have relatively limited knowledge about the content of possible alternatives, and perhaps limited access to information about alternatives. Similarly, the range of choices will be limited by restrictions imposed by parents, schools, and community groups, based in part on what is considered age-appropriate behavior. That some adolescents may try to circumvent these restrictions in the interest of experimentation in itself points to an aspect of the identity search specific to adolescence.

The social pressures placed on early and middle adolescents about identity issues are different from those exerted on individuals at later ages. Because in most instances these adolescents are residing with their parents, parental expectations have a particular salience in adolescent thinking. Adolescent rebellion, which may or may not involve identity questions, is frequently a reaction to the explicit, implicit, or imagined demands of parents. Other social pressures on adolescents are exerted by their peer group. The psychological importance that adolescents place on conforming to peer standards and on receiving peer support has ramifications for both the probability of an identity search and the content alternatives that may be considered.

Perhaps most significant for understanding the role of identity questions for the development of early and middle adolescents is the distance between their present age and the time when they will have to act on any decisions that they now make. Being aware of the myriad events that could thwart their plans or entice them from their choices, the commitments of these adolescents are more tentative than those of persons at later ages. Not that an adolescent cannot have commitments—rather, realism may dictate some modesty in their expression.

In comparison, individuals in late adolescence (youth), particularly those attending college, are at a time in the life span most suited to exploring identity concerns. In college a person is likely to be exposed to a very wide range of alternative career goals, belief systems, and lifestyles, both in classes and in the campus community. Experimentation with various possibilities is often actively encouraged. Social support for persons going through an identity crisis usually is readily available from faculty and from other students undergoing similar experiences. Further, the consequences of rejected identity alternatives generally do not extend beyond the college setting. In terms of the defining criteria for the identity statuses, higher standards for both knowledgeability and activity can more meaningfully be applied to late than to early or middle adolescents.

The patterns of social pressure are markedly different by the age of youth. Many, perhaps most, individuals have substantially reduced contact with their parents, thus lessening the influence of parental expectations on identity formation. Peer conformity pressures are also likely to be lessened at this time. On the other hand, the expectations and preferences of a steady dating partner and potential spouse may take on great importance for identity development.

The subjective experience of time often inspires in youths a sense of urgency to form identity commitments. The span of the college years is seen as quite limited and they feel a need to be prepared to meet the challenges of the "real" world upon leaving school. This perception contributes both to the seriousness of exploration of those alternatives considered and to the desire for certainty and stability regarding the choices made.

Adolescents and youths are concerned about whether chosen identity elements will live up to expectations, but adults are living with the consequences of their choices. This difference generates a scoring expectation for still higher levels of knowledgeability and activity. It also contributes a different emotional tone to the interview than is found at younger ages. Adults must come to terms with what they have discovered to be the negative as well as the positive aspects of their identity commitments. They may also feel wistful or curious about identity alternatives once considered but set aside. Where identity choices have not worked out well, adults may undergo an emotionally distressing mid-life crisis. We must determine to what extent such crises are primarily emotional, reflecting disillusionment, or if they are true identity crises involving efforts to make new, potentially more rewarding identity choices.

Because most adults have achieved relative emotional and financial independence, social expectations and pressures are less influential in structuring and maintaining a person's sense of identity. However, a factor unique to adulthood that may be given substantial weight during a mid-life crisis is the consequences that any changes in identity choices may have for one's spouse and children. Also, their expectations will have an influence. In some instances, these may work against change, but in others they may contribute to it.

The adult's time perspective will have a differential effect on identity status categorization. Because many of the formative events in an adult's identity development will have occurred many years prior to the interview, the resultant identity scoring will depend on the accuracy of memory for those events. What would seem greatly significant to an adolescent or youth going through an identity crisis, and therefore have been reported in an interview, may not seem so important from the perspective of the adult years, with the result that the information is not discussed. This change may occur most frequently for identity alternatives that were explored during an early identity crisis but were never subsequently acted upon. For this reason the rates at which adults are placed in the Identity Achievement status are very likely to be underestimates.

Age-related differences in the identity interview and shifting defining criteria for the identity statuses with various age groups pose a methodological problem for conducting and utilizing identity research. For studies in which only one age group is employed, the scope of the problem is limited. The same interview and scoring standards are being applied to all members of the research sample so that identity status groups within the sample can be meaningfully compared. Even though the results of research may be generalized to other groups of the same age level, the applicability of findings to other age groups may be questionable.

In developmental research, where several age groups are studied, the methodological problem is most acute. Cross-sectional studies across wide age spans become difficult to interpret. Differences in distribution of the identity statuses could reflect either true developmental trends or merely the use of shifting definitional criteria for the statuses at the different ages.

In longitudinal studies, the problem is similar. Shifting criteria may create changes in identity statuses when the content of the interviews does not change. Such a conclusion is appropriate so long as it is recognized that identity status is an age-relative construct. Also, shifting criteria may create some of the instances of anomalous changes from the Moratorium or Identity Achievement statuses into the Foreclosure status. Evidence of a crisis that was given great weight at an earlier age may appear less significant at a later age if the person did not act on the alternatives considered or on a resulting commitment but rather turned to an alternative strongly influenced by identification figures.

The strengths of the longitudinal technique, however, allow for overcoming many of the difficulties associated with shifting criteria. Because full data are available on each respondent at several times, careful listening to the tapes can help determine whether any apparent changes are a function of (1) actual ontogenetic development, (2) age-related shifts in the scoring criteria applied, or (3) interviewer errors. Most important, the question of what happens in the identity development of adolescents or youths 5 or 10 or 20 years later stands on its own merits provided uniform defining criteria for the statuses are applied *within* any wave of data collection.

Identity in Males and Females

As discussed in preceding chapters, when Marcia (1964) initially developed the identity interview, it was intended for male college students. Subsequent efforts to extend the research to female college students resulted in an interview including some new content areas in addition to those used with males. Since then it has generally been recommended that research with both sexes involve an interview that is structurally the same (see Chapter 4).

Even when every effort is made to employ the same interview with males and females, differences in the content of questions relating to crises and commitments are likely to appear within the domains. Given the different cultural expectations placed upon men and women in contemporary society, some identity contents are more likely to be chosen by men and others will be more frequently chosen by women. For example, there are sex-typical differences in vocational choices and in gender-role expression. Notice that these are differences in frequency, not kind, and an interviewer must remain flexible, not assuming sex-typical divisions of identity contents.

Differences are found in the actual interviewing done with males and females, but none exist in the defining criteria for the identity statuses. Exploration and commitment have the same meaning for both sexes. Thus, the methodological problem in comparisons of different age groups does not apply to comparisons of males and females.

Approaches to Data Analysis

The information obtained in an ego identity interview can be coded to yield category and/or continuous measures. The type of scoring procedure chosen will be a function of the hypotheses under study and the investigator's preferences.

Category (Nominal) Measures

The ego identity statuses as formulated by Marcia constitute a nominal typology. Each status is uniquely defined by the combination of placements on the dimensions of exploration and commitment. There is no way in which the four statuses can be ordered into a meaningful sequence representing an "increasing" sense of identity. A clearly articulated self-definition is found equally among individuals in the Foreclosure and Identity Achievement statuses. Only the processes by which the identity elements are established are different.

It may also be misleading to consider the identity statuses as falling into a natural developmental sequence. An individual may enter adolescence in either the Identity Diffusion or Foreclosure status, thus making it difficult to assign a developmental priority between these statuses. Further, as is evident from the developmental model in Chapter 3, movement among the statuses can and does proceed in either direction among almost all pairs of statuses; the only exceptions involve movement from the Moratorium and the Identity Achievement statuses into the Foreclosure status.

An important decision that must be made in applying the category approach is whether the global or overall identity status for the individual is of interest, and if separate identity status scores for each domain are important. In the early identity studies, only global status scores were reported, but in more recent research either global or domain identity status scores or both have been used.

Five guidelines can be used in arriving at an overall identity status judgment for an individual summarizing all the information presented in the interview.

1. Weighting should be given to whatever identity status the respondent shows in that area of the interview which he or she considers most personally important.
2. Weighting should be given to the clearest, or most easily recognized, status shown by an individual in any domain.
3. Weighting should be given to the Moratorium or Identity Achievement statuses if shown in any domain because these constitute evidence that the person is capable of exploring alternatives and is seeking to establish an identity different from early identifications.

4. Weighting should be given to the identity status observed to be used for the largest number of domains in the interview (including both primary scores and secondary elements).
5. Weighting should be given to the intuitive impressions of the scorer, for inevitably identity status scoring is a clinical judgment task.

The final determination of a global identity status score should reflect a combination of all the guidelines listed above.

The principal advantage of the global score is that an individual's standing with respect to identity is neatly summarized with one descriptive label. As with any global typology, this approach results in a loss of any information inconsistent with the dominant or central tendency generating that person's category label. In identity research, such inconsistent information includes the identity statuses in specific domains that differ from the overall score.

A focus on separate identity status judgments for each domain of the interview preserves more information and allows for establishing an identity status profile. As discussed in the next section, separate content-area scores can be used to generate continuous, frequency measures of the identity statuses.

The nature of category data severely limits the number of statistical procedures that can be employed. Most commonly, global identity status scores have been used as the independent variable in analysis of variance designs. Such a procedure allows for comparisons among the identity statuses for psychological and behavioral correlates. The descriptive portraits from such research have been used to evaluate our theoretical understanding of the identity construct and to establish the discriminant validity of the identity status interview. Although content-area identity status scorings can similarly be used as an independent variable in research designs, this has seldom been done. It entails conducting several analyses (one for each interview domain), thus increasing the likelihood of generating significant results by chance. More important, there generally has been no reason to assume that identity status in one content area should be related to a dependent variable more than identity in another content area. Where differential hypotheses can be generated, however, the use of separate identity status scores clearly is appropriate.

Schenkel and Marcia (1972) used domain status scores to determine whether adding a new domain to the interview enhanced the utility of the interview by allowing greater discrimination between the statuses on the dependent variables. With the tendency for content domains to proliferate, thus lengthening the interview, this procedure appears particularly useful in deciding whether the benefits from adding a new topic are worth the costs in added research time.

A second approach to statistical analysis with identity status category data involves the use of nonparametric statistics. The nonparametric procedures employed will depend upon the hypotheses under investigation. Also dependent on the research hypotheses will be the choice of whether to use global identity status scores or identity status judgments separately by content area. Again, a global score is indicated when the objective is to make comparisons among individuals in the various identity statuses. However, in research comparing males and females on the distribution of the identity statuses, employing identity status scores separately for each content area will yield far more useful information (see Chapter 3). The same applies to comparisons between any sets of groups differing in background characteristics. In developmental research involving a longitudinal design, it is possible to identify the domains in which change is occurring by using separate domain scores in the McNemar test for the significance of changes (Siegel, 1956).

Finally, some researchers, notably Josselson (1973) and Donovan (1975), have used global identity status scores in generating detailed clinical portraits of persons in the various statuses. In neither of these instances were statistical analyses employed.

Continuous Measures

Because of the relatively limited power of nonparametric statistics, there have been several attempts to generate scales for the identity statuses with at least ordinal properties. Unfortunately, this task has proven to be difficult. The simplest procedure is to assign numbers to the statuses on some hypothetical basis such as level of developmental sophistication. For example, Identity Diffusion could equal 1, Foreclosure 2, Moratorium 3, and Identity Achievement 4. Such an approach is *not* appropriate, however, because the underlying conceptual ordering is not meaningful. A Foreclosure is not something more than a Diffusion in the same way as a Moratorium is more than a Foreclosure. These are differences in kind, not degree. The meaning of a mean score for an individual would of necessity be ambiguous. For example, a mean score of 2 could be obtained either by being Foreclosed in all the areas covered in the interview or by being in the Identity Diffusion status in half the areas and in the Moratorium status in the other half. Similarly, comparisons between groups using such a scale could not be meaningfully interpreted. Each status is different from every other status in nonmetric ways; that is, they are nominal categories.

Two approaches involving continuous measures have, however, been demonstrated to be useful, although each has its drawbacks. The first involves generating separate continuous measures on the dimensions of exploration and commitment. The other involves obtaining frequency measures for each of the identity statuses across the content domains covered in the interview.

Matteson (1974) was the first researcher to have judges generate scores on the *degree* to which a respondent had explored alternative potential identity elements and the *degree* of strength with which commitments were held. Each dimension was scored on a four-point scale, in this form:

Exploration (Crisis)	Commitment
1 = limited	1 = limited
2 = some	2 = some
3 = considerable	3 = considerable
4 = very strong	4 = very strong

These continuous-scale ratings are ordinal and can be used in correlational research or as the dependent variable in t-test and analysis of variance designs, or in other designs using parametric statistics. Their use permits determination of whether exploration and/or commitment are differentially related to other variables being studied. The principal drawback in this approach is that the uniqueness of the identity statuses is lost in arriving at the scores on the exploration and commitment decisions. Both Identity Achievers and Moratoriums will gain high scores on exploration. Both Identity Achievers and Foreclosures will have high scores on commitment. But inferences on the identity statuses can often be made by carefully analyzing and interpreting the patterns of results obtained on the two dimensions.

The procedure for obtaining frequency scores for the various identity statuses was developed by Waterman (Waterman, Kohutis, & Pulone, 1977). With an interview covering four content areas, an individual's frequency scores for each status can range from 0 to 4, depending on the number of domains in which the person is in each status. For example, if someone is an Identity Achiever in vocational plans, a Foreclosure on religious beliefs and gender-role attitudes, and Diffuse on political ideology, that person would receive a score of 1 on Identity Achievement, 0 for the Moratorium status, 2 for the Foreclosure category, and 1 for Identity Diffusion. The advantage of this procedure is that each status scale has interval properties and permits use of parametric statistics. The identity statuses can thus be treated as the dependent variable in analysis of variance designs. However, the four status scales are not statistically independent. If one is frequently in one status, the scores for the other statuses are automatically low. Also, this frequency score procedure treats all content areas as if they are equally important to a person's self-definition, a circumstance that will not often apply. It may be possible to adapt this procedure so as to give greater weight to the more significant content areas, as is done in arriving at a global category judgment for identity, but this adjustment has not been tried.

Choosing a Scoring Technique

The most important determinant in selecting a procedure for scoring ego identity interviews is the nature of the hypotheses to be tested. These guidelines can be useful:

1. For testing hypotheses about differences between persons in the various identity statuses, the clearest presentation of results is afforded by using global identity status category judgments. The identity status groups can be used as an independent variable in analysis of variance designs, with comparisons between specific pairs of statuses tested in a series of post hoc comparisons. (Example: assessing differences between the identity statuses in anxiety or authoritarianism.)
2. For testing hypotheses about differences between two or more existing populations in the frequency of the identity statuses, scoring for identity status in each of the domains covered in the interview seems most appropriate. This technique would allow for using either analyses separately by domain or for t-test or analysis of variance comparisons of the frequency scores present in the various statuses. Alternatively, ratings for the dimensions of exploration and commitment may be obtained for each domain and the data analyzed with either t-tests or analyses of variance. (Example: comparing males and females in the probability of presence in the various identity statuses.)
3. For testing hypotheses about developmental changes in identity or for assessing the effect of some intervention program on identity, scoring for exploration and commitment and/or for identity status separately by domain would be indicated. This approach allows for identifying the nature of the changes occurring. If identity status category judgments are used, then the McNemar test for the significance of changes can be employed. If a continuous measure is utilized, then either a repeated measures t-test or analysis of variance can be conducted.

Scoring for the various category and continuous measures are not mutually exclusive. It therefore seems appropriate for the interview scorers to make all the necessary judgments and ratings.

The Scoring Manuals

The issues of scoring and methodology discussed in this chapter should be kept in mind when reading the sample scoring manuals for the different age groups. Chapter 8 gives material for early and middle adolescents, specifically junior and senior high school students. The material for late adolescents, particularly college students, is presented in Chapter 9. Chapter 10 gives the sample scoring material for adults. In these chapters only three domains are discussed in detail: (1) vocational choice, (2) religious beliefs, and (3) family-career priorities. Sample interview schedules covering seven domains for each age group are presented in the Appendix.

8
Identity Status in Early and Middle Adolescents: Scoring Criteria

SALLY L. ARCHER

Adolescence is the stage in the life span that Erikson designated the first in which the task of identity formation becomes salient. It is during adolescence that individuals first question the values, goals, and beliefs of their "significant others." Having traversed the earlier psychosocial stages of development with more or less success, adolescents enter this fifth phase of life, more or less (1) cognizant of personal strengths and weaknesses, (2) eager to initiate a search for purpose and direction, (3) in the context of and yet separate from people who are important in their lives, and (4) confident in themselves and others that they can effectively resolve the tasks in this final stage of preparation for adulthood.

Because identity formation is a complex task that is gradually resolved, it is useful to separate adolescence into several phases to document the development and refinement of self-definition. The first two phases, early and middle adolescence, are addressed in this chapter; late adolescence is the focus in Chapter 9.

In this chapter, "adolescents" refers to individuals between ages 12 and 18. Reference to early adolescents typically means respondents between sixth and ninth grade (the middle-school years), approximately 12 to 15 years of age, whereas "middle adolescents" pertains to individuals between tenth and twelfth grade (the high school years), about 16 to 18 years of age. Some researchers will find it more appropriate to define their sample by age; others, by grade. Sometimes it is more meaningful to categorize by age because one is granted particular privileges at that time, such as a driver's license; at other times grade level signifies more, such as graduation from junior or senior high school.

One should realize that 12-year olds respond to the interview simplistically relative to 18-year-olds. Also, within a given age group substantial differences in approach to identity activity also can be found. Adolescents may be in different identity statuses in different domains at the same time. Individuals may be strongly invested in some domains while they are exploring alternatives in others. At the same time they may choose to disregard still other potentially self-defining domains. (See Chapter 7 for an elaboration of this point.) Explanations for scoring adolescents' identity interviews will include early and midadolescent examples from several domains, or content areas, to demonstrate the variability one should expect to encounter.

In the next section of this chapter the processes of identity formation, comprising of the dimensions of exploration and commitment, are examined as implemented by early and middle adolescents. Five criteria of exploration and six criteria of commitment provide the foundation for scoring for the identity statuses.

The Meaning of Exploration and Commitment in Early and Middle Adolescence

Exploration

Exploration (crisis) pertains to the examination of alternatives with the intention of establishing a firm commitment in the near future. It is documented at one of three possible times: (1) the present, (2) the past, whether it led to a commitment or not, and (3) never. The criteria that are used to judge whether exploration has occurred in enough depth to warrant this scoring are: (1) knowledgeability, (2) activity directed toward gathering information, (3) considering alternative potential identity elements, (4) emotional tone, and (5) desire to make an early decision.

Knowledgeability

The amount of information one is accumulating and understanding about potential alternatives is called knowledgeability. Given this age group's limited experience and cognitive sophistication, accuracy may be less than one would like. Personal interpretation may be weighed heavily because it is fairly characteristic that adolescents color their understanding with personal, concrete experiences; thus, simplification or distortion may result.

For example, a sixth-grader may be trying to choose between family and career priorities. Their knowledge may amount to feeling that babies are cute but lots of work and mothers should be home for them until they go to school. About career, the adolescent may want to be a teacher, because teachers have summers and holidays off and don't work such long hours. Furthermore, one can always get one's job back as a teacher. But one's sister is a mother of a two-year-old and is a teacher. If she can do it, will this sixth-grader be able to do it when she grows up? By contrast, the high school senior might be able to address such complex issues as the woman's biological clock, education, securing a job, and economic security. By the same token, the college senior may have learned about tenure and politics affecting careers, further complicating the parenting issue.

Activity Directed Toward Gathering Information

Adolescents must demonstrate sufficient activity to allow them to gather information that will provide the knowledge necessary to ultimately arrive at a decision between viable alternatives. Again, early adolescents are often limited in their opportunities for exploration, whereas midadolescents may engage in part-time jobs, apprenticeships, travel, or interaction with a widening circle of potential models, living a variety of life-styles.

When experimentation is minimal or the primary models to observe and talk with are limited to parents, siblings, neighbors, and teachers, one may be less able to venture into avenues that could be more personally expressive if only they could ever be encountered. The media, especially books and television, may provide sufficient exposure to alternatives to trigger further activity, allowing one to become more knowledgeable about options that cannot be experienced directly. Identity activity may include personal introspection; observing others; talking with a variety of sources such as parents, siblings, friends, teachers, and clergy; reading; watching television; working in relevant jobs; and pursuing related hobbies.

For example, an early adolescent pressured into dealing with the sex-role issue of being a tomboy may challenge her parents, talk to her friends, and look at *Seventeen* magazine, whereas midadolescents contemplating femininity may prefer personal introspection, talking to a revered teacher, or watching soap-opera stars enact feminine roles.

Considering Alternative Potential Identity Elements

Adolescents, lacking cognitive sophistication, may have difficulty weighing the advantages and disadvantages of several identity pathways. However, this is a necessary criterion for exploration. Younger adolescents may provide fewer contrasts with less depth but the process must be the same.

When several alternatives are considered at the same time, one is using a simultaneous pattern in considering alternatives. Early adolescents, who may be seriously engaging in identity activity for the first time, are likely to use this pattern. Older adolescents may have examined alternatives several times over and may now be engaging in a sequential pattern. At one time, an alternative was chosen; later, another option arose that contrasted with the previous consideration. The old choice is subsequently discarded for a more personally expressive option.

Some adolescents will explain that they are committed to one alternative and yet identify another as a backup. If the first option has always been accepted as the preference, the second is not considered an alternative. Exploration is therefore not credited based on these two options because they are not "alternatives" being considered as potential identity elements.

For example, a tenth-grader may have decided to be a professional baseball player when in seventh grade. By the ninth grade, he discarded this possibility and decided he would make an excellent computer programmer. In tenth grade, he continues to maintain this plan but also states that he could always take over his father's insurance agency if computer programming didn't work out. The baseball-player and computer-programmer considerations are an example of the sequential pattern; taking over his dad's insurance agency is an example of a practical backup (not self-defining, at least at this time) should his present choice not work out.

Emotional Tone

Emotional tone may or may not be a strong cue of exploration for adolescents, in part because some of their exploration does not require a decision or implementation in the near future. Therefore, the "test" of implementing one's choice may be postponed for some time, decreasing the potential for excitement or anxiety.

Early exploration is often characterized by an open, excited, curious tone of voice, although we must remember that some individuals are inclined to intellectual, rational decision making. As exploration continues, older adolescents are especially likely to express subjective discomfort about potential choices as they become increasingly pressured by significant others, such as parents or teachers, to conform to their aspirations for the adolescent. Also, older adolescents may sound "leisurely" as they slowly learn how to sort through the advantages and disadvantages of options.

For example, respondents who are feeling the pressure of decision making may all but wail, "I don't know what to do," "If only," "Suppose that won't work," and "Why is this so hard?" "Don't rush me, I'm thinking about it." Rational decision makers may say, "I've made a list of the pros and cons." Younger adolescents may sound like this, "I think I like this idea better but that sounds pretty good too, hmmm."

Desire to Make an Early Decision

This is the one criterion that younger adolescents will often not volunteer for some domains, particularly those in which the choice cannot be implemented with any rigor in the near future. Most respondents, it is assumed, will want to make a decision as soon as possible in order to act in a personally expressive and consistent manner. The state of indecision should therefore result in discomfort for them. One must remember, however, that adolescents may not be able to enact a choice for a substantial period. Knowing this, they may feel it appropriate to allow an open-ended feeling to their preferences, which adults keep informing them will change anyway.

When adolescents are asked when they plan to resolve their dilemma, they may say, "Soon would be nice." But speed is not necessary, and as adults suggest, not advantageous. There may be a "tentative" quality to the adolescent's approach to making a decision. An important indication of an adolescent's exploration is the use of the present tense when discussing activity and persistence in discussing the issue.

For example, choosing a college major or career may be very different for a 13-year-old in junior high school than for a 17-year-old applying to colleges. Yet choosing to become a member of a religious organization may be implemented immediately by a 12-year-old or a 17-year-old, depending, of course, upon the religion. As a result, in this second case, their desire to make an early decision may be comparable.

In summary, for adolescents, exploration must be examined in terms of the limited personal and social-environmental contexts in which alternatives can be experienced. It is most often characterized by (1) their ability to enumerate alternatives from which they plan to make a choice, (2) their generation of advantages and disadvantages for each choice, (3) their investment in activity to procure this knowledge, and (4) their continued effort, because this is an important area of their life.

Commitment

Commitment refers to a stable investment in one's goals, values, and beliefs evidenced in supportive activity. The criteria that are used to determine whether a commitment is held firmly enough to represent an investment of one's identity in a domain are: (1) knowledgeability, (2) activity directed toward implementing the chosen identity element, (3) emotional tone, (4) identification with significant others, (5) projection into one's personal future, and (6) resistance to being swayed. Each will be elaborated in terms of expectations for the adolescent age span.

Knowledgeability

Again, knowledgeability refers to the amount of information accrued and understood about the chosen commitment. It might be acquired from family members, peers, teachers, the media, and personal experiences. Again, taking into account this age group's lack of experience and cognitive sophistication, information may be limited, simplistic, inaccurate, or distorted by personal interpretation.

For example, sixth-graders may select a science career and not realize the amount of education required or the specific skills needed for job performance. They may choose to be veterinarians because they love animals, but their emphasis may not include the medical aspects of the profession. With older adolescents, one should expect a more sophisticated and detailed understanding of the aspects of a career choice. In the example cited, one would need to hear an older adolescent weigh likes and dislikes for animals, science courses, and expectations to perform medical feats. Yet the high school senior's comprehension of an area will be influenced by fantasies and expectations and should be less realistic than that of a college student taking courses in the area of study, or the high school graduate directly employed in the relevant area.

Adolescents already participating in a field in which they have made a commitment obviously demonstrate greater knowledge than do those not yet able to become active. This difference is easily understood in the vocational area, where the adolescent may be awaiting college or employment. It can apply to other areas as well. Individuals choosing a "liberated" gender role, marriage, or parenting will not truly have the opportunity to understand the implications of their choices until implementation in the adult world is made possible.

Activity Directed Toward Implementing the Chosen Identity Element

Adolescents invested in an area must demonstrate some activity supportive of their personal commitment. Acceptable activity may include talking with people knowledgeable in the chosen area, reading, visiting relevant places, becoming friends with people of similar orientations, practicing, obtaining summer or part-time employment appropriate to this choice, or pursuing a relevant hobby. In many instances, adolescent behavior will represent preparation for a role. For example, babysitting can enhance knowledgeability about parenthood, day-care, or childhood education careers, just as becoming a member of a political youth organization teaches one about appropriate behaviors in which one might eventually engage as a politician or an informed voter. In other instances, adolescent activity may be demonstrated by actual day-to-day involvement. As a new church member, the adolescent may read religious writings, such as the Koran or the Bible daily, pray, attend services, and talk about religious issues with religious friends.

Emotional Tone

The emotional tone of the committed adolescent is usually quite different from that of the individual who is engaged in exploration or is uninvested. Usually, there is a calm, secure, stable, satisfied firmness to the voice and manner of the respondent.

Exceptions include the following. Those who are pleased with their choices but anxious about their ability to implement them, will, of course, not fit the calm and stable description. Adolescents whose parents or others have instilled in them fear that choices are not tentative but permanent may also sound anxious. Last, individuals whose decisions were difficult, perhaps causing conflict with others important in their lives, or who felt that one choice meant, perhaps naively, never experiencing something else very important to them, may sound tense, sad, or wistful when describing their plans or activities.

For example, a female who has chosen to be a feminist may feel like an outcast among her traditional family and may fear that her career orientation may mean that she will never be able to have a family life of her own. On the one hand, she is challenged and enthusiastic about her career plans; on the other, she is wistful about her old secure family ties and hesitant about the implications of her career choice for her long-range future.

The emotional tone of uncommitted individuals who are not exploring alternatives may sound quite different. They are often apathetic, flat in voice tone, and lethargic in energy. Some are alienated from investment in a given domain and voice their anger. Others are avoiding commitment, or marginally interested, and convey an easygoing, engaging manner that belies the potential importance of the domain.

For example, an adolescent who chooses to remain single may generate flippant remarks about playing around, being unattached, and looking over the field, instead of projecting into the future and introspecting about their own personality and goals that would make being single the more appropriate choice. Thus, the emotional tone can distinguish the committed from the uncommitted, as well as the exploring from the non-exploring, uncommitted adolescent.

Identification with Significant Others

Models are important sources of information for adolescents, providing alternatives through direct imitation or contrast. This criterion often characterizes Foreclosures who establish commitment without considering alternatives. One typically finds that a model influenced these adolescents to follow a pathway. Among this age group, parents are the most common models, although teachers, media personalities, peers, siblings, clergy, and so on may also serve this purpose.

Identity Achievers may also identify models who have strongly influenced their choice of commitment. The difference is that Identity Achievers often extract aspects of different models, that they then combine in new and unique ways to be useful to their individual development.

For example, a 15-year-old Foreclosure, discussing his liberal democratic leanings, acknowledges that his father is also a liberal democrat and that they probably think a lot alike. A 15-year-old Identity Achiever, discussing his liberal democratic leanings, may mention several teachers, a parent, and a political figure who influenced his choice to be a liberal democrat rather than a conservative republican. He may have agreed with some models' positions, developed a contrasting perspective with others, and been impressed by still others' dedication to particular issues.

Projection into One's Personal Future

Midadolescents are able to tentatively project their plans into the future in broad and simplistic sketches as far as the mid to late twenties. Early adolescents are vague, providing some ideas up to the point of high school or college graduation. As long as there is a sense that their plans mesh with other aspects of their future life as they envision it, and they are concerned about the important implications of this decision for the future, then the adolescents are given credit for this criterion for commitment.

For example, a 17-year-old male explains that he plans to go to college, get a job, get married about four years after graduation to establish economic stability, and also play around until it's out of his system. Maybe he will have a family when he's in his mid-30s or 40. It has to be done in that order at about that pace or he won't be able to handle it.

Resistance to Being Swayed

When adolescents have a lot of time before their choices can be implemented, they may sound less resistant to being swayed than one might expect. Flexibility is expressed, conveying the realization that a lot could happen between now and then. The key to giving credit to this criterion, however, is the adolescent's inability or unwillingness to generate an alternative that is thought to be better. Some adolescents will suggest ideas about other directions that could be taken, but when pressed further about the likelihood of change, say it's not likely.

The Foreclosure often sounds more resistant to being swayed than the Identity Achiever. This reluctance may appear because Achievers have considered alternatives and may be more cognizant of other possibilities. Thus, they can convey the impression of being more open and flexible about change. But again, for this criterion, though they recognize the feasibility of other alternatives, they resist being swayed from their choice if they are genuinely committed.

For example, a 13-year-old girl may indicate that she plans to be a nurse. When asked if she would change her mind if something better came along, she said she could become a dancer. How likely is it that she will switch from nurse to dancer? Not likely.

In summary, for adolescents, commitment is most often characterized by their ability to (1) clearly state a choice, (2) discuss its advantages and disadvantages, (3) describe activities they engage in to support this commitment, (4) resist change, and (5) project into the near future this choice's implications for the next decade or so of their life. Foreclosures and Identity Achievers may be comparable in the strength of their commitment. The distinguishing factor between these two statuses is whether exploration of alternatives has taken place. If alternatives have been assessed, the individual will be Identity Achieved; if not, Foreclosed.

Scoring Complications for Early and Middle Adolescence

Separating Identity Crises from Emotional Crises

Adolescence is often described as the time in one's life span in which normative crises are numerous. When being interviewed in any domain, emotional crises pertaining to independence from parents, idealistic romances shattering, pressures for sexual activity, and such other moral dilemmas as drugs, stealing, and lying may appear. The scorer must separate such emotional crises from identity crises. Only where emotional crises lead to identity crises should they become a factor in scoring for identity status.

A 16-year-old rejects any plans to marry because his parents divorced with lots of anger and hatred. Because he cannot discuss the pros and cons of marriage for himself, his rejection could not constitute an identity commitment not to marry. Rather, it is seen as an emotional crisis, resulting in alienation, hence Diffusion.

Separating Identity Crises from Changes for Personal Gain

A second scoring difficulty pertains to adolescents discarding their values, beliefs, or goals for personal gain or convenience. For example, an adolescent reared as a strict Catholic may encounter frustration because the Pope opposes abortion and the use of many forms of contraceptives. She or he chooses to replace Catholicism with a personal religion. This negation of Catholicism results from personal inconvenience, not a religious identity issue. Only if she or he subsequently discovers and describes how a personal religion is more satisfying than an organized religion in terms of personal religious needs might this be scored as an identity change in the domain of religious beliefs.

Identity in Males and Females

Contrary to popular opinion, males and females follow similar pathways to their identity development (Archer, 1989b). Each sex is as likely to use any of the four identity processes in most domains. To date for early and middle adolescents, the only domains in which the sexes have been discriminated have been family and career priorities (Archer 1985a) and friendships (Grotevant, Thorbecke, & Meyer, 1982). In each case females demonstrated significantly greater sophistication in their decision making. Sexuality is the other domain in which significant sex differences have appeared (Waterman & Nevid, 1977). This domain has not yet been used with early or middle adolescents.

Most sex differences pertain to the specific issues or content addressed within the domains. For example, males are often more concerned with status or monetary gain to be had in their career, whereas females are more likely to express a desire to engage in a career that is personally stimulating and helpful to others. Moreover, males more frequently challenge religion from a scientific slant, females from concern for compatibility of religious beliefs with life experiences of self or family members.

The other noticeable difference between the sexes is the complexity of elements that the older female adolescents bring into play when making their decisions compared to that of males (Archer, 1985a, 1992). For example, career decisions for females not only include likes, dislikes, abilities, and perhaps status, but also how the career fits into other demands of life such as spouse, children, and her biological clock. Males do not tend to introduce relationships with others into their decision making. Also, the number of elements taken into account by males tends to be fewer and less complex. Therefore identity formation should be less difficult for the adolescent male.

The Identity Status Domains

In early and middle adolescence many individuals will be scored Identity Diffuse or Foreclosed regardless of domain. During these years, however, initial curiosity may arise, as well as dissatisfaction with identifications made during childhood. Within an age, too, there is substantial variation in adolescents' way of approaching the process of identity formation. Examining the manner in which the criteria are expressed may provide valuable predictors for later successful resolutions of potential identity crises, or their lack.

Vocational Choice

For adolescents, the broadest basic question leading to vocational choice is whether to pursue employment, and/or marriage and/or family, and/or additional education subsequent to high school graduation. For scoring purposes, establishing one's vocational identity requires selecting a specific form of these options. If one plans immediate employment, the form of work should be specified, such as secretary; if marriage, the style to be enacted, such as conventional or dual family and career; if college, majors considered, such as physics or music. The more immediate choice of high school curriculum track is in part influenced by this expectation.

The degree to which the earlier Eriksonian industry versus inferiority stage was successfully resolved should influence adolescents' approach to vocational choice. During this earlier stage, particularly through the educational process, work skills are acquired and constantly assessed. Developing awareness of one's strengths and weaknesses, likes and dislikes, should have enhanced the adolescents' ability to narrow career choices. A plethora of career options may arise from parental preferences, suggestions from teachers or counselors, and exposure to the media. The opportunity to select from among many such alternatives appears advantageous except for adolescents unable to recognize and assess their skills accurately. Such individuals would find it difficult to categorize options in a personally meaningful way and hence may be unable to limit choices to a workable number. Consequently, they may withdraw from or avoid the task.

Older adolescents should have advantages for generating more realistic assessments of career options. They are more likely to have sophisticated cognitive skills and increased opportunities for exposure to various vocations through summer employment, part-time jobs, and interactions with individuals involved in careers of potential interest.

In some instances, vocational decision making may be hindered by limited exposure to career alternatives. Some parents may attempt to prevent exploration in the hope that their adolescent will pursue the parent's preference. The cross-fertilization of ideas that can often grow from peer clique sharings may be lost for individuals who choose or are forced into isolation. Some school systems may not provide adequate career counseling or work programs. Media alternatives may appear more fictional than realistic.

Societal and individual flexibility should enhance participation in the task of vocational exploration. For example, if important societal members convey the message that early commitments are permanent and unalterable, rather than tentative, fear of a lifelong mistaken career choice could render some individuals unable to cope with this pursuit. Furthermore, the attitudes of significant others about the job market and the feasibility of advancement may also color the adolescents' motivation for investing identity energies in the vocational area.

Identity Diffusion

The typical vocational Identity Diffusion expresses lack of commitment to any career. Little or no urgency is felt about a time by which one might make such decisions; thus, activity directed to that end is minimal. For some adolescents, no careers have yet been considered. For others, especially older adolescents, barriers may have been encountered, blocking access to their choice. Barriers might include failure in relevant school subjects, nonacceptance into colleges, and physical limitations or societal discouragement. Rather than pursue simpler lines of work in a similar career or explore entirely different fields, the Diffusion withdraws from career exploration altogether, at least temporarily. Adolescents not pursuing previously desired careers may now demonstrate knowledge, but lack enthusiasm and hope.

Example

(Female, 18) Delores had planned to be a nurse since she was 6 years old. She had applied to nursing programs, although her science grades were only average. She was not accepted into any schools. She felt keenly disappointed and dismayed. When asked about her vocational plans, she expressed bewilderment. She had no ideas about what she might do. She had never considered anything but nursing. She would probably take any job she could find for the next year. Right now, she hurt too much and was embarrassed about her inability to follow through with her plans.

Comment

Delores was initially Foreclosed. She had expressed a lasting commitment supported by activity in the form of appropriate high school course work and applications to nursing programs. Her bewilderment about the school rejections revealed her limited knowledge about academic standards as well as her own inaccurate assessment of skills necessary for entrance into the program. Her emotional tone shifted from confidence to dismay and hopelessness. If she had rallied by seeking a similar career, such as lab technician, she would have continued as a Foreclosure. Perhaps due to her limited knowledge about the medical fields and/or her emotional state, she did not select that route, nor did she then begin to consider entirely different career avenues, in which case she would have become a Moratorium. Rather, she temporarily withdrew from identity activity, and so became Identity Diffuse.

Foreclosure

The adolescent Foreclosure expresses a genuine commitment to one vocation without ever having seriously considered other possible vocational directions. This selection is often made at an early age, as during elementary or junior high school. The individual will usually reinforce this choice by exposure to relevant books and television programs, along with fantasy play and oral assertions. Their emotional tone is one of assurance as they discuss their anticipated implementation of this vocational plan. Because they tend to restrict their activities and knowledge to this chosen field from an early age, these adolescents are labeled prematurely committed. Through their own lack of exploration they miss opportunities to explore potentially more personally expressive vocations. In most instances, a significant model figure is identifiable, such as parent, teacher, or media personality.

Example

(Male, 12) Fred plans to be a baseball star. He has participated in Little League. He describes his baseball skills as the best on the team. His father participates in a local softball league. When questioned about the likelihood of becoming a professional ball player, he acknowledges that it may not be possible, although somebody has to make it to the big leagues. His second choice, however, is to become an accountant and take over his father's accounting business. He indicates that math is his best subject in school, and so he'll probably be a pretty good accountant.

Comment

Although Fred identifies two distinct vocational possibilities, he prefers the first, and the second serves only as a backup. Furthermore, both career choices have Foreclosure routes, with his father as the model for each of them. This exceptionally articulate sixth-grader has knowledge about baseball as a direct result of his participation in the game. About each vocational option, he assesses his skills and concludes that these are appropriate choices for him. His emotional tone is confident as he projects into the future about his vocational alternatives: A; if not A, then B.

On rare occasions, an individual with two vocational choices, each with identifiable Foreclosure routes, may be scored a Moratorium or Identity Achiever. Such scoring requires evidence of very serious, anxiety-provoking, and involved self-evaluation about the appropriateness of one choice over another. If the decision is difficult due to the need for approval from each Foreclosure route, then the individual still would be scored Foreclosed.

Moratorium

Moratoriums are simultaneously or sequentially selecting from among several career alternatives. At present, a commitment is absent, but one is anticipated in the near future. The individual is weighing the advantages and disadvantages of several vocations simultaneously. With sequential considerations, the adolescents have seriously considered one career option only to discover that it didn't seem right. Subsequently, they have attempted others. For each pattern of decision making, the knowledge and activity should be comparable. The adolescents should be able to assess their skills in the context of the needs of the job. It must be realized that adolescents who have not had direct exposure to vocations idealize or express a naive understanding of vocational requirements. For this age group personal impressions, unless grossly in error, are considered acceptable knowledge. Appropriate exploration might include discussions with parents, teachers, counselors, and peers; visits to colleges or potential employers; relevant reading; or active participation via summer or part-time employment.

Anxiety will probably be more prevalent among older than younger adolescent Moratoriums. Important societal members, such as parents and teachers, often increasingly pressure adolescents, during the later high school years, about family, employment, and/or college orientation. The individual's internal timetable may also initiate increased anxiety. The younger adolescents will usually have the luxury of longer periods before choices need to be enacted; therefore, their moratorium will often be characterized by leisurely reflection on the advantages and disadvantages of vocational alternatives. An exception may be selection of high school curriculum tracks or, for a pregnant female, which of several options to pursue. She might see an abortion as the only option that will permit her to continue with her schooling or pursue a career subsequent to high school. Yet her greatest desire may be to be a parent, although her preferred implementation date may have been much later, perhaps after establishing a career in the work world. Weighing such important alternatives could cause the adolescent female much anxiety.

Example

(Female, 17) Mona is presently debating whether to go to college or find employment after high school graduation. She thinks she may favor motherhood above all other career possibilities. This choice is surprising to her because her own mother had stayed home to raise six children and Mona had decided at an early age that she would not follow in her mother's footsteps. Subsequent to her junior year, she had taken a summer day-camp job working with preschoolers. She loved the children and this turned her thoughts around about motherhood. If what she wanted was family roles, immediate and temporary employment, rather than college, might make more sense. No particular jobs interested her. She could, however, be an early childhood major in college, which would be compatible with her love of children. Simultaneous with this struggle, her art teacher was suggesting that she major in art advertising in college because she had very fine art skills and job opportunities were open in this field. This possibility too intrigued Mona. She expressed concern about the difficulty of making her decision, which, she felt, must be made by December in her senior year. Exciting as her future appeared, she also felt anxious about making the best decision.

Comment

Mona is a classic example of a Moratorium. She expresses two distinctly different alternatives: working with children, as their mother or school teacher, and art advertising. She needs to make a decision in the near future. Her emotional tone is one of excitement and anxiety. She is aware of her skills in working with children and in art, through her activities in the day camp and in the art classroom. She does not receive credit for the employment subsequent to high school alternative because she has not given much thought to job possibilities. Motherhood and the early childhood major are not treated as separate choices because they have a common identity theme: her love for preschool children. Had she expressed other intrinsic (e.g., her desire to teach) or extrinsic (e.g., monetary) reasons for her college major, it might have been treated as an alternative separate from motherhood. Pursuing a career choice in common with her mother would not have warranted a Foreclosure because her choice resulted from her own experiences subsequent to a contrast identification with her mother. Consideration of a second field, art advertising, also eliminated the possibility of the Foreclosure status.

Identity Achiever

The Identity Achiever has successfully resolved the moratorium and is presently committed to the vocational alternative that feels most personally expressive. Enticements toward "better" career options are resisted, although flexible statements are typically made, representing willingness to change if something better came along. The genuinely committed individual is, however, unable to generate a better choice, "better in their own terms." Their emotional tone often exudes confidence, as well as relief, that the decision has been made. Some adolescents will continue to express anxiety because they are concerned about their ability to carry through with their preference effectively. Many adolescent Identity Achievers are able to recognize that their choices are tentative and may not ultimately be implemented; some have selected backup courses of action, should their first choice prove inappropriate. Some Achievers who are less flexible may see their choices as unalterable, and hence are more likely to experience anxiety about the successful implementation of their choice.

The Identity Achievers should be able to discuss the pros and cons of their expected career as well as those discarded. They should be able to relate these career alternatives to their own abilities, likes, and dislikes. Again, the scorer must keep in mind the amount of exposure early and midadolescents could have had to these careers. Key phrases of commitment include the difficulty of the choice, as well as the seriousness with which the task was approached. Some Diffusions can discuss a number of career choices and be presently planning to implement one of them. However, they will demonstrate cheerful willingness to shift to other possibilities and refer to the commitment as not difficult to make.

Adolescents are often in the peculiar situation of not being able to implement their choices until later. For example, the high school sophomore who has chosen a college major cannot begin this college commitment for several years. But activity directed toward increasing knowledge about the area, perhaps through hobbies, part-time or summer jobs, and/or increased communication with "like individuals" warrants appropriate activity for the Identity Achieving adolescent.

Example

(Male, 16) Arnold expressed relief about his recent decision to become a psychologist. His father had placed a lot of pressure on him to become a business administrator, insisting that the job market for psychologists was nil. The boy talked to some administrators his dad knew, read college bulletins, and tried to imagine himself in this role. He decided that it just didn't feel right. His friends were frequently seeking his advice about their problems. He enjoyed listening, thinking, and then helping them decide what to do. The psychologist idea kind of grew on him. When a psychology professor from a nearby university came to the school to talk about careers in the field, he knew this was what he wanted. When asked if any other options had ever been seriously considered, he said yes. Before the idea of psychologist came up, he had thought about becoming a veterinarian because he loved animals. He decided, though, that he couldn't handle the medical aspects of the career, especially because chemistry and biology were two of his weaker subjects in school.

Comment

In this instance, three alternatives were seriously considered. Two were generated from within, based on Arnold's assessment of his own likes and abilities; one, from without, as his father's preference. For the latter, he attempted to gain knowledge about the field by talking, reading, and thinking about business administration. His emotional tone became one of relief and confidence as he discarded the options that felt wrong or required skills he did not aptly demonstrate; namely, business administration and veterinarian. The visiting psychologist became an important figure with whom Arnold could relate. The boy heard about career possibilities that were compatible with his much enjoyed "peer counseling" activities. His career direction was chosen.

The sequential considerations of veterinarian and psychologist were sufficient to warrant the Identity Achiever scoring. If, however, only the two career choices of psychology and business administration had been considered, it would have been crucial to listen and find whether the father's preference was seriously considered as a personally expressive option. If the boy had merely "gone through the paces" of exploration for his father's approval, then the scoring would have been Foreclosed on psychologist. If a substantial amount of anxiety had been incurred over the personal appropriateness of each of these choices, the Achiever status could have been warranted.

Religious Beliefs

Early and middle adolescents would have difficulty addressing religion as an example of a larger ideological framework. Early adolescents will typically address this domain in terms of whether they do or do not have a "religion" to which they belong in line with family beliefs and practices. Middle adolescents become more interesting as some of them question, approach, or withdraw from structured religions. Late adolescents are more likely to contemplate a broader belief-system framework.

Adolescents express numerous reasons for attending religious services, some reflecting commitment, some a lack of personal investment in religion. Among the committed, the most common theme represents acceptance of the faith from an early age. Participation is continued because they believe in God, religion is important to their lives, it teaches them how to distinguish good from bad, and leaves them with a positive feeling after attending services or praying. Among the uncommitted, common themes include parental demand for attendance, parental approval obtained through (noninvested) participation, or opportunities for social interaction with romantic partners and/or friends. When asked about the value of the services, the uncommitted often give such cursory responses as "it's okay," "it's dumb," or "I don't really pay much attention to it."

Questioning, doubt, or change in religious beliefs arise from many sources. Frequent religious questions center on the existence of God, heaven and hell, life after death, and the credibility of religious stories. Further questions arise, especially for middle adolescents, from the dichotomy between Bible stories and the theory of evolution advanced in science courses, and from unexplainable phenomena "scientifically explained" through the media, including such sources as *Chariots of the Gods*.

Doubt often arises among adolescents who seek to understand how their God could allow tragedy to befall a loved one or deny a crucial request, sought through prayer. Some older adolescents contemplating interfaith marriage are disillusioned by the hypocrisy between the disapproval generated by clergy and parents, who also proselytize love and understanding among humankind. Conflict between doctrinal issues and self-serving positions in such controversial areas as abortion, contraceptives, and consumption of alcohol give rise to questioning, doubt, and sometimes, for some older adolescents, withdrawal from religion. That withdrawal is also an excellent medium for rebelling against religious parents should one need to assert one's independence.

Adolescents may join or renew their faith for varied reasons. An initially social reason for attending services may be replaced by a personal investment for individuals who discover that religion can be an expressive way of defining themselves. Adolescents who identify strongly with their parents may choose to become religious because their parents at mid-life discover religion. Some adolescents turn or return to religion because they fear loss of control over their own lives, especially for self-defined immoral excesses in such areas as sexuality and drugs. They may feel that only the love of a forgiving God can save them and provide them with hope for the future.

Religious commitments can be exemplified by identifying with atheism, cults, or traditional organized religions. Atheists and agnostics, to be scored committed, must be able to understand their stance on religion, and include a present moral or universal ethic. If their identification is based on default, apathy, or alienation, they should not be scored committed. Cult members who participate for social rather than religious reasons would be scored uncommitted as well. Individuals may be scored committed if they maintain a personal religious ideology that reflects their morality and/or provides them with an understanding of their position and purpose in the universe. Some older adolescents shift from organized religion to a personal religion, usually characterized by extensive reading of scripture and prayer. Questions of social responsibility, morality, and their place in the universe frequently arise.

Identity Diffusion

In general, Identity Diffusions show little or no interest in religious matters. Interestingly, they will often state that they believe in God. They may also identify themselves with a religion. These two statements represent a need for social approval or an assumption that everyone must give at least a nod in the direction of religion. The scorer will notice, however, that religion itself does not occupy much of their day-to-day thinking. Attending services twice a year and praying on rare occasion for personal needs does not qualify as sufficient activity for commitment. Nor does weekly attendance at services for social motives, as opposed to devotional motives, warrant being scored for commitment. Attendance at religious observances in response to parental pressures also fits this category. Although knowledge of religious tenets and their rationale typically is limited, we sometimes observe greater knowledge without its having personal meaning to the respondent.

Example

(Male, 13) Dirk stated that he believed in God, attended church every once in a while, and prayed when he got really scared. When asked why he believed in God, he said because you're supposed to. When asked what he got out of believing in God and attending church, he said he had never thought about it. When asked why he prayed when scared, he said he just did. When asked how important religion was in his home, he said not very important.

Comment

This is a classic example of Apathetic Diffusion. Little information is provided and little is generated spontaneously. The socially appropriate statement, "I believe in God" (because, like everyone else, I'm supposed to—the characteristic theme of Diffusion) does not warrant commitment, nor does his activity level, attending church every once in a while.

Foreclosure

The majority of adolescent Foreclosures have continued to participate in their parents' religion. They have never successfully considered any other faith, although they may occasionally attend different religious services with friends or romantic partners. They are able to discuss the basic beliefs of their faith. The younger adolescents often do so through Bible stories or their equivalent. The older adolescents can often explain their preference for an organized or personal religion as well as why the tenets of their faith are preferred to those of another. Services are attended regularly, in the form of children's (e.g., Sunday school) or adults' observances. Daily religious thought and regular devotional reading or prayer would signify appropriate activity for adolescents committed to a personal religion. Participation in youth organizations for social purposes does not warrant activity representing a religious identity.

Where an adolescent changes his or her religion due to pressure from another significant identification figure, the scoring is still Foreclosed, unless the adolescent undergoes a great deal of stressful, personal evaluation before being able to make the change. Some individuals will become religious for the first time during adolescence. When no previous religious commitment existed, the individual would be scored Foreclosed.

Example

(Female, 17) Francine has a Jewish father and a Methodist mother. The parents agreed to rear her in the Jewish faith. Her paternal grandparents too have been instrumental in developing her appreciation for her Jewish cultural heritage. She has been quite involved in her temple. She recently established a romantic relationship with a Mormon. He encouraged her to attend his Church of Latter Day Saints. She temporarily drew away from Judaism as she thought about joining his faith to be with him. She broke off the relationship when she discovered that her Jewish background was more important to her.

Comment

This respondent was a classic Foreclosure because she had been reared and committed to only one faith. Both her parents have been significant identification figures for her. The introduction of the boyfriend as an important identification figure complicated this scoring. Because she thought about joining his faith to be with him but subsequently remained committed to her own faith, she remains Foreclosed. Her interest was in her affiliation with the boyfriend, not the religion itself. Had Francine expressed serious interest in Mormon religious ideas with appropriate exploration and subsequently returned to her own faith, she would have been scored an Identity Achiever.

Moratorium

Moratoriums may be questioning whether to remain religious or eliminate religion from their lives. They may be strongly challenging the religious tenets with which they were reared. They may be contemplating a change in organized religion or deciding whether to participate in one or pursue a personal faith. They may be weighing the merits of religion and science, determining whether to choose between, accept, or reject both.

Also accepted as moratorium behavior is contemplation of reorganizing one's belief within a faith if the individual perceives real change in religious identity because of it. Although unusual for this age group, it tends to occur more commonly among Catholics who cannot imagine themselves being other than Catholic, yet cannot abide the Pope's position on certain issues or accept some of the tenets of the faith. While attempting to resolve any of these dilemmas, the adolescent typically experiences a great deal of anxiety and seeks an answer in the near future.

Example

(Male, 15) Martin has a strong commitment to his Baptist church. He attends services every Sunday, is an officer in the youth organization, and reads his Bible nightly. Science is his strongest and most enjoyed academic field. He has recently become very uncomfortable because of the conflicts that have appeared to him between the teachings of the Bible and scientific evidence about evolution. He has talked to his minister and several high school teachers. His reading of the Bible has become more intense, yet thoughtful. He spends long hours talking with friends about the issues that most concern him. His discomfort has caused him to lack pleasure in both areas. He is eager to resolve this dilemma: Can he be religious and still pursue a science career?

Comment

Martin exhibits all the criteria appropriate for a Moratorium. He is knowledgeable about religion and science through his church activities and coursework. His emotional tone is one of concern, anxiety, and eagerness for an answer in the near future. He engages in activity to that end, namely, talking, reading, and thinking. His alternatives pertain to his belief in Bible teachings versus science, which could more broadly affect the roles of religion and science, possibly as career alternatives, in his life.

Identity Achiever

The anxiety of the Moratorium is replaced with a calm and comfortable emotional tone in the Identity Achiever. A religious position appropriate at that time has been chosen. The adolescents can discuss the reasons for the choice. As appropriate, weekly attendance at services, prayer, scripture readings, and so on are demonstrable. The importance and role of religion in their lives can be articulated without difficulty. They can anticipate the role religion will play in their future. Older adolescents, with more sophisticated cognitive abilities, should be able to consider factors that might influence their religious stance, such as an interfaith marriage, and elaborate upon what they would do under such circumstances. Committed adolescents will resist being swayed from their religious orientation. At the same time they may express flexibility by recognizing that other faiths may be more appropriate for other people.

Example

(Female, 16) Alice discussed her recent conversion from Catholicism to a personal religion. She had been reared very traditionally by her Catholic mother. The girl had accepted Catholicism and enjoyed the social interactions planned by the youth organization. She attended mass every week. During her high school years, however, she became increasingly angered by the Pope's position on abortion and contraceptives. This conflict led her to question the church's role in dictating her morality. Ultimately, she questioned the role of religion in general in her life. She decided that she believed in God and needed to pray and commune with a personal "father" figure who could guide her in her decision making. She felt that her morality should be determined from within herself. She disliked the structure and limited opportunities for individualism afforded her by organized religion. Against her mother's wishes, she terminated her participation in the Catholic Church and turned to her personal relationship with God.

Comment

Alice initially demonstrated commitment to religion through her weekly attendance at mass, participation in church youth activities, and general acceptance of Catholicism. Her questions about abortion and contraceptives were self-serving, not identity issues, and did not warrant Moratorium status. These questions, however, triggered religious identity questions about her morality, the place of morality in religion, and the role of religion in her life. She resolved these questions to her satisfaction. She chose a commitment that was personally expressive. The importance of resolving her religious identity at that time was demonstrated by her questioning and subsequent commitment, particularly in the light of her mother's opposition.

Family and Career Priorities

The primary purpose of this domain is to clarify the priority of self-definition between family and career roles. Is neither important? Is one of greater importance, or are both crucial for self-fulfilment? If both are greatly significant to the individual, a potential for conflict arises, for both roles can place great demands on one's time and energy.

Family can pertain to spouse or children or both, with each being contrasted with career. When addressing the family aspect of this potential area of conflict, most adolescents assume that the question pertains to the conflict between children and career. Hence, the interview was deliberately separated into spouse/career and parent/career sets of questions to provide the opportunity to distinguish the two for content analysis or separate identity scorings if desired.

Spouse and career are not usually seen as a potential conflict. Most adolescents feel that husbands and wives can both be employed without conflict. The majority of both sexes expresses the expectation that both partners will work to at least secure a financially stable foundation for a subsequently expanding family. However, when asked, "If spouse and career roles did conflict, which would you give priority to?" males typically choose career, expecting their wives to understand. Females usually choose their spouse, stating that they could always get another job, but not another person like the individual they chose to marry. Girls anticipating a substantial investment in career also include a comment to the effect that they plan to marry someone who will understand that their career is important to them.

The majority of both sexes, especially among older adolescents, place children before career. However, many younger male adolescents and some older males as well, state that because they are the primary bread-winner, the children will have to understand that their father's career may have to come first. They'll spend what time they can with their children. Many males are Foreclosed in this area, some choosing career as their priority, others choosing family. Males are also far more likely to be Identity Diffuse in this domain than are females. A number of males anticipate no conflict and have given no thought to this area. The reason most often given is that they consider themselves responsible for children in the breadwinner capacity only. Individuals must express a priority and justify it to be identified as committed in this area.

Among the females, this is one of the most difficult domains in which to choose a commitment. They often feel primary responsibility for children, evidenced by their willingness to take time off from work for their preschoolers and statements of concern about caregiving when their children are ill. In neither instance do the majority of adolescent girls even suggest that their spouse should maintain partial responsibility for these tasks. Many females also feel the need to personally express themselves through employment. They do not wish to be full-time homemakers. Conflicts can arise for females who express the concern that day-care centers often are of poor quality. If no family members can offer to take responsibility for the children during her working hours, she is left with no perceived support system. Lacking personal or professional support, these girls ponder how to fit both career and family into their lives. Although they attempt to weigh alternatives, some important long-range factors are not even considered. For example, many girls are unable or unwilling to consider the question of whether taking time off from work will be detrimental to their careers. For those who plan to withdraw from the labor force when their children are young, there is a tendency to assume that they can settle back into their careers once their last child is in school. They don't consider the possibility that their work skills or jobs may be obsolete or that they may not be hired back. Nor do they consider how much time might be taken off from work due to the number of children they plan to have, spacing between the children, and the age of children at which these girls would be willing to return to work. In fact, there is a substantial lack of reality about the costs involved in dual priorities or choosing either role to the exclusion of the other. However, individuals who struggle to resolve issues, regardless of the naiveté involved, are credited with sophisticated identity activity within their age group.

Knowledgeability and activity in this domain should be represented by examining the importance of career and family to one's self-definition. Dividing one's time and energy between the areas is a vital issue. Career counseling and family life courses often do not address the potential conflict between these two possible life goals. Moreover, models may be limited primarily to parents, teachers, and friends' parents who do not think to discuss such issues with this age group. In males, the emotional tone is often indifference or calm, whereas in females, anxiety is prevalent. Females are very likely to be concerned and naive. Little opportunity is afforded them to realistically examine the pros and cons. Scorers must keep in mind that these girls' best source of information in this domain is often their own parents' unresolved struggles with these issues.

Most adolescents do use their own parents as models for "prioritizing" the domains of family and career. The parents' satisfaction with their own life-style and its effect on the children are the justifications most often cited for the adolescents' choices. For example, boys who feel deprived of attention because their mothers work tend to want their wives to stay home while the husbands attend to career. Those who emphasize getting ahead monetarily want their wives to contribute to the family income. Girls whose mothers work outside the home and are responsible for most of the homemaker tasks will probably have the most precise future plans about priorities and expectations for how they will be implemented.

Identity Diffusion

Identity Diffusion is more characteristic of younger adolescents who may sense the possibility of conflict but lack enough information or interest in either area to invest their energies in assessing potential conflicts. Apathy is the most prevalent form of Diffusion expressed in this domain, especially by males who describe their parenting role in limited ways and consequently anticipate no conflict between parenting and career.

Among females, however, Identity Diffusion may represent inability to resolve what appears to be an unresolvable dilemma—a full-time career and primary responsibility for children. It is more characteristic of the older girls to have elaborated on their desires and attempted to fit together the pieces with no satisfactory solution. Hence, they have put aside the issue. Perhaps at some undefined future date they will again attempt to examine possible alternatives.

Example

(Male, 14) David anticipates that there could be a conflict between the time needed to play with his kids and time needed for work. He plans to play hockey professionally and won't be home much. When asked how he would resolve this conflict, he shrugs and says he doesn't know. It'll just have to be the way it has to be.

Comment

David does not take a clear stand on his priorities. Although he recognizes that a conflict could arise, he plans to flow with the path of least resistance—things will be the way they have to be. There is no tone of concern, no projecting into the future, no consideration of people involved.

Foreclosure

The classic Foreclosure anticipates no conflict between the options of family and/or career. Often, one priority is easily identified, with the second domain indeed playing second fiddle. For others who plan dual priorities, there is a calm expectation that the several domains will mesh without difficulty.

Usually, a parent or older sibling models the choice successfully in the eyes of the adolescent. Foreclosed males typically identify career as their priority, with father modeling this role. Foreclosed females often choose parenting as their primary priority, although nontraditional mothers demonstrating dual priorities often contribute to the adolescent's choice to pursue both avenues. If the mother or father is comfortable with dual-priority roles, daughters, and possibly sons, will follow this lead without doubts. In such situations the dual priority would have been chosen through a Foreclosure route.

Example

(Female, 17) Felicity is the mother of a nine-month-old baby. When she graduates from high school this year, she plans to go on to college, majoring in computer programming. After college she plans to make a career for herself. She says there is no conflict because either her mother, her sister (who has two children of her own), or a babysitter will be available for her children. It's working now while she's in high school, and so there is no reason for her to doubt that she can continue in this way through college and into her career. The one difficulty is that she is tired. When she gets home she spends all her time with the baby until she goes to bed; then Felicity studies, does laundry, and cleans the house. She'd like to have some free time for herself, but her career and baby are more important.

Comment

This adolescent girl already knows what it takes to be a parent, and she is implementing dual priorities. She expresses a clear commitment to following the path she has already undertaken. She is not seeking other alternatives, although she does regret not having time for herself. She demonstrates knowledge, activity, projection into the future, stability without considering alternatives; she is Foreclosed on dual priorities.

Moratorium

Family and career are important roles for the Moratorium who is trying to resolve which domain takes precedence. Some adolescents contemplate resolving this issue by changing priorities at different times in their life. Others consider the importance of their potential spouse's attitude toward implementing one plan over another—compromise and understanding being two important descriptors older adolescents may generate.

Females are very likely to use sophisticated identity activity in this domain. Tension is common in the girls' voices as they talk of juggling biological clocks, education, establishment in careers, financial stability, marriage, and children. Males appear to be most concerned about the pressures of careers, which they often identify as the most important domain for self-definition. However, some older adolescent males give thought to what they mean by good family relationships. Their conflict is often focused on society's expectation of success in career, regardless of the outcome's effect on the family. The more family-oriented males, who are affected by this pressure, may feel anxiously torn between these potential priorities, one from within self, and one from without by significant others. Among males who anticipate conflict between these domains, many are inclined to think little about it at this age. Some of the older adolescent males, who have experienced important romantic relationships, are inclined to address this issue directly. For a Moratorium scoring, one must hear genuine recognition of conflict with the weighing of alternatives, not Diffuse statements such as "they'll just have to put up with it" or "it's only for a few years."

Example

(Male, 18) Max expresses interest in a career as a firefighter. He also plans to marry and have several children. The conflict is that for some years he'll be on rotating shifts as a firefighter, which will be a hardship for his family. As a firefighter, he sees no alternatives. Rotating shifts is simply a fact. Asking his family to understand, placing much responsibility on his wife's shoulders, not seeing his kids, are major drawbacks to the career. No other career, however, holds the same allure for him. He really wants this career; maybe he shouldn't even have a family. He ponders what to do.

Comment

Max is scored Moratorium because he is presently trying to make a decision, "pondering what to do." He delineates the issues of his conflict: being a firefighter with rotating shifts places a burden on his family; thus he would not be a good family man. Does he become a firefighter? Does he become a husband and father? Which, or both? Could he possibly find an equally desirable career that would not interfere with family roles? As long as he is seriously contemplating these alternatives, his behavior is characteristic of the Moratorium.

Identity Achiever

This status is represented by individuals who previously considered the alternatives of making family or career their priority. Perhaps they thought one way earlier in their lives and now look at it differently, or they may have weighed the advantages and disadvantages of prioritizing each area simultaneously. They may have chosen to become invested in (1) only one of the two areas; (2) both areas, one being of greater importance; or (3) both areas, attributing comparable importance to each.

Because respondents usually have already been interviewed in the domains of vocation, marriage, and parenting, this domain can be brief for those who have resolved the family and career conflict. Many of the issues may have arisen in the earlier sections of the interview. Therefore, information previously given should be taken into account when determining any of the statuses in this domain. Do so especially for the Moratorium and Identity Achiever, however, because their responses to the family and career domain are often the most complex, riddled with inconsistencies not fully resolved. The scorer must be prepared to distinguish between issues of self-definition and issues of implementation when determining if a respondent is an Identity Achiever in this domain. Struggles about whether and to what degree one can fit each priority into one's life are deemed identity issues. How to make self-chosen identity components work are implementation issues that Identity Achievers may be grappling with.

Females are far more likely than males to be sophisticated decision makers about family and career priorities. They are reared to expect that children are primarily the woman's responsibility. Adolescent females are cognizant of this point. It is the ramifications of this assumed responsibility which they often do not anticipate and which trigger conflict when barriers are identified. Males who choose to value family more highly than career but who are surrounded by significant others who believe career should be the most important goal, may also become Identity Achievers after they unravel the pressures, advantages, and disadvantages of each priority, and come up with what is most personally expressive.

Example

(Female, 17) Ada has her heart set on being a paramedic. However, she also wants to be a parent of at least three children. She tried to resolve the dilemma first in favor of one choice, then the other. Something was always missing. Her friends weren't very helpful. They suggested that she just do what she wanted to do. But Ada knew that children took a lot of time; being a paramedic, she'd have to be on call. She finally decided that they'd have to realize at work that she could only take night shifts so that she could get home in time to feed her children breakfast, get them off to school, then get to sleep herself, houseclean, prepare dinner, put the children to bed, then go to work. Then she felt relieved; it had been a very serious issue for her to resolve. She felt that the pieces had fallen into place.

Comment

Ada's willingness to consider career versus family represented Moratorium behavior. She assessed difficulties that each would bring to bear on the other. She sought advice from friends. The emotional tone of discomfort, followed by relief, signaled the end of Moratorium. Her resolution is, at least for the time being, satisfactory for her: a dual priority. Although her plans are unrealistic, she is scored as an Identity Achiever because she considered alternatives to the best of her knowledge and made a decision that felt personally expressive.

9 Identity Status in Late Adolescents: Scoring Criteria

JAMES E. MARCIA AND SALLY L. ARCHER

Introduction

The scoring criteria presented in this chapter are intended for use with late adolescents, aged 18 to 22.[1] The dual processes of exploration and commitment are the primary scoring considerations. The criteria are somewhat more stringently applied for this age than for early and middle adolescence. The reasons for this difference are directly related to the developmental theory of identity formation. Early adolescence may be seen as a period of *destructuring*, wherein previous cognitive, psychosexual, and physiological accomplishments undergo transition to a more pre-adult form. Middle adolescence can be construed as a *restructuring* phase in which new organizations of old and new skills are formed. Late adolescence, in contrast to the two earlier periods, is seen as a period of *consolidation*, of discernible identity composition, and of testing in the world the newly constructed identity. Hence, late adolescence is the period in the life cycle when for most persons identity "gets done" for the first time.

The four identity statuses are based upon the presence, absence, and degree of two processes: exploration (once called "crisis") and commitment. The areas or domains within which these variables operate are less important than the underlying processes. The assumption is that genuine exploration of personally meaningful alternatives followed by selection of a general direction for one's interests and abilities is the basic indicator of identity formation. A further assumption is that the structure formed as a result of this process will be adaptively assimilative for a limited time, after which it will become disequilibrated and another exploratory period will ensue, to be followed by subsequent commitment (accommodating). Hence, the variables of exploration and commitment are intended to account for identity formation, change, and reformulation.

---

[1]The authors wish to thank Kim Bartholomew and Joyce Nicholls-Goldsmuid for their help in selecting some of the interview fragments in this chapter.

The Meaning of Exploration and Commitment in Late Adolescents

Exploration

In late adolescence, exploration is both cognitive and behavioral, although the cognitive aspect should always be observable in some behavioral manifestation. A person may say that he or she "thought about" alternative religious views while pursuing the childhood faith, but continued to practice undeterred. One would expect a genuine exploration to have had disruptive effects such as decrease or cessation in religious ceremonial observation, questioning of religious authority figures, and discussions, perhaps disputes, with family and friends. Even if exploration were primarily cognitive, the respondent should be able to discuss, in some depth, the alternatives weighed, and be able to refer to some hiatus in traditional religious observance. Following are some criteria to be used in assessing the presence, absence, and degree of exploration.

Knowledgeability

By late adolescence the individual should have made a fairly accurate assessment of personal needs and abilities and have a realistic picture of available societal opportunities. A college student who is committed to going into the law ought to know that most of the first year in law school is spent in the library, not the courtroom, and that few lawyers have practices like that of Perry Mason. A psychology major ought not to expect to hang out a psychotherapy shingle upon completing the B.A. with a psychology major. One is looking for more than a superficial understanding of the details in the education or apprenticeship necessary to a vocation as well as some knowledge of day-to-day activity in the vocation. Similarly, for the ideological areas of religion and politics, a mere label (e.g., Protestant, Liberal) is insufficient to indicate exploration of the domain. The interviewer is looking for knowledge of alternatives as well, and, beyond that, for some information about comparisons and contrasts that indicate a respondent's thoughtfulness about the ideas underlying the labels.

Activity Directed Toward Gathering Information

Here we are assessing essentially the legwork necessary to obtain information about alternatives. Knowing for certain that one wants to be a dentist because that is what one's parent does, or being certain about one's views on sexuality without ever having been in a relationship where sexuality is an issue, does not indicate much explorative activity. On the other hand, speaking with representatives of several vocations, discussing alternative religious views with proponents of those views, self-directed reading about nontraditional sex-role alternatives—all indicate explorative activity. The important matter here is some self-initiated, in-depth searching.

Considering Alternative Potential Identity Elements

Most persons as they grow through childhood become aware of different aspects of themselves, each of which, if pursued, would take them in different life directions. Adolescence is the period in the life cycle during which, at least for some persons, experimentation is tolerated and sometimes encouraged. Not to exploit such an opportunity is to purchase a small measure of security at the price of a large measure of self-restriction. At late adolescence, the time remaining before confronting the harder realities of adulthood dwindles, and the world begins to become less patient with the adolescent's experimentation and active consideration of alternatives. When one speaks with late adolescents at age 22, then, one is most likely to probe for previous consideration of alternatives; by contrast, 18-year-olds may be in the middle of such considerations. Whether one looks at present or previous considerations, the primary issue is the authenticity of that consideration. It is one thing to remain ensconced in a childhood vocational or ideological niche while peering out for an alternative: it is another to leave the niche and to actively explore different paths commensurate with one's interests and abilities. Whether or not the original directions are returned to is not relevant for the determination of identity status; the relevant aspect is that attention has been paid to alternatives and that the consequences of their pursuit have been weighed.

Desire to Make an Early Decision

Direction is an especially important facet of exploration in *late* adolescence. The goal is not exploration for its own sake, as it may well be earlier in adolescence, or even during subsequent identity crises in adulthood. The goal of exploration in late adolescence is to determine the best-fitting vocational, ideological, and interpersonal alternatives with which to begin young adulthood. One type of individual, characterological Moratorium, seems able to maintain the tension of active struggle, especially among ideological and interpersonal alternatives; however, this person requires a fairly rarefied supportive environment, and not everyone can work in a university. In general, then, one expects emotionally directed exploration, not just careless "fooling around." The former would characterize a Moratorium; the latter, an Identity Diffusion.

In summary, exploration may be nonexistent, previous in time, or current; and it may vary in the breadth of alternatives considered and the depth of consideration. The issue of the extent of exploration is particularly important in discriminating between Foreclosures and Identity Achievements.

Commitment

Commitment becomes more important in late adolescence than it was during earlier periods. Before one can really *be* an adult, one must assume the role and its associated behaviors: entering or preparing for a vocation, espousing some coherent view of oneself in the world (a "philosophy of life"), and deciding how one is going to define one's adult sexual relationships. No one pretends that this first version of adulthood is the real thing—that one's grownupness is much more than skin deep. But one must begin somewhere. And that first constellation of vocational, ideological, and interpersonal commitments at late adolescence is a beginning. The meaning of commitment is close to what Erikson describes as the virtue of this psychosexual stage: Fidelity. Commitment, like fidelity, refers to a definitive choice among possibilities and adherence to the chosen direction in the face of distracting and inviting alternatives. This choice does not mean imperviousness to change, but it does mean reluctance to abandon easily a path set out upon. Following are some criteria for assessing presence, absence, and degree of commitment.

Knowledgeability

Stated simply, the adolescent who is committed knows what he or she is getting into. This knowledge is based upon the results of behavior consistent with one's stated commitments. One mistrusts the depth of a respondent's commitment when he or she claims to want to go into business, yet has taken no commerce courses nor engaged in entrepreneurial enterprises. The wish to make money is not enough to warrant commitment; one must have explored and been able to articulate how one intends to go about it, and why. Knowledgeability is related to articulateness. One usually has difficulty speaking clearly about something of which one knows little or has thought little. An additional assumption is being made: if one is knowledgeable and thoughtful about an area, one will talk about it in an identity status interview. Are we claiming that Identity Achievement is a function of one's ability to articulate one's story? Yes. One may have a Foreclosed identity without being able to articulate the details in its formative process. However, to have achieved (constructed) an identity means to have thoughtfully examined aspects of one's life; and in most instances the results of this thoughtfulness will be orally communicated in an identity status interview.

Activity Directed Toward Implementing the Chosen Identity Element

To know what one is getting into, one must acquire relevant experience; one can do only so much in one's head. Hence, one aspect of commitment involves behavior in commitment-related areas. For example, one may espouse nontraditional sex roles, but unless one has actually tried behaving in nontraditional ways, that commitment is suspect. Similarly, one may claim to adhere to a political philosophy, right or left, that clearly calls for activism; yet, if no evidence is found of direct political activity, commitment is assumed to be minimal. In assessing the activity aspect of commitment, one is asking in what ways the respondent is "making it real." Having stressed activity, a clarification should be made. Often, much identity work gets done internally with few visible signs. The general scoring rule is that if almost all the work is internal, then the person tends toward Moratorium; if some external indications of exploration and commitment are evident, then the person is likely to be an Identity Achiever; if there are obvious behavioral indications of commitment, but exploration is questionable, then a Foreclosure categorization is given. In other words, behavioral indicators are important, but well articulated beliefs, betokening significant internal work, are good evidence for at least a beginning of Identity Achievement.

Emotional Tone

Essentially, one finds five predominant affective tones among the identity statuses: the solid self-assuredness of the Achievement; the inflexible self-righteousness of the Foreclosure; the struggling, intense, somewhat anxious demeanor of the Moratorium; the breezy insouciance of the playboy /playgirl Diffusion; and the sad, wistful, or remote quality of the more isolated Diffusions. Just as no one of these characteristics (i.e., knowledgeability, activity, and so on) is, by itself, sufficient to indicate presence, absence, or degree of commitment, neither is emotional tone. Some Achievements may seem smugly inflexible; some Moratoriums are not really suffering. But in general, the presence of commitment seems to produce poised self-confidence; and its absence appears to lead to self-doubt, as well as the extremes of loquaciousness and taciturnity.

Identification with Significant Others

The presence of significant role models as ideal figures is less important at late adolescence than at early adolescence because by this time the ego ideal has already undergone its major modification. At late adolescence, significant figures have a direct and realistic role as teachers, mentors, validators, and exemplars of the possible consequences of vocational or ideological decisions. In other words, what important others do with and for the late adolescent individual in *reality* is more important than who they are or what they stand for in an idealized sense. Usually, the more identity work an adolescent has done, the less he or she wants to be "just like" a role model, and the more he or she can discriminate positive (emulatable) and negative (avoidable) aspects of significant others. The less identity work has been done, the more the individual either wishes to copy exactly an admired figure or despairs of ever living up to a model (projected) standard. In short, identification at late adolescence passes from idealization to realistic, self-interested appraisal.

Projecting One's Personal Future

As in the preceding section, the emphasis is on realistic projection of one's personal future. One of the hypothesized criteria for identity development in early adolescence is "the ability to construe alternative futures" (Marcia, 1983) with little emphasis on the realistic aspects of those futures. At late adolescence, however, the result of thoroughgoing exploration and firm commitment should produce a somewhat reasonable five-year plan. One interview area especially sensitive to this issue is that of sex roles, for here one may deal with questions of career versus marriage priorities, child-rearing values, and spousal division of labor. Realistic projection into the future relates directly to commitment. Firm commitment to a particular direction should lead to behavior consistent with that direction, and the resulting accumulation of experience should produce some ideas about what is and is not possible and/or likely to occur. Lack of commitment leads to either truncated experience or scattered, diffuse experience—"kicks."

Resistance to Being Swayed

"What would happen if something better came along?" the interviewer asks. "What do you mean, something better?" the respondent replies. "What would be better in your terms?" the interviewer rejoins. This bit of dialogue occurs repeatedly in identity status interviews. Responses range from willingness to enter almost any field, endorse any belief, and consider any sexual–interpersonal alternative, to rigid insistence upon one vocation, one belief system, and one set of sexual standards. Between the easy vacillation of the Diffusion and the intransigence of the Foreclosure lie the strong flexibility of the Achievement and the bound uncertainty of the Moratorium. A response that indicates advanced identity formation usually has three aspects: (1) acknowledgment of the possibility of change, (2) linkage of possible change to the individual's abilities and societal opportunities, and (3) reluctance to change except under fairly pressing circumstances. As a rule, the respondent high in identity can articulate some of the conditions under which a change would occur, but usually shows little enthusiasm for it.

In summary, commitment is a crucial element of identity formation in late adolescence. For many late adolescents, the problem is not saying "yes" to one direction, but saying "no" to others. There is an Italian saying that "he who leaves the old life for the new one knows what he leaves but not what he enters." To a certain extent, this is the predicament in adolescent commitment, and many Foreclosures and Diffusions would prefer to "bear those ills they have, than fly to others they know not of."

Foreclosures, because they are committed, may seem inappropriately included in the comment above. Foreclosures do not *make* commitments, however, any more than do Diffusions. Foreclosures simply are, or find themselves, committed in an almost inexorable movement from their past to their present.

Scoring Complications for Late Adolescents

Validity of Exploration

Determining whether or not a genuine exploratory period has occurred within an identity domain is probably the most difficult scoring issue. It is also where the interview method is at its strongest and questionnaire methods at their weakest. The problem here lies not so much in the scoring as in the interview procedure. The interview gives flexibility to probe, and it is this area concerning the validity of a crisis that the interviewer almost always has to probe, sometimes rather creatively. One cannot score what is not recorded on the tape, and so an interviewer must be sufficiently cognizant of the scoring criteria before entering the interview to ensure that sufficient questioning is undertaken to determine the validity of exploration.

During identity formation, having undergone an exploratory period, one can return to an initial commitment. Hence, the presence of the same commitment content in an individual in early and late adolescence is not prima facie evidence for Foreclosure. Nor is a change in commitment content prima facie evidence for Identity Achievement. In the former, alternatives must have been actively and effectively considered; there should be evidence of a behavioral departure from the initial direction before a subsequent return to it. In the latter case, one must be certain that the changed commitment content is not just a reflected-upon variation on a childhood theme. For example, moving from a parentally encouraged Marxist political view to a strong socialist position without much consideration of alternatives does not indicate sufficient exploration. If the Marxism had been temporarily abandoned, though, some real-life experiences had intervened, the person had reflected on the discrepancies between experiences and previous beliefs, and *then* arrived at a committed socialist position, an Identity Achievement score would be indicated.

Multiple Status Scoring of Areas

Very few persons are in the same identity status across all domains. Most will be in the same status in at least several areas, thus making most overall status decisions nonproblematical. There are no specific scoring rules for arriving at an overall status given an unclear split among the domains (e.g., Identity Achievement in two domains, Moratorium in two, and Diffusion in one). Here, one must rely on the overall tone or flavor of the interview. However, one scoring method that yields additional information employs a subsidiary status indication for each domain. Just as few persons are in the same identity status across all domains, similarly, identity status within each domain may not be "pure." One may decide that an individual is Diffusion in, say, religion, but that there is also a possibility of Moratorium. Recording the alternative status for a particular area preserves this information. One way of preserving it is the following: a predominant status for a domain is scored, for example, *F* (Foreclosure); an almost equally strong possible status as *F*, say *IA* (Identity Achievement), combined with the *F* would yield *F*, *I*A. To reiterate, if one is fairly certain that the individual is, say, Foreclosure in a domain, score *F* alone. If the person is likely to be Foreclosure, but may very well be Identity Achievement, score *F*, *I*A. If the person is very likely to be Foreclosure, and Identity Achievement is only a possibility, score *F*(*IA*). In the example above, the 2–2–1 split could be much less problematic if the scoring by domain were *A,M*; *A*(*M*); *M*; *M*(*D*); *D*(*M*). Here, the decision to call the respondent Moratorium overall is clear.

The Importance of Process over Content

Most persons giving identity status interviews are likely to have a broadly common outlook. Most will be in the social sciences and will tend to have similar liberal and nonauthoritarian values. Hence, identity status interviewers may begin with a bias as a result of the content of their own identity formation process. Sometimes it is quite difficult to see a traditional, highly authoritarian respondent as in a high identity status, although this may be the accurate designation. Even more difficult is scoring a nonauthoritarian, liberal respondent as low in identity. Interviewers must keep in mind that it is the *process* of identity formation, not the content, that is being assessed. There may be a relationship between process and content; going through an identity formation process may make certain content more likely and other content less likely. However, we have no research on that subject as yet, and until we do—even, perhaps, when we do—we may always be on safer ground to keep the issues of process and content separate and to score the process alone.

Identity in Males and Females

In general, women appear to have interpersonal issues more in hand than do men. The sexes are comparable in commitment to occupational issues. Women seem a bit more advanced in religion, men a bit more in politics. Also, men tend to take a more serial approach to identity issues—one domain at a time. Women tend more to try to make an organized whole from many elements. Hence, the commitment pattern for males is often characterized by intraindividual scatter among the areas. The commitment pattern for females is frequently marked by integration of commitment among several domains. Bearing these expectable differences in mind, the researcher should be somewhat stringent in scoring exploration, a process that definitely should have taken place in the past seven or so years of the adolescent's life. The researcher should be somewhat more lenient in scoring commitment, a newer arrival on the identity formation scene.

The Identity Status Domains

The process of establishing values, beliefs, and goals can be assessed in many areas of an individual's life. During late adolescence an individual may be examining self-definitional attributes in domains such as vocational choice, ideology, sexuality, family roles, and/or sex-role preference. Three potentially salient domains are addressed in this chapter to exemplify scoring status by domain issues. The domains discussed are vocational choice, religious beliefs, and family–career priorities.

Vocational Choice

Whether the late adolescent is in college or in the workplace, we are looking for a psychosocial meshing between an individual's capabilities and needs on one hand and society's demands and rewards on the other. The individual is expected to have assessed his or her abilities and interests, investigated possible societal opportunities, and made a commitment that is being acted upon. This commitment may take several forms: domestic (homemaking, childrearing); vocational (secretary, plumber); or educational (apprenticeship, college major). These forms may also be combined. But the person must have accomplished the transition from a receptive (child) to a productive (adult) orientation, and have done so in a self-reflective manner accompanied by a behaviorally consistent life-style.

There is a problem with the occupational area as a criterion for identity formation. Social conditions can limit, sometimes severely, educational and vocational alternatives. In difficult economic times, just getting a job—any job—is important, with the result that exploration and commitment become luxuries. If there is not much room for variability within an identity interview area (e.g., political ideology in a totalitarian state), then that area becomes disqualified as an indicator of Identity Achievement—not as an indicator of identity, per se. The achievement or construction of an identity requires important life areas in which choice is possible. If no such areas exist in a society, or if the only areas available are relatively trivial, then the modal identity status for that society will be, at best, Foreclosure, at worst, Diffusion.

Another issue that has arisen with respect to vocation, and may arise again, is the possibility that ideological commitment will preclude a vocational one. During the Vietnam war era in the United States, many young people became committed to an ideology of nonparticipation in the majority culture. A part of that ideology was that to occupy a vocational niche in society was to lend support to an establishment that was acting immorally; hence, no "vocation," as typically defined, was acceptable. These individuals were called "Alienated Achievements" and the quality of their performance on dependent variables was similar to, and in some cases exceeded, the more conventional Identity Achievements. The general point is that identity, at its most meaningful level of conceptualization, is organizational, synthetic, and gestaltlike. Domains may be scored separately, and one may speak of a "vocational identity," but ego identity, which this research began as an attempt to measure, refers to a more or less organized whole. Interviewers should be watchful for integrating themes running through the individual domains. For example, there are vocations that a Marxist could not legitimately choose; and there are beliefs about sex roles and sexuality that an Orthodox Jew could not espouse. Yet both of these persons may have an overall Achieved Identity. Sometimes it is useful, after one has scored the separate domains, to reflect upon the whole person who has just been listened to and attempt to summarize with one of the identity statuses the overall tone or flavor of the individual's identity structure.

Identity Diffusion

There seem to be three types of Diffusion in vocation. The first might be called the "opportunist." This individual will latch on to whatever looks profitable and not too difficult at the moment; if computers are in, then it is computers; if ergonomics is the field of the year, then ergonomics it is. The enthusiasms are short-lived and a declaration of commitment in the interview is fairly easily swayed by an astute interviewer who can suggest equally attractive, and possibly more easily achievable, vocational directions. A second type of vocational Diffusion seems to be just drifting, waiting for some occupation to choose them. Such persons tend to make other pursuits their immediate focus; such as "partying." There is a naive faith (with, perhaps, an underlying despair) that something will happen, something will come along. A third type of Diffusion in vocation reflects some psychological disturbance. Here, the vocational choice is based upon a rather megalomanic fantasy, incommensurate with the reality of the individual's achievements or occupational preparation. Aspiring to be a clinical psychologist in private practice with a "C" average in undergraduate psychology courses, or setting out for a career in ballet at age 21, are examples of the fantasy-based approach.

All these types of Diffusions have in common a lack of commitment, or, at least a lack of realistic commitment that leads to vocation-relevant behavior. They may or may not have experienced an exploration period. If they have done so, it is usually superficial and brief.

Examples[2]

A. (female)

Interviewer (I): Why did you come to SFU?

Respondent (R): It's close; that's about it.

I: Why did you choose English as a major?

R: It's the easiest course there is.

I: What do you plan to do with it?

R: Teach.

I: How willing do you think you would be to change your plans if something better came along?

R: Yeah, I'm all willing. Not all willing, but I don't really know what I'm interested in, so if I find something else really interesting I'll go into that. It depends how well I'm doing in the course.

B. (male)

I: How did you happen to come to SFU?

R: They don't have a first-year language requirement. That's it.

I: What do you plan to do with a degree in psychology?

R: God knows. I don't know. I want to instruct in a prestigious university and do research and write books . . .

I: What seems attractive to you about that career?

R: You make lots of money, relatively large sums of money. . . . A lot of prestige.

C. (female)

I: Why did you pick the area of business or commerce?

R: Well, it's got to do with career sorts of things and money expectations, where people are hiring. And I really didn't know what was left, that kind of thing. 'Cause you've got your basic areas, for me anyway, as far as business and that goes.

I: What are you getting out of your education right now?

R: I think I'm basically here because I know I want a university education and I don't really want to work right now. And I guess I really don't know what else to do, where else to go.

---

[2] The following are interview fragments selected from recent full transcripts. They illustrate either exemplary or problematic types of responses. Often, too little information is included in a fragment to make a valid rating. After reading a number of responses, however, the reader should have a clear enough idea to be able to begin to score identity interviews.

D. (male)

I: How did you happen to choose economics as a major?

R: Because of my surroundings, I guess. Surroundings such as meeting the kind of students that are sort of streamlined into one field. And they happen to be in economics. So I had an association with my friends who were in before I started my post-secondary education. I picked up the goal from them.

E. (male)

I: So, did you ever seriously consider anything else or did this [criminology] always seem most interesting to you?

R: Well, I've never considered anything else. But being in university now—well, I'm on academic probation right now—I'm finding it tough. And if things don't improve considerably, I'm thinking of, we'll say, taking a couple of years off.

I: Do you know what you might do?

R: No. Just, I guess, labor work probably, maybe for a while.

I: If you decide to take a year or two off, would it be with the intention of coming back or would it be up in the air?

R: It's hard to say. It's hard to say what job—it depends on the job. And if I was satisfied with the work I was doing, I don't think I'd come back. But today you either have to have an education or a trade, one of the two. Well, that's the way I feel, anyway. And with the job selection now, they're picking the cream of the crop. Or actually, it's who you know too, which helps me quite a lot.

Comments

A. This person chose to attend a particular university and selected a particular major as a matter of convenience. If something else appears that is both interesting and easy, she will probably go in that direction.

B. B also chose to attend the university as a matter of convenience. What attracts him about his current major does not seem to reflect a thoughtful integration of his abilities and some potential vocation, but the (unrealistically) perceived prestige and power of that vocation.

C. This individual wants to get a job, and thinks she will get a better one if she goes to a university. She is probably right, but it is the marketplace that will vocationally define her, not herself.

D. This is a fairly good example of a vocation finding a person. There is a Foreclosure quality to the response; but it is so offhand, and is occurring so relatively late in adolescence, that one suspects the depth of commitment. It is likely that if there were new friends, there might be a new major.

E. There is a possibility here of a development out of Diffusion. The academic probation may result from the kind of lack of motivation that can change with some experience in the work world. There is not a sufficient sense of struggle to call the respondent a Moratorium, but the willingness to accumulate experience and the general tentativeness suggest possible future movement.

Foreclosure

The Foreclosure is certain about vocational direction, and this has been an important identity element for him or her for a number of years. Usually, a discernible parental or other authority's influence is in the background. Even if one cannot determine a specific figure, if the vocational direction was determined very early, and little thought was given to alternatives, then Foreclosure is the only appropriate designation. The assumption is that any vocational decision made during latency is heavily influenced by adults, and that if this effect continues unmodified into late adolescence, the work of identity construction has not taken place.[3]

Examples

A. (male)

I: How did you decide on law as a career goal?

R: I grew up on law. I've always had an interest for it. I guess I've grown up with it. (His father is a lawyer.)

I: Did you ever consider going into to something other than law?

R: Ya—there's all sorts of things I've considered, but they're not really plausible for me. Law is the only thing that I've seriously considered.

I: Is that wrapped up with the fact that your father is in law?

R: Most definitely. Of course, he'd like to see me get into it, but I don't think that's necessarily the reason I'm doing it. I think he would be happy whatever I did.

I: Do you have any ideas of what branch of law you'd like to go into?

R: No, I'm fairly easy on that.

B. (female)

I: Did your parents have any career plans for you, something they'd like to see you go into?

R: No, but I think they're really happy with what I'm doing now.

I: What if they said, "No, [accounting] is a terrible profession and you'd be unhappy at it." How much weight would that have?

R: Probably quite a bit because we're a pretty close family. So I probably would have sat down and really thought about it

[3] Foreclosure on an occupation does not mean that the individual will necessarily be less successful in that occupation than one who is in the Identity Achievement status in the same field. This qualification particularly applies to the arts; Mozart comes to mind.

then [to decide] if that's really the right . . . thing for me. But they didn't do anything like . . . that.

C. (female)

I: What would you like to do with [a bachelor's degree in nutrition]?
R: I'm in the area of dietetics and so I would be working as a dietician, preferably in a hospital.
I: When did you decide upon that as a career choice?
R: Last year.
I: What about prior to that?
R: Prior to that, I knew that I liked working with food and . . . I also was looking for something. Something science-oriented and I just more or less combined the two and figured that was what I wanted.
I: In high school, did you have any set career plans?
R: No, I just more or less knew that I wanted something . . . science-oriented, so I took the sciences.
I: What about your parents? What kinds of jobs or careers have they been doing?
R: My mom's a nurse and my dad's a dentist.
I: Was there [any] influence about the health sciences as . . . you were growing up?
R: There was no direct influence . . . but there more or less was the influence, if not directly, it was indirect, just . . . by their being who they were.
I: Was there ever a time when you felt a fair degree of indecision or conflict about your interests, academic . . . and professional?
R: Yeah, there was. There was a time when I wasn't too . . . sure whether I wanted to go and get a linguistics degree . . . preferably leading to audiology and speech sciences. I took a few linguistics courses, but I found that it . . . wasn't what I wanted to [do] . . . take a program. I wouldn't have wanted three or four years of it. So I decided that I should return [to] something that I was initially interested in.
I: What attracts you to being a dietician?
R: First, it's a helping profession and that in itself is one of the major things that attracts me to it . . . the degree part of it attracts me, too. It could lead to further programs. . . .
I: What other things do you think you might possibly diverge to?
R: If I had to? I would think microbiology and . . . maybe medicine. I've also always wanted to get my music degree, which is something I may work on next year or the year after.
I: How certain or tentative are [your] plans?
R: About 70 percent.
I: What about staying within the sciences, health sciences in particular?
R: Very certain. I would always look for something in that area.

Comments

A. A is an almost classic example of a Foreclosure. Although he says he considered "all sorts of things," the ease with which this idea is dismissed, as well as its nonspecificity, disqualify it as a statement indicating exploration. Frequently, Foreclosures, like this person, deny that they are going into an area because of their parents' wishes. It is not especially fashionable to admit this choice. However, when an exploratory period is absent, and the individual's choice is strongly similar to the parents' wishes, then Foreclosure can be assumed.

B. This segment is presented because it illustrates two things: some creative probing by the interviewer, and the tendency of the Foreclosure individual to lapse into the first person plural ("we") when speaking of herself or himself.

C. Example C presents a difficult scoring issue. Was there a genuine exploratory period in linguistics? Did taking courses in this area represent a real divergence from earlier parent-supported childhood directions? Two aspects of this interview fragment lead to a scoring of Foreclosure: the individual's statement about her parents' "indirect" influence, and her persistence in health sciences—even linguistics would have led to audiology and probably to speech therapy. (The music area should have been pursued further by the interviewer.) Based upon this fragment, a scorer would be wise to record a possible element of Identity Achievement. Hence, the suggested scoring is *F*(IA).

Moratorium

Moratoriums are engaged in exploration, which their tendency toward greater verbalization reflects. Often, one has the feeling of watching a conceptual tennis match as one alternative gets played off against another almost equally attractive option. Especially at late adolescence, however, Moratoriums are usually not all over the occupational map; they tend to be committed within a general area. Nor are they always intensely struggling; sometimes they are simply rationally considering alternatives and attempting to reach a resolution. Nevertheless, to be called Moratorium, they must appear concerned and they must be actively exploring alternatives with the aim of arriving at a vocational commitment.

Examples

A. (male)

I: Do you have a clear goal of what you want to do?

R: Not a specific goal. It's broad. I haven't narrowed it down and determined it, but part of going to university was to try to determine what I want to do. I have specific interests—I've declared a major in communications. So I think I'm going to stick with that. I have a real interest in things like public relations and advertising right now. I'm also doing this 100-level psychology course and have developed an inkling of an interest in psychology. And so, who knows, I may pursue a minor in psychology or may even switch over and do that. I can't determine that just yet. I want to be in the academic environment, at least through my under-division classes, and then by the time I get into third and fourth year, I'll have a clearer objective in mind in terms of what I want to get out of university.

Comments

A. Moratoriums' responses tend to be lengthy. This fragment is taken from an eighty-minute interview. This example has most of the features of the Moratorium in vocation. He is vaguely committed within the general area of social sciences; he has some notion of the major leading to a future vocation; and he has constructed the broad outlines of a relevant plan. He is undecided, which one can observe in his back-and-forth style of response.

Identity Achievement

Identity Achieved persons will have seriously explored at least one viable alternative to their chosen occupation and will have begun to think of themselves as a *something* (e.g., a teacher, an engineer). They are not merely "going into" a field; their chosen occupation will have begun to be part of their identity, their self-definition. They emphasize more what they are going to *be* than what they are going to *do*. As a rule, this change is manifested in their already having sought work or volunteer experience in their vocational field.

Examples

A. (female)

I: When did you decide on your plans to take a master's degree in social work?

R: Last year.

I: How did that happen? How did you make that decision?

R: Just by volunteering and working in the social-work field. I have my social-work certificate, just from a B.A. level. I was in retail [sales] for a while and decided to go back into social work.

I: What has your experience been in that field?

R: I worked on a crisis line for about 3 years and I've done some marriage counseling and therapy, and I've also worked in a senior citizens' house for about a year now.

I: And so you feel fairly happy with that as a choice?

R: Yeah, pretty competent. It's just a matter of getting in and getting accepted now, and that's it.

I: Do you think your career plans now are very different in their goals than perhaps they were in high school?

R: Yeah, they are. They've changed a lot . . . they've changed from the sciences; I was going to go on for lab technician, and I was going to study biology—now I'm going into a helping profession just because of the experience I've had in it.

I: What led you to those experiences—that is, volunteering for a crisis line and other jobs?

R: I heard about it through college when I was first taking university transfer courses at the college level, about their needing people, and I just wanted to fill in maybe an extra eight hours a week . . . and then I really enjoyed it.

B. (female)

I: When did you decide to pursue computer technology?

R: I'm 30 years old now. . . . When I was 25 I started saving avidly to return to school. I realized I didn't want to be a secretary for the rest of my life. Working as a secretary, I had opportunities to learn various word-processing systems. In fact, I've learned four. I'm now teaching on a system that's quite sophisticated—a shared-resource system with a central processing unit. And so it's more than just word processing; it provided me with an introduction to microprocessors. And I seem to have an aptitude for it. And I thought, well that's a step if I do go back to school to do a business degree—a natural major may be computer science. . . . Another thing you have to consider when you go back to school late is that you have to pursue something that's going to be marketable. I can't afford the luxury of obtaining a degree in Canadian history or something. That's unfortunate.

I: Was there any planning or ideas from your parents to do something like this?

R: No. Unfortunately, my parents were of the school that a woman graduates from high school, gets married, and has babies. And so education wasn't necessary. It's unfortunate that I didn't get much encouragement from them, and that led me to go into secretarial college and become a secretary, because they more or less pushed me in that direction.

I: What do you envision doing in the future?

R: Well, I thoroughly enjoy teaching. I enjoy teaching a technical subject. I think that, given the growth of this technology, there will be room for people who enjoy teaching others how to operate various systems. For instance, I could see myself working for a vendor such as IBM or Xerox as, not a salesperson, but as a marketing support person.

Comments

Both A and B are examples of individuals who have made career decisions based upon experience with both their chosen career and alternatives. They are somewhat older than the usual upper-level college student; hence, they have had more opportunity to garner real-life experience. The elements of the Achievement process remain the same, however: a significant departure from earlier directions and a subsequent commitment, manifested behaviorally, in either a new direction or an old, reformulated one.

Religious Beliefs

Neither religion nor politics, per se, are the primary issues in this portion of the interview. These areas were chosen because they were the most likely to provide access to an individual ideology. One of the assumptions in psychosocial developmental theory is that as one moves from being a "taker" (childhood) to being a "caretaker" (adulthood), a shift in ideological framework occurs. Religious and political beliefs formulated in childhood are assumed to be relatively nonfunctional in adulthood. Even primitive societies provide rites of passage whose function is to update and confirm an earlier imposed identity. One can have an ideology that does not include religious *beliefs* but that resolves *questions*, such as the existence of God and standards for deciding moral issues. Asking questions about religious beliefs is a fairly easy entrance into the ideological realm; and responses indicating thoughtfulness about religious issues are taken as evidence for the ideological construction assumed to accompany identity formation. However, having or not having a religion is not the criterion for Identity Achievement; considering ideological issues in some depth is the criterion.

Here, as in other areas of the interview, content is not relevant for determining identity status. Whether or not one has a religion, per se, or what the content of that religion is, is not relevant for judging identity. The relevant issue is the depth and breadth of consideration the individual has given to ideological matters. Without a rationale, however, an individual is rated as higher in identity if he or she can specify a religious belief. When one listens to the religious portion of the identity status interview, the questions to be asked are: "Does this person have a coherent belief system?" "Is it identical with the one he or she adopted as a child?" "Has there been an exploration period—a time of weighing alternative outlooks?" "Is the person's current life behaviorally consistent with the stated beliefs?"

Sometimes, the individual interviewed grew up in a kind of ideological vacuum. A general decision rule says that if you spent your childhood in a diffuse context and you are currently diffuse, then you are scored Diffusion, not Foreclosure. There is also a possibility that an individual coming out of a diffuse context may "get religion," in some form, around late adolescence. How this change is seen depends upon the person's knowledgeability and commitment. If the respondent is both knowledgeable and committed, then a rating of either Achievement or Foreclosure is given depending upon the degree of rigidity shown. For example, if there has been no exploration of alternatives and none can be genuinely contemplated, then a rating of Foreclosure is given; however, if there appears to be a willingness to explore alternatives and the beliefs are somewhat flexibly held, the individual is scored Identity Achievement.

Another issue that arises about religion is the difference between a belief system and a cultural tradition. This distinction becomes especially important with respondents whose religions are closely tied to ethnic origins. If you say you are Jewish, the appellation can refer to religious beliefs, to ethnic origin or allegiance, to adherence to traditions, or to any combination of the three. The interviewer must determine what "being Jewish" (or being "Ukrainian Catholic") means to the subject. Even if the religious ideological aspect is missing, adherence to ethnic traditions may be sufficient to provide a sound basis for an identity.

Identity Diffusion

Diffusions are notable for their lack of thoughtfulness about the whole ideological realm. Often, they tend to see philosophy-of-life issues as a waste of time. They find nothing in the contemplation of such matters to be gratifying—thinking about the meaning of life is not much fun. Often Diffusions will have constructed a façade of an ideological system that they would like others to believe they espouse. That is, the stated ideology becomes a kind of currency they exchange for signs of respect and even affection from others. When this belief system is challenged by an able interviewer, however, its shallowness becomes obvious.

Typically, Diffusions' responses to questions in the religious domain are notable for their brevity. Often the interviewer will try to push to elicit more content, only to find that, in fact, "nobody's home." Another Diffusion pattern is a kind of oral smokescreen, throwing out complicated pseudo-sophisticated jargon ("I'm a pantheistic humanist."), in hopes of having it taken for knowledgeability. An interviewer must always ask for the content of a belief system and not just a label.

Examples

A. (male)

I: Do you have any particular religious affiliation or preference?
R: No.
I: Do you ever think about religious kinds of issues?
R: Occasionally.

I: Do you talk to people about it?
R: No, hardly ever. Unless there's some reason. I've taken a couple of philosophy courses, philosophy of religion. Just for interest, though. Not . . .
I: Did that answer any questions for you at all?
R: No, but it gave me a way to sort of think about it.
I: How does it come together for you, then?
R: I don't really have a belief or anything. Just—I don't know.

B. (female)

I: Do you have any particular religious views or philosophy of life?
R: No, it's hard to say. I'm taking a social psychology course right now that covers that. I'm not sure. I haven't really . . . I'm not against it, either. Like, I . . . really respect people with—people's religious views. . . . And, um, I don't know. I'm just kind of actually trying to decide for myself what—if I have any particular beliefs or not. Nothing that I know of. I like to keep an open mind, though, and kind of look at everything.

C. (male)

I: Were you brought up in the church?
R: Yeah, I was brought up in the Lutheran Church. . . . I went through confirmation and all that stuff when I was 14—at 14 you get confirmed—I was boarding and I was allowed not to go; I didn't have to go any more. And so that was just great; I didn't bother going any more. I don't have strong beliefs at all.
I: Did you ever have any particular feel for the whole thing?
R: I'm not religious at all. I know lots about it. . . . I have friends who are "born again" and all that. I've always kept a pretty open ear to it. If someone wants to be religious, that's fine with me . . . just don't knock at my door.
I: If you had children . . . ?
R: Oh, I'd probably put them through the Sunday-school program just to let them know a little bit of what's happening, rather than other people I've known who've grown up never having gone even to Sunday school, who are just total airheads on the whole.

Comments

A. Those unacquainted with identity status interviews may find the paucity of A's responses hard to believe in a college student. This type of ideologically impoverished response is much more frequent than one would like to believe.

B. This subject's emphasis on "openness" reminds one that the word can mean "empty" as well as "receptive."

C. C had the ingredients for a Foreclosure or Achievement, in that some early structure was provided. However, his current diffidence indicates Diffusion.

Foreclosure

Where Diffusions tend to be vacant on ideology, Foreclosures, especially in religion, are usually firm believers in the faith of their childhood. Almost all committed persons, Foreclosure or Achievement, say that their beliefs are different from their parents' and different from the beliefs they held as children. It is up to the interviewer to determine the validity of these claimed differences. If respondents say their beliefs have changed significantly since they were younger, then they should be able to articulate major departures. If a Roman Catholic has decided that the Virgin Birth is questionable, this choice does not indicate a major shift. However, if you were brought up Roman Catholic and have questioned the church's social policy and find yourself favoring birth control, abortion, a Marxist political stance, but denying the Pope's authority, then these positions do indicate a significant shift. Similarly, if a respondent says that his or her beliefs are different from the parents' beliefs because the respondent is more "liberal," this statement does not indicate a significant departure. An individual who can cite a period of major difference from the parental faith, such as disbelief or commitment to another religion, however, would not be scored Foreclosed.

Sometimes, one finds a respondent claiming the same religious beliefs as his or her parents held, but with very weak commitment. Here, as in the preceding section, the lack of commitment takes precedence over the lack of an exploratory period and the individual is called Diffusion, not Foreclosure.

Examples

A. (female)

I: Are you active in the church right now, in any type of religion?

R: Yeah, I'm Roman Catholic, and before I went to UBC I'd be going [to church] once every week.

I: Is your Catholic faith an important part [of your life]?

R: Yeah, it is . . . and I wouldn't give it up, and if I had any children I would hope that they would be religious. I guess I couldn't push it on them, but I would . . . try to influence them. I think it leads the way to a right way of life, better living.

I: You were exposed to the church when you were young and went to the catechism?

R: Yeah, for six years.

I: Are your parents still fairly religious right now?

R: My Mom is more religious, if you can measure religion at all, than my Dad. My Dad is Anglican and my Mom is Roman Catholic. She was an orphan when she was younger and was brought up in a convent . . . my Dad is religious; he attends church and doesn't say much about it. My Mom will say something about it if something needs to be said.

I: Was there ever a time when you seriously questioned or rejected your religious beliefs, the Catholic Church, and so on?

R: If I ever did reject my religious beliefs, I wouldn't be very happy with my life. I wouldn't have that focus or that basic ground. I have questioned it in a way.... I've always ended up criticizing [others'] points of view [on religion]. I don't think I'd ever give up my religious point of view.

I: Is there much indecision or conflict right now [about your beliefs]?

R: There's no conflict. I'll always believe that way. I will always be stable... you can't measure or judge some things. Some things have to be experienced. Some things just are, and there's nothing that you can do to say "this isn't right," because you can't actually see or measure [them]. Some things just are.

B. (male)

I: Do you have a particular religious preference or belief system?

R: Yes, I've been brought up in the Lutheran Church since I was little. I was in a church school in elementary school. And I did catechism and confirmation, and everything. I've been brought up and so that's my preference. Just because of the way I was brought up.

C. (female)

I: Do you have any religious preferences or beliefs?

R: I'm Roman Catholic by birth.

I: What does that mean to you?

R: I believe mostly everything that they teach me in my faith (although) there are some things that I'm kind of doubtful on... a few little technical things like they say that during the Mass the bread that they have is changed actually into the body of Jesus Christ, and I'm not so sure about that.

I: What do you do when you have these kinds of questions or you feel skeptical about some issues? Do you try to resolve the issues or just keep them in mind?

R: I just keep them in mind. I [sometimes] discuss it with my friends [but] most of them are really strong R.C. and they think that I'm silly for even thinking about things like [that]. Sometimes I discuss religion with my parents; they're really strong R.C.s too, and so if I go into anything in any detail at all, they get nervous.

I: Are those issues very important for you, or are they very minor issues?

R: They're minor issues.

I: Are you very active in going to church?

R: I go to church every Sunday and I do volunteer work with my church.
I: Do you think that your views are the same as they've always been?
R: Yeah . . . there's not been much change at all.

D. (male)

I: Do you have any particular religious beliefs?
R: We're Sikhs.
I: Has there ever been a time when you questioned [your beliefs] or thought about doing something else?
R: No, I haven't thought about doing something else.
I: If you had children, how would you bring them up?
R: I guess I would teach them the same things I learned in my religion.
I: Do you think there's any chance that in the future you'd start to question [your beliefs] or change your mind about them?
R: No.

Comments

A. Although somewhat lengthy, A is included because her "absolute" beliefs are typical for Foreclosures. "Believing" is equated with "stability"—probably referring to psychological health.

B. B illustrates the embeddedness of the Foreclosure in his or her family. To be a member of this person's family is to accept their brand of Christianity: not accepting that might lead to ostracism from the family.

C. C furnishes a picture of what Foreclosures do if they have religious questions. First, the questions are not especially major (such as transubstantiation here); second, doubts are usually discussed with adherents of the same religion, so that one is fairly certain of a supportive rather than a confrontational audience.

D. D is included because of the respondent's immediate lapse into the first person plural when the question calls for an answer in the first person singular.

Moratorium

It is probably in the ideological area that the intensity of the Moratorium's struggle is most evident, and the interview is almost always interesting, although sometimes wearing. The possibilities considered can become fairly esoteric ("flaky" is a more accurate, though less kind, description). But one can usually distinguish the seriousness of the Moratorium's endeavor from the verbal smokescreen thrown up by an articulate Diffusion. Again, there should be *some* boundaries around the belief system and a movement toward resolution in the future.

Examples

A. (female)

I: Do you have any particular religious affiliations or preferences?

R: No, a particular nonaffiliation perhaps. I don't really believe in churches. It's funny, but religion to me all through our time has been the cause of the greatest conflict in the world. And for that reason I almost don't believe in it. (But) . . . I think people need, I think people naturally create their own beliefs, just for security. I think everybody sort of fears what's going to happen. So if they don't believe in God, as in whatever their church says God is, people tend to make up their own image of some sort. . . .

I: How does your own belief system work?

R: It's sort of . . . um. Well, it's very confused actually. And it's sort of always changing. Within my family, my brothers and sisters and that, we discuss it a lot . . . but I guess there is an all-over spirit, but it's not an "it." And it's within, it's ourselves. How to explain this? And so we are all part of this spirit.

I: Do you think your ideas will continue to change?

R: I think they'll probably continue to change. Every once in a while I think that what I think is so far out, probably compared to a lot of other people's religious beliefs. And therefore, I haven't completely formulated it and therefore, it's sort of combinations of discussions rather than reading. But I don't think I'll ever adopt a "Christian" religion.

B. (female)

I: How would you describe your spiritual beliefs?

R: Well . . . they don't at all conform with those expounded by most churches.

I: What are your beliefs?

R: It's hard to pin them down and get them out. It's a lot of a mixture of Zen with some . . . basically, it's more a belief in humanity rather than God. I don't think there is [a God], I think there's a certain degree of fate, but there is no "grand Master" up there playing us like a chess game and that you basically get what you deserve; that there must be some kind of tabulation going on as to how well or how poorly you are as an individual, how bad you are, and that you eventually pay for it in some direction or another. As to hereafter or heaven or whatever, I don't believe in any kind of a wonderful ending to it all, pie in the sky kind of thing. But I think there is some continuum after life. I don't think this is "it." I don't think it can be "it."

I: How did you decide that?

R: Just reading and speaking with people with strong religious beliefs, especially Christians.

I: So your parents' beliefs would be different than yours? Would they be more traditional?

R: Yes.
I: When did you start thinking about that or taking on that belief system?
R: It's been a gradual thing. You grow up with the Judeo-Christian ethic and you start to question it when you hit puberty; you find flaws in it . . . and then things have just expanded from there.
I: Do you feel confident in your position now, or are there still uncertainties for you?
R: I think there are areas of uncertainty but I'm confident that . . . I refuse to say that I'm right because there are so many religions that claim that they're right that I don't even think there even is one particular correct theory or view on religion. It's more or less a personal theory that you form yourself . . . but in what I believe, I think I'm fairly confident in it.

Comments

A. This is a fairly good example of a Moratorium in the midst of formulating a belief system. She has a vague idea about what it will look like when finished, and she differentiates it from Christianity. She is clearly involved in the exploratory process.

B. B is a bit further along than A in articulating a belief system. Both A's and B's ideas about religion have a do-it-yourself quality typical of Moratoriums. The in-process nature of the Moratorium is also evident in B's responses.

Identity Achievement

Persons who are called Identity Achievements have considered seriously at least one belief system different from their own, or have departed significantly from the belief (or no belief) position of their childhood, and have now located themselves within a definable structure to which they exhibit some behavioral commitment. They are not usually as definite about raising their children in their chosen faith as are Foreclosures. However, neither are they as laissez-faire as Diffusions or Moratoriums. They are not usually as interesting to listen to as Moratoriums; one hears more about the end of a process with Identity Achievements than about the process itself. There is a self-assuredness and comfortableness about their current position, but this is not the inflexibility or self-righteousness of the Foreclosure.

Examples

A. (male)

I: What do you believe in?
R: I definitely believe in the God of the Judeo-Christian Bible.

I: And your parents?
R: No particular belief—I suppose a humanistic world view, but not very consistently.
I: How did your beliefs come about?
R: I had rejected the whole tradition [as a young teenager]. At 18, I started going through some real questions about why I was doing what I was doing and whole-life issue questions . . . [such as]: "Where do we get our acceptance of others from?"; "How can we judge good and bad?"; and "Who am I?" My uncle presented me with the existential point of view. I was fairly attentive to the thinking I had unconsciously accepted as I grew up. Then I picked up the Bible and started reading it, and it seemed to be answering the questions that the other ones weren't.

B. (male)

I: Can you tell me about your religious beliefs?
R: I decided at this point that I'm agnostic. When people talk about God . . . and their belief in God, they deal with it in terms of a fear and I don't see it that way and I will continue to profess that, as Christians say God is supposed to be representative of love . . . you don't fear love. Until Christianity recognizes the inherent contradiction, I'm not prepared to accept it as my religion. It may even be a self-contradiction that even though I profess to be an agnostic, I believe that if, in fact, there is a God that we just have various levels of His acceptance of us or our acceptance of Him. I don't think that as Christianity preaches that if you don't accept Him as your eternal savior that you're condemned to the fiery depths of hell. If in fact God exists, He encompasses all people . . . I'm a very spiritual person, there's no question about it, but it's an individual or interpersonal thing.

C. (female)

I: Was there ever a time when you doubted or questioned your religious beliefs?
R: Yes, I would say by the time I was in high school I started questioning Christianity. . . . When you're a child, you think that Christianity is the only faith that exists, because in North America that is what is promoted. But then you find that half the population of the world follows some other kind of religion and you realize how relative it all is. I mean, does that mean that only the Christians are going to heaven, that the Moslems and so on are not? So you start asking a lot of questions about it. So for me, religion is more a guideline to being a good person and conducting your life in a brotherly fashion.
I: How did you resolve these questions?
R: Well, I did some reading. I read about the Moslem faith, and I did some reading about Buddhism. Then I realized that no one is going to know for certain what the right road to follow is, but that you can get something from them all. I think that

in life you can never go wrong adopting a certain code of ethics or morals that you can follow, and hopefully whatever God is up there—whether He be a Moslem God or a Christian God or whatever—is going to recognize that.

Comments

The examples presented illustrate three ways of arriving at an achieved position.

A. A had rejected traditional beliefs, and an "existential" authority figure, finally choosing what appears to be a fundamentalist, Bible-oriented position.

B. B defines himself as an agnostic, in opposition to establishment Christianity, but retains the ethic of Christian love. Defining oneself "in opposition" has a Moratorium quality to it; however, B. seems too committed to be scored as Moratorium. Probably an *IA*(*M*) scoring would be appropriate here.

C. C is a little vague about her final resolution, which sounds somewhat Universalist-Unitarian, although not labeled as such. However, it is clear that she has left her childhood position and that she does not seem to be struggling to achieve a resolution. In the absence of more information about the structure of her belief system, one might score this fragment *IA*(*D*).

Family/Career Priorities

Due to the recent upsurge in dual-career families, three additional identity domains have been developed (Archer, 1985a,c). These pertain to the roles of (1) spouse, (2) parent, and (3) the priority of family versus career. With extensive outside employment for women, changes in attitudes and behavior have been demanded of both sexes. As a consequence, these three domains have heightened salience for both males and females of this age as they invest in career preparation and romantic intimacy. The domain of family versus career prioritizing is elaborated here.

Because the majority of individuals in our society plan to be parents and the majority of women, while parenting, now work as well, the conflict of juggling these two time-consuming major life activities has created intense identity issues. Neither sex can easily evade the potential dilemma, because a conflict for one partner will lead to consequences for the other. The issues are whether one plans to pursue family and career goals, and, if so, do they have equal value? Or one goal, and if so, which one? What happens if one's partner has different values pertaining to the priorities of these goals? Because responses typically are very different when confronted with conflicts between being a spouse and having a career, and conflicts between being a parent and having a career, the interview was designed to ask these questions separately. The researcher has a choice: (1) score these two identity domains (spouse/career; parent /career) separately, (2) score one conflict only, or (3) use the more sophisticated of the two scorings if they differ. In essence, there is flexibility in the use of the family/career priority domain, affording a number of research questions about this area.

Commitment requires a clear statement of priority, which can be to (1) spouse/parent *or* career or (2) a dual priority of spouse/parent *and* career. One can use the knowledge obtained from the separate, more detailed spouse and parenting domains as well as vocational choice to enhance accuracy of scoring. Inconsistencies between what is said in this domain relative to the three domains mentioned earlier should be carefully recorded. The interviewer should have recognized and probed any lack of congruence among the areas. For example, the content of a respondent's parenting domain may be filled with examples of planned dedication to children. And yet, the content of the subsequent family/career priority domain for the same respondent may reveal career priority with expectations that the children will cope somehow.

Priorities should be supported with knowledgeable statements about the effort to be invested in each of the domains. Respondents should be able to project into the future how they will live out their priority. Although implementation of these priorities may not be feasible in the present, their activities in preparing for adulthood should be consistent with the expressed priorities. Furthermore, although some uncertainty may remain about their ability to carry through with their plans, they should be basically satisfied with the priority chosen.

Exploration is exemplified by activity in the present directed to acquiring knowledge in order to understand and choose realistic priorities. Respondents should at least be able to provide a sketchy outline of perceived conflicts. Again, the emotional tone should denote genuine desire to resolve this dilemma in the near future.

Scorers should keep the naiveté of the respondents in mind. Lack of experience in most of these domains easily results in unrealistic notions about implementing several goals at the same time. Also, egocentrism of youth may result in unrealistic and unfair assumptions about the roles a partner may pursue that would negate the necessity of conflict.

Identity Diffusion

Males are more typically Identity Diffuse in this area than are females. Usually, no sense of possible conflict between the roles is articulated. For those who recognize the potential for conflict, the assumption arises that it is the partner's problem, not theirs. For the most part, Diffusion in this domain takes the form of apathy.

In some instances, there may be marginal concern. If these areas are not to be dealt with directly for a number of years, however, the issues may not prompt investments of energy relative to other more immediate life concerns and goals.

Examples

A. (male)

I: Do you think there will be any conflict between being a husband and pursuing a career?
R: No.
I: If you were confronted with a conflict, which would you give priority to?
R: Whichever mattered more at the time.
I: Would it be difficult to decide which mattered more?
R: No.
I: How about between parenting and career?
R: Same thing goes.
I: How much concern have you had about this?
R: None.

B. (female)

I: Do you think there will be any conflict for you between being a parent and having a career?
R: No, a job is a job. And I don't know if I want kids or not.
I: If you were confronted with a conflict, what would you do?
R: Depends. If I have to work, I have to work. If the kid's real sick or something, then I have to take care of him.
I: Would it be a difficult decision?
R: No. You do what you have to do.

C. (male)

I: Do you anticipate any conflict . . . ?
R: Why should there be conflict? She does what I expect and there's no problem. I'm the breadwinner and she'd better take care of the kids. They're her problem.

Comments

A. The cursory answers with no attempt at elaboration make the apathy of the respondent apparent.

B. This respondent lacks enthusiasm for either role. She intends to do what is most necessary at the time.

C. Occasionally an Alienated Diffusion emerges. In this case, there is no genuine discussion of the advantages and disadvantages of different perspectives. Rather, the respondent dictates demands, placing all responsibility for undesired tasks elsewhere. We hear no acknowledgment of the potential consequences of expectations.

Foreclosure

This is perhaps the most common approach to the conflict domain for both sexes. The commitment typically comprises placing the highest priority on children. However, some adolescents choose either a dual, spouse, or career priority. Significant others often play an important role in this domain. Typically, a spouse or potential spouse, as well as the adolescent's parents' perceived approaches to such conflicts strongly influence the respondent's choice.

For Foreclosures, conflict is rarely anticipated because a priority has been determined and will be honored. That priority has never been questioned by the respondent. Playing devil's advocate as an interviewer seems to annoy many Foreclosures about this domain. As they project their plans into the future, there is no wavering from the perceived plan. Interestingly, potential barriers are simply not acknowledged or tolerated. The tendency is to shrug them off.

Examples

A. (female)

I: Do you think there will be any conflict between being a wife and having a career?
R: No.
I: If you were confronted with a conflict between your responsibilities as a wife and your work responsibilities, which would you give priority to?
R: My husband because he's more important than my job.
I: Have you ever been concerned that there might be such a conflict?
R: No.
I: Do you think there will be any conflict between being a parent and pursuing a career?
R: No, that will be my career.
I: How would you compare your ideas with those of your parents?
R: About the same. They always thought we came first.
I: How do you feel about that?
R: Your children should come first. If they don't, you shouldn't be a parent.
I: How does the person you're presently in a relationship with feel?
R: The same.

B. (male)

I: If you were confronted with a conflict between your responsibilities as a husband and your work responsibilities, which would you give priority to?
R: My wife. A job is a job and there's always one out there. I can switch from field to field, but my wife is, she's it.
I: . . . conflict between being a parent and pursuing a career?
R: Not yet, no.

I: Do you foresee any?
R: I really couldn't say.
I: How would you compare your ideas with those of your parents?
R: My mom was always there. The family comes first, she always said. The roof over the head has to be there and food always has to be in the stomach. I always agreed with that.

C. (female)

I: Do you think there will be any conflict for you between being a wife and pursuing a career?
R: No, because R stays home now and takes care of the housework. I know that if we both worked, we would share things that had to get done around the house. I don't think he would ever object to me having a career.
I: Do you think there will be any conflict between being a parent and pursuing a career?
R: If I got to that point, that R . . . gave me an ultimatum between being his wife or having a career that I wanted, I think I would choose the career. I have my own mind and I know I would never stop him from having the career he wanted and I feel he should do the same for me.
I: How have you arrived at this conclusion?
R: Just by always getting my own way and knowing that I'm my own person. I have just as many rights as anybody does to make decisions for myself.

Comments

A. This is a very typical Foreclosure dialogue. Straightforward, clear objectives are stated without hesitation. No conflict is anticipated. This is no surprise because she is surrounded by people of similar perspective.

B. Although B seems to sense a possible conflict upon the arrival of children, he has no intention of pursuing that potential thought. Also, it is interesting that family comes first, yet the content agreed to is "roof over the head and food in the stomach." Considerations about the extent of time spent on family versus job to make money for the roof and food isn't even generated. As with Respondent A, the voice is firm and determined. Again, we find agreement with significant others, namely the parents.

C. This female expects remarkably smooth sailing. This is what I want, what I typically get, and that's the way it will continue to be. She assumes reciprocity—that is, if I don't interfere with your plans, you won't interfere with mine. Notice that, when asked the parenting question, she heard it as a spouse issue.

Moratorium

Females are more likely to be in Moratorium about this conflict than are males, particularly upper-class females. As the realities of career and family appear, females are more likely to begin to plan a timetable for various goals. Male college professors who are fathers appear harried infrequently. But the female college professor model, juggling career and family, typically does. Also, female models are more likely to openly discuss these kinds of difficulties with students than are male models. Furthermore, students are more likely to address such concerns or curiosities to married professional women. It is a conflict addressed in Psychology of Women and Sociology of the Family courses. Therefore, it appears to be a female issue.

In the context of home, working mothers are still more likely than fathers to be seen cooking, cleaning, *and* doing their homework if they have returned to school. They are also likely to complain and resent their exhaustion. Men who are attempting equitable sharing of parenting and home responsibilities exemplify similar pressure but, unfortunately, they continue not to be the norm.

The typical conflict is, "Can I do it all?" Without having experienced "all," it is difficult to realistically judge this conflict. The knowledgeability demonstrated by youths about this area is therefore typically unrealistic. Those whose mothers have dual priorities sometimes better understand the juggling. But it is interesting how little youths appear to attend to their parents' activities and difficulties.

As indicated, primary activity directed toward gathering information includes talking with individuals who have chosen different priorities, taking such courses as Psychology of Women or Sociology of the Family, reading articles on the topic, and observing individuals who are in the situation.

To be scored Moratorium, individuals should be able to discuss the elements of the priority issues that concern them. As in the other domains, a decision in the near future should be desired. The primary concern is typically between parenting and career. Spouses can manage on their own, but children are dependent on you. Some concern is also expressed about the quality of day care. Once children are in a regular school program, concerns for them decrease dramatically. For example, latchkey issues are addressed among adults today but atypically by late adolescents.

Spouses, too, can be of concern to this age group. Remember that many males and females, as youths, are trying to establish successful intimate relationships. They may express concern about jeopardizing such partnerships for the sake of careers that they have not yet begun.

Examples

A. (male)

I: Do you think there will be any conflict for you between being a husband and pursuing a career?

R: I have been in conflict about that for some time. It's the kind of thing in which I have to decide which is more important. If something good came along now, would I decide to get married right away and jeopardize my career or would I go on with my career and hope that something else came along?

I: How do you think it will interfere?

R: I really don't have any concrete answer for that yet. But other people keep talking about it so it's got me worried. I'm not one for getting married today and finding myself divorced tomorrow because of my career.

I: Do you think there will be any conflict between being a parent and pursuing a career?

R: I don't think there would be much of a problem with parenting and a career. To be a parent, I would pretty much have to be a husband.

B. (female)

I: Do you think there will be a conflict between being a spouse and pursuing a career?

R: No. You're both adults. You know you need the income from both of you. I might have to compromise and take a lesser job if a problem arose like relocation. But I think he would help me find work that suited me. He knows how much I enjoy art advertising.

I: Do you think there will be a conflict between being a parent and pursuing a career?

R: Lord, yes! I'm petrified. Who's going to take care of a little baby, so helpless and dependent on you. I don't think I could bear to leave it. And yet I don't want my career jeopardized if I found something I really liked. You see, I figure by the time I have a baby, I'll be well into my career. I've probably invested three or four years of my life in it. I can see taking maternity leave. I'd like that. But then what? Day care, nursery schools? Am I a rotten mother? Suppose he cries when I try to leave him off. I've seen my sister's child try to cling to her. She puts her down, says good-bye, goes out to the car, and cries. I dread this.

C. (female)

I: Do you anticipate any conflict between being a parent and having a career?

R: Well, I'm a mother now. And yes, there is a lot of conflict. I love my son. When he grins up at me, no matter how ornery he's been, my heart melts. But frankly, I'm going crazy home all the time. I take a course here or there. But I don't want to stay home forever. I really want a career like I had originally planned.

I: How do you think you'll resolve this conflict?

R: I don't know yet. I mean, I'll probably have one or two more kids. Where do I fit in school or work? Stopping and starting gets you all messed up. But I'll be so old by the time I'm ready for a career, who would take me? Do you know how hard it is to juggle school and a kid? I listen to other 21-year-olds. Boy are they in for a shock. And if there are more kids . . .

I: When do you think you'll resolve this issue?

R: I'm not sure. But I need to soon. I've got to plan carefully if I'm really going to try for both. I just don't know. . . .

Comments

A. This male respondent's anticipated conflict is between spouse and career but not between parent and career. His statement, "it gets me pretty worried" is a sign of Moratorium. However, the scorer should then look for activity directed toward resolving that dilemma. The "other people keep talking" could be construed as one such sign of his listening to the problem for possible resolutions.

B. This female has the reverse conflict. Her sister is apparently functioning as a dual-priority model who experiences stress over the process. As the respondent projects into her future, the conflict arises over a young infant-preschooler's care once her career is well established. She seemed willing to negotiate with her husband about relocation but perhaps she is reflecting flexibility early in the relationship, which decreases as career involvement increases. Interestingly, she identifies no support system for her future.

C. This mother has realistic information because she is already juggling parenthood and part-time school. Does she push her schooling and opt for a career and/or have more babies? As she assesses her timetable, she is overwhelmed about her ability to fit it all in. Notice that she, too, volunteers no support system to help her.

Identity Achievement

To be Identity Achieved in this domain, respondents should be able to discuss knowledgeably the pros and cons of the alternatives that have been considered and justify the option they chose as most personally expressive. They should be engaged in behavior that is congruent with this option, even though the priority may not be implemented until some later time. The emotional tone should be somewhat relaxed, although if a dual priority is chosen, there may be apprehension about its feasibility. Respondents should also be able to project their plans into the future, revealing the time line for the occurrence of whichever priorities are chosen.

Models may play a significant role in the choices, but assessment of alternatives is essential to Achiever status scoring. In other words, doing as advised by a model, without considering options, would generate Foreclosure status scoring.

Examples

A. (female)

I: Do you think there will be any conflict for you between being a wife and pursuing a career?

R: No.

I: If you were confronted with a conflict between your spouse and work responsibilities, to which would you give priority?

R: Except in cases of illness, my career. I've realized that I must marry someone of like mind, i.e., career oriented, or I won't marry.

I: How did you arrive at this decision?

R: Actually, I was in a muddle for a while. My parents were hassling me about marriage and kids. I was expending energy on my courses, talking about my plans to become president of a corporation. For a while they had me feeling guilty and selfish. But when I really looked at myself—what I enjoy, what I'm good at, it fell into place. Marriage and children are their priority, not mine. I was really relieved when I figured that one out. Now I just ignore my parents and am happily preparing for my career.

B. (male)

I: Do you think there will be any conflict between being a parent and pursuing a career?

R: I didn't use to think so. In fact, I didn't give it a thought. I just planned to do what my folks did. But here at the college, a couple of my professors, some of the guys, have been talking about parenting/career conflict. Two of them even brought their little kids to class. At first it ticked me off. But then I kind of got into seeing their pleasure with the kids. They even canceled class when their kids got sick, explaining that their wives stayed home last time and it was now their turn. Hearing the girls talk, appreciating what these profs were doing, made me sort of reverse roles and think from their perspective. At some frat parties, we actually got into heated debates about who's responsible for what.

I: How much concern do you have about this?

R: Lots. I realize now that the only way having a career wife is going to work is if I pull my weight at home. I expected to do some cooking and cleaning. I do that now. But it's a lot more than that. I don't want to be bored with a housewife. My mom doesn't do anything. Dad sits in front of the TV. No, that won't do now. I'm even rethinking my career goals. I mean if I get really invested, keep reaching, I could lose cvcrything. I've got to find the right balance of things. It looks tricky.

I: When do you think you might have this conflict resolved?

R: Well, outside of figuring the balance out, I know what the priorities are going to have to be. I've got to make time for

> my wife and kids. I'd like my wife to stay home with the kids when they're real little, but if it would hurt her career, we've got to work out some compromises like my profs have.

Comments

A. This college woman has chosen to make career her priority. Her own parents triggered her conflict over marriage and parenting versus career for her. "For a while they had me feeling guilty . . ." and "I was really relieved . . ." signal the conflict and its resolution. Her introspection, "really looked at myself . . ." exemplifies appropriate activity. She now projects into the future with a positive and enthusiastic emotional tone.

B. This respondent should receive a primary scoring of Achiever although there are secondary elements of Moratorium. He has resolved the major issue of priority, "I know what the priorities are going to be . . ." but he has continued concerns about implementation, which may include some minor identity issues yet in another domain—"If I got really invested, keep reaching. . . ." Initially, he had opted for his parents' approach. Models of a different perspective caused dissonance. He engaged in activity to assess the pros and cons, such as "heated debates" and has subsequently changed his orientation.

10
Identity Status During the Adult Years: Scoring Criteria

Alan S. Waterman and Sally L. Archer

According to the identity theory developed in this book, the stages of adolescence and youth are the times in the life span when identity formation is of principal concern. The adult years are viewed as the time when the identity decisions reached earlier are implemented and the individual experiences most deeply the rewards and costs of the commitments that have been made (or the lack thereof). As adults, our self-definitions are repeatedly tested and few if any of the elements comprising our previously established sense of identity are likely to survive unmodified. Identity research with adults is of particular interest on two accounts: (1) to learn the long-term consequences of utilizing the various identity processes during the previous stages in development, and (2) to understand the circumstances leading to reappraisal of previously established identity commitments during the adult years and the differences between the ways in which identity crises are handled by adults compared to adolescents and youths.

For the purposes of this chapter, the adult years are considered to extend from the mid-twenties until the late fifties or early sixties. The fate of identity among the elderly is not considered here, and would undoubtedly require its own scoring manual. Even a span of three-and-a-half decades is almost certainly too broad for one scoring manual, but the extent of the research that has been carried out with adults does not now permit the finer distinctions that should become possible in future years. Still, the statements in this chapter should be interpreted in the context of where in the adult years a respondent falls.

The Meaning of Exploration and Commitment in Adulthood

Exploration

In scoring identity interviews with adults, it should be recognized that relevant crisis can occur at any time from adolescence to the present.

When a past crisis occurred during the high school or college years, the scoring criteria pertaining to the identification of crises during those stages should apply (see Chapters 8 and 9, respectively). As described here, when an identity crisis occurs during the adult years, it will differ in marked ways from those experienced earlier in the life span.

The shifting criteria for the meaning of exploration with increasing age poses an important problem for understanding the Identity Achievement status. The definition of the Identity Achievement status involves a history of exploring alternatives leading to the formation of personally meaningful commitments. No qualification is made as to how recently any past crisis may have occurred. For example, an individual of age 45 could be considered an Identity Achiever whether the crisis occurred at age 16, 26, or 36. It may at first seem incongruous to give the same status scoring in each of these instances, for the quality or subjective nature of the crisis experience is likely to have been quite different depending on the age at which it occurred. Nevertheless, the *process* of identity formation is the same and therefore the same status scoring applies. At the same time, it is appropriate to make note of differences in the timing of identity crises because comparisons can appropriately be made between adult Identity Achievers whose crises occurred early in life with those whose crises occurred at a later age.

There is one exception to considering an early identity crisis as relevant to the placement in the Identity Achievement status for an adult. Because that which is important for scoring purposes is the origins of the person's goals, values, and beliefs, we must ask whether the early crisis contributed meaningfully to the current commitments. If the questions forming the content of the crisis have little or no bearing on the current commitments, the crisis should not be viewed as having scoring significance.

As mentioned in Chapter 7, scoring for identity crises at earlier times in an individual's life will depend upon the respondent's memory for prior events having implications for identity formation. Of particular importance is that what was seen to have great significance to an adolescent or youth at the time, may in retrospect seem to have been of little consequence. As a result, it may not be reported in the interview except under careful questioning. Thus, both when conducting identity interviews with adults and when scoring, one should, to the extent possible, try to gain an appreciation of the meaning of events in a person's life at the time at which they occurred.

Recognize too that an individual may have experienced an identity crisis within a particular domain on several occasions. Normally, this experience will pose no problem for arriving at an identity status scoring. However, as with the timing of an identity crisis, the presence of multiple crises should be recorded because it will allow for comparisons between individuals having multiple crises and those having only one.

In the material that follows, the focus is on the criteria for identity crises, as these are observed to occur during the adult years.

Knowledgeability

Higher standards for knowledgeability can more appropriately be applied to adults than to high school or college students. Their broader life experiences and the longer time they have had in which to accumulate information should be translated into greater specificity in their descriptions of the alternatives they are considering or have previously considered as adults.

Activity Directed Toward the Gathering of Information

Here too, higher standards may be seen as applying to crises during the adult years. Adults have had the opportunity to learn more about how to acquire relevant information and can be expected to be more efficient in their efforts to learn what may be helpful in resolving a crisis. Where a person appears to be emotionally distressed but is taking no useful action in working toward a resolution, there is reason to believe that the emotional reaction itself is serving some psychodynamic or sociodynamic purpose (e.g., as an excuse for failure or a bid for sympathy) and that the issue is not, at its center, an identity crisis.

Evidence of Considering Alternative Potential Identity Elements

Both the patterns of simultaneously available alternatives and the successive exploration of alternatives observed at earlier ages are found to characterize adult crises as well. About the latter pattern, for adults there has been more time in which different options may have been acted upon. Whenever the person appears to have gone through several distinctly different phases in life with respect to a particular domain, it should be presumed that this represents the previous exploration of alternatives. This would be the case even when there appears to be no focalized crisis in which the person was trying to make important life decisions in a self-reflective manner. (Although we recognize that this conclusion is somewhat troublesome, it seems more appropriate than defining someone Foreclosed who has acted in very different ways at varying times in his or her life and now possesses clear commitments.)

Emotional Tone

Where identity crises during the stages of adolescence and youth may be initially exhilarating and the process of exploration enjoyed as one's horizons expand, this will seldom be the case for adults experiencing a mid-life crisis. During the adult years, identity crises usually involve overturning established patterns of activity, giving up the known for the unknown. Although the old goals or values are seen as no longer fitting the individual in current circumstances, the prospect of having to find new options is more likely to generate anxiety than enthusiasm. Adults usually feel that they should already have established viable answers to identity questions. Indeed, the necessity for change may be expressed as representing some personal failure in life rather than the opportunity for personal growth. With the successful resolution of the crisis, however, adults will often report that in retrospect it was a valuable, if sometimes painful, experience.

Commitment

Adulthood differs from adolescence and youth in that it is a time for implementing the decisions that were made during the earlier stages. The commitments of high school and college students are largely anticipatory, focused on the assumed rewards, both intrinsic and extrinsic, of any commitment. In contrast, adults are living with both the real rewards and the real costs that derive from putting their goals, values, and beliefs into practice. As a consequence, the descriptions of commitments made will be more balanced and, in some circumstances, ambivalent. In concluding whether a goal, value, or belief warrants being called an identity commitment, the scorer should decide whether it is indeed personally expressive for the respondent.

Knowledgeability

As with the criteria of knowledgeability discussed for exploration (crisis), a higher standard for knowledgeability for commitment exists at this stage than at previous stages. However, recognize too that a high level of knowledgeability can exist with no sense of personal commitment in the area about which the person is so knowledgeable. For example, an abstract understanding of political concepts can exist without any felt investment in a particular ideology.

Activity Directed Toward Implementing the Chosen Identity Element

Again, because adulthood is a stage when implementation of goals, values, and beliefs is to be expected, a higher standard for activity should be employed here than in previous stages. It is hard to maintain that a belief is indeed a personally expressive aspect of the respondent's identity where statements of beliefs are made without supportive activity.

Emotional Tone

Among adults, the emotional tone associated with commitment may range from the enthusiastic to the matter-of-fact. The excitement of anticipation often found among adolescents and youths may have been replaced by a calmer sense of centeredness. The person has been doing what he or she wants to do, perhaps for an extended period, and is well acquainted with both its benefits and its drawbacks. This type of balanced assessment does not detract from the quality of the commitment to the chosen course of action, provided it is perceived that the benefits clearly outweigh the costs. In contrast, where matter-of-fact description of current activities appears to reflect the unthinking carrying out of routines, it is doubtful that an identity commitment can be said to exist. Similarly, where the costs of an activity outweigh the benefits, even when the activity is of long standing, it cannot be viewed as personally expressive and, therefore, its duration does not indicate commitment.

The interpretation of self-critical statements is relevant for scoring identity commitments. Among adults, the wistful expression of missed opportunities when accompanied by general satisfaction with one's choices does not reflect the absence of commitments. "If only . . ." and "If I had it to do over . . ." statements may reveal only the individual's capacity for learning from experience. The same types of statements, when more extreme in tone and in the absence of expressed satisfaction with one's life, contradict commitment. Self-criticism ranging in intensity from moderate to severe also constitutes evidence for the absence of commitments. When the person is taking coherent action to redirect the pattern of living, this act suggests placement in the Moratorium status. However, in the absence of such activity, scoring in the Diffusion status is more appropriate.

Identification with Significant Others

Identification figures generally do not play a major role in commitments formed during the adult years; there are, however, exceptions. Perhaps the person most frequently serving as a source of potential identity commitments is the respondent's spouse. Differences between marital partners in goals, values, and beliefs may become a stimulus for rethinking ideas that had previously been established or developing commitments for the first time in an area that had not, until then, been a source of personal concern. Other potential model figures are college professors for respondents returning to college, mentors encountered in connection with their employment, and spiritual leaders of religious organizations with which they are affiliated.

Although the presence of strong identification figures is suggestive of a foreclosure process in the formation of identity commitments, the situation is complicated by the older age of the individuals involved. If the circumstances are such that the respondent had never previously expressed serious concern with the domain in question, then scoring in the Foreclosure category is indeed warranted. If, however, the person has a history of established beliefs in the area and, as a function of exposure to the model, those views are markedly changed, then scoring for the Identity Achievement status may be more appropriate. The greatest confidence in such a conclusion will exist where the respondent discusses the experience of conflict in the renunciation of the old belief and the adoption of the new. Where the new belief system is taken over fully formed and without serious questioning, the Foreclosure scoring may still be justified. (Because these conditions are most frequently encountered in connection with religious conversion, we refer you to the discussion of the religious domain later in this chapter for elaboration of this problem).

Projection of One's Personal Future

Because, as we have seen, adulthood is a stage of implementation, the criterion of projection into the future may hold less relevance. The sense of continuity from past, to present, and into the future should still be evident in the interview. However, in the adult years, once decisions are made, it is not usually necessary to delay for any substantial time their implementation. In that sense, it can be said that adults live more in the present than do either adolescents or youths.

Resistance to Being Swayed

Of all the age groups, adults with identity commitments should be the most resistant to attempts by the interviewer to undermine the goals, values, and beliefs that have been expressed. Because they are presumably acting upon the identity elements they have established, any wavering by adult respondents in response to challenging questions probably implies that the views offered were either not well thought through, or are not particularly personally expressive, or both.

Scoring Complications for Adults

Among the scoring problems encountered with adult respondents, four require special attention: (1) the development of foreclosure during the adult years, (2) the nature of mid-life crisis, (3) the presence of self-serving commitments, and (4) sex differences in the expression of the criteria.

Adult Foreclosure

It is usually assumed in identity research that Foreclosure commitments arise early in an individual's life, most often in conjunction with parental behavior and attitudes or the parents' aspirations for their children. The earlier the ideas arise that form the content of identity commitments, the more confident the scorer can be in the appropriateness of the Foreclosure category. However, there are instances in which the goals, values, and beliefs to which the person is committed first arise during the adult years and yet scoring in the Foreclosure status is still warranted. This scoring will be appropriate when the views adopted represent the first time in a person's life that he or she has held commitments in the domain in question. For example, for many men who were mustered out of the armed forces following World War II, having entered the military directly from high school, the choice of employment was based not on reflection of vocational interests and abilities, but on happenstance. They went to work for whatever company happened to be hiring at the time they began looking for work. Many of these men were not particularly interested in the work itself when they began but after five or ten years found that the work became personally expressive and then represented a vocational commitment. Because there was no history of a vocational identity crisis and because these men became committed to the first alternative they seriously considered, scoring in the Foreclosure status seems most appropriate despite the age at which the commitment occurred.

Nor is this phenomenon of "late Foreclosure" limited to the domain of vocation. It can arise in any area to which only superficial thought is given during the stages of adolescence and youth and in which a strong interest develops during the adult years (e.g., parenting roles for many males, political ideology frequently for both sexes). If the person appears to have been in the Identity Diffusion status up to adulthood and now has strong commitments, it must be determined how much consideration of competing alternatives went into the process of forming the present views. Where the commitment is reported to have emerged naturally, without significant reflection, and particularly when there is an identifiable identification figure, then the person will appear to have foreclosed on his or her identity. Where the respondent reports going through a period of uncertainty or speaks of investigating an option before committing to it (even if only one option is discussed), use of the Identity Achievement status may be more appropriate. In the latter instance, it seems reasonable to conclude that the individual has made a personal decision and has not taken over goals or beliefs in an unreflective manner.

Mid-Life Crises in Relation to Identity Crises

Much has been written about mid-life crisis but little of it has been relevant to determining whether it is or is not an identity crisis. The common theme in discussions of mid-life crisis is the rejection of goals, values, and beliefs with which the person had been living up to that time. Naturally, such a rejection of well-established life patterns will be accompanied by substantial emotional distress. For purposes of identity status scoring, it is essential to know how the person is endeavoring to cope with this crisis. If the reaction is primarily emotional and no constructive action is being taken to find new goals, values, or beliefs worthy of a commitment, then scoring in the Identity Diffusion status is most appropriate. On the other hand, where the respondent is engaged in serious attempts to reorder priorities or finds a renewed sense of direction or purpose, then the Moratorium status scoring appears warranted. Based on what we currently know about mid-life crises, it can be hypothesized that a mid-life crisis starts as an emotional crisis that may or may not evolve into an identity crisis. It is hoped that identity research with adults will expand our knowledge of the nature and course of such crises.

Self-Serving Commitments

As at the other stage levels, the problem arises with respect to self-serving commitments in adulthood. Such beliefs should not be considered as having identity implications, because their function is generally to achieve personal advantage, rationalize particular behaviors, or further personal convenience. They are usually isolated options, not integrated into a larger ideological framework, giving direction or meaning to a person's life. Such self-serving commitments are most frequently encountered in the political domain (e.g., favoring a tax cut, farm subsidies, or import restrictions) but could also occur in a variety of other areas.

Identity in Males and Females

As stated many times in this volume, there are no differences between males and females in how the identity statuses are conceptualized. The defining criteria of exploration (crisis) and commitment are the same whether one is scoring an interview with a male or female respondent. The data on the relative frequencies of the identity statuses for males and females within various interview domains during high school and college years indicate only limited sex differences (see Chapter 4). To date, few identity status studies with adults have been structured in such a way as to allow for sex comparisons; thus no conclusions can yet be drawn for this age group.

It can be hypothesized, based on the research with adolescents and youths, that although in most interview domains no sex differences will be found in the relative frequencies of the identity statuses, differences may exist in some areas for which greater salience exists for either sex. Specifically, there is reason to believe that the domains of family and career priorities and parenting roles may be of more salience to females than to males. In contemporary society, women are expected to have primary responsibility for child care, even when they are employed outside the home. Thus women may be more likely to address questions about whether to become a parent, at what age to do so, and how to express themselves as parents than are their husbands. Correspondingly, women may also be more likely to make conscious decisions about the relative priorities to place on the family and career aspects of their lives. This likelihood should be reflected, in turn, in their use of the various identity status decision-making processes.

It should also be recognized that males and females may differ quite widely in the content of their identity elements. Such differences may be expected to be greatest in the domains of vocation and sex-role attitudes, and to varying degrees in the other interview areas. However, the content of identity elements is not a determining factor in identity status scoring and so does not bear on the question of the relative use of the identity status by males and females.

The Identity Status Domains

The scoring of identity status for adults in the various interview domains will depend on the unfolding of events beginning even before the onset of adolescence. Identity status commitments, whether Foreclosure or Identity Achievement commitments, may be carried into adulthood without major modification. For this reason it is important that in identity research with adults, scorers become thoroughly familiar with the scoring criteria as they apply to high school and college students as well as to adults. In the sections that follow, we focus on aspects of identity formation that are specific to the adult years.

Vocational Choice

Most adults interviewed in the area of vocation will have been working in their chosen field for some time. This greater level of experience should result in a more detailed description of the work and its advantages and disadvantages. The emotional tone in this section of the interview may be more balanced or matter-of-fact, in contrast to the excitement of anticipation often seen in younger groups. In assessing commitment to the chosen field, it should be determined whether the respondent feels the work continues to be personally expressive, or that the rewards of the work are sufficiently important to maintain a psychological investment in it.

A particular problem encountered by adults with respect to employment is layoffs. Where a layoff is temporary and the respondent expects to return to work relatively soon, this event may have no marked effect on a person's vocational identity. However, where the layoff is long and may be of indefinite length, then it will be hard for the person to maintain a vocational commitment in the area. The stress of prolonged unemployment is likely to undermine the sense of self-esteem and give rise to anxiety, depression, helplessness, and other negative emotional states. In the process, the person's vocational identity shifts from that of worker to that of someone out of work. The identity status scoring shifts in a corresponding fashion from a committed status (Foreclosure or Identity Achievement) to an uncommitted status (Moratorium or Identity Diffusion). The respondent may defensively persist in the use of the old vocational label, such as, "I'm an unemployed steelworker," but in the absence of realistic hope about a return to work, the identity cannot be viewed as personally expressive.

Another problem experienced by adults in the vocational area is burnout. Whether because of the lack of opportunities for further advancement, work-related stress, or conflict with supervisors or coworkers or both, work that had at one time been personally fulfilling is now undertaken without enthusiasm. Instances of burnout are easy to identify in identity interviews because of the negative emotional tone with which the vocational domain is discussed. Emotional expressions of frustration, anger, and apathy are common. However, even with this negative emotional state, many respondents may not be contemplating any career shift. In these instances, scoring in the Identity Diffusion status is indicated because the vocational commitment does not represent a positive statement of identity. Presumably, the person would change fields if he or she could be assured of comparable income, security, prestige, and so on. Where a career shift is contemplated, scoring in the Moratorium status is warranted only when the ideas considered are sufficiently advanced that some concrete steps have been taken to change fields. In the absence of action, the thoughts about change may be no more than pipe dreams.

Many adults find it necessary to undergo a career change or job retraining as a function of being laid off, job burnout, or early retirement. Respondents undergoing such an experience may sound quite similar to high school or college students attempting to choose a career for the first time. A variety of options may be considered, investigation of job opportunities after completing the necessary education, and uncertainty about whether one really has the potential to be successful in whatever career is chosen. Some adult respondents may express embarrassment over their needing to start over in a new field and others will be relieved that they have finally gotten out of a field about which they had negative feelings.

If the individual accepts a first offer for job retraining without much reflective appraisal of its implications, it seems probable that he or she is following a path of least resistance and therefore is Identity Diffuse. Where the respondent is still making new career decisions or when the decisions made are described as tentative, placement in the Moratorium status is appropriate. Where a firm commitment has been made, the person should be considered as in the Identity Achievement status, provided the new career can be said to be distinctly different from the previous one. If the new career appears to be a variation on the theme characterizing the former field, a primary scoring in the Foreclosure status is indicated, with a note that secondary Identity Achievement elements are present.

In the evolution of an identity scoring system for adults, one of the more difficult questions to resolve was how to consider the activity of homemaker in the context of career. (The problem here arose in part because a later domain in the interview taps questions of family versus career priorities and there was a desire to avoid double-counting crises.) As presented in Chapter 7, the main question in this area is the choice of one's life work. Thus, vocation is not equivalent to work outside the home and homemaking activities can appropriately be considered a career. As with other vocations, distinctions should be made about whether or not the homemaker role is personally expressive and whether it was adopted in a reflective or nonreflective way. Where the choice of a homemaker career can be seen as conforming to the expectations of others, without personal investment in the role, the respondent can be said to be Identity Diffuse. In contrast, where the work is seen as a statement of personal choice, where no options involving work outside the home were seriously considered, the Foreclosure scoring is most appropriate. The Identity Achievement status is the appropriate scoring when a reflective decision was made to commit to the homemaker role after the possibility of seeking outside employment was actively explored. It is not necessary that any outside careers have been investigated to place a respondent in the Identity Achievement status.

One variation on the homemaker career choice is particularly common. Many women plan to work prior to having children, then to stay home with the children while they are young, and return to full-time employment after the youngest child is in school. In these instances, it is important to determine whether the primary identification is with the role of homemaker or with work in the employment field. If it is the former, the respondent may indicate the need to resume employment because there will not be enough work that needs to be done at home while the children are in school. If the latter applies, the respondent is likely to speak of taking time out to take care of the needs of the children and there will be an active desire to return to the chosen field. Either way, scoring for the presence or absence of commitment should be made in terms of the primary work role (homemaker or outside career), not the secondary role. If no conflict was experienced over adopting the scenario described here, then no crisis can be said to exist (even though both the homemaker and outside career roles are being enacted). Correspondingly, struggle over whether or not to adopt this life plan would constitute evidence of a vocational identity crisis.

Identity Diffusion

Identity Diffusions with respect to vocation often sound bored, frustrated, or alienated from the work they are doing. The expression "it's a living" is a sign that the work being done is not personally expressive. Even when a respondent has been employed in a field for a long time and does not anticipate making any changes, the lack of work involvement carries the implication that vocation is not a meaningful aspect of personal identity.

One of the more difficult situations for vocational identity scoring particularly relevant for the Identity Diffusion status occurs with respondents who are more interested in their work than as just described, but where the level of involvement is still marginal. Such individuals like the work they are doing, feel competent at it, and do not plan any changes. Yet when questioned about their willingness to change, they express openness to other possibilities if they were to arise. This casual attitude toward change suggests that the present work activities represent a path of least resistance rather than a true identity commitment. In deciding whether a commitment is present or not, pay attention to both the degree of pleasure expressed for the current work activities and the range of other options that might be considered. The less the pleasure is expressed and the broader the range of options, the more appropriate is scoring as an Identity Diffusion.

The relationships of job burnout and chronic unemployment to placement in the Identity Diffusion status have already been discussed.

Example

(Female, age 23) Debby has been working as an x-ray technician for several years following completion of her Associate of Arts degree at a community college. She enjoys the work but plans to continue with it only until she starts a family. She is currently engaged with preparing for her wedding, planned within the year. Debby expects to stay home with the children while they are young but is not sure if she will find that too confining after the freedom she is now experiencing. If such a conflict does arise, she does not know how she will handle it, because she does not see it as feasible to be a mother and have a career. If she were to return to work, it probably would not be in her current field because the hours are not sufficiently flexible to meet family obligations. Right now she is not too concerned with these questions because having children is not an immediate prospect.

Comment

Debby appears not to have a vocational commitment to being either an x-ray technician or a homemaker. Though she currently enjoys the work she is doing, she is not projecting herself into the future in that career. Similarly, there are no indications that she anticipates that the homemaker role will be personally expressive. The negative aspects of parenting are described but not its positive aspects. Although there is evidence that she is aware of a potential crisis, she is not giving the issues serious consideration at present so that Moratorium scoring is not appropriate. On the basis of the information available, Debby should be scored as a Pre-Crisis Identity Diffusion.

Foreclosure

In most instances, Foreclosures in the domain of vocation will have selected their career choice early in life. The distinctive feature of these interviews is the consistency of the career trajectory followed by the respondents. It is not to be expected that an adult Foreclosure in this domain will be engaged in precisely the type of work first envisioned, but rather that there exist thematic lines that draw together all the respondent's schooling and work activities. Thus, the person may discuss changes of employers or even of career direction without these necessarily constituting a vocational identity crisis, provided that all the options considered are clearly related. The themes identified must be felt to be personally expressive of the respondent and the work performed must be described as rewarding.

Although most vocational Foreclosures will express a desire to continue with their current type of employment, exceptions do occur. Just as a Foreclosure may speak of past changes in the direction of his or her career, so too there may be anticipation of future changes. If any potential change is contemplated in the short term, a Foreclosure scoring is warranted provided the person remains within the established thematic lines. For example, individuals in the field of engineering may expect to shift from work in product design or production to management, usually with the same employer. Similarly, in education, a person may expect to go from classroom teaching into school administration. These career patterns represent established routes for continuing professional advancement within the chosen fields.

If change is not anticipated until a much later date, such as retirement, this outlook does not undermine the presence of a current vocational commitment, even if the move contemplated is in a quite different vocational direction. Here the person's vocational identity can be said to be currently stable, with recognition that at some future time, it may no longer be situationally or psychologically appropriate.

The phenomenon of Foreclosure commitments appearing for the first time during the adult years has been discussed. Though not common, this change does occur in the domain of vocation. For example, a person in the military may be assigned, perhaps arbitrarily, to a form of technical training and come to form a strong commitment to that field, whether in the service or in civilian life. Others may have bounced around from job to job without real interest in anything until they find one type of work especially rewarding and commit to it. Here it is important to distinguish between those whose changes are part of a conscious plan of career exploration and those whose job changes were a matter of convenience or happenstance. In the former instance, the presence of current career commitments would imply Identity Achievement, not Foreclosure. Still another example of a Foreclosure commitment established in adulthood is the person who has never found the homemaking role personally expressive (and therefore was Identity Diffuse) and who, perhaps after the children are of school age, forms a true vocational identity commitment to the first type of paid employment undertaken outside the home.

Example

(Male, age 52) Ferris is a senior vice president for real estate investment with a major commercial bank. He attended college without a clear career objective, majored in political science, and graduated with average grades. Following graduation he went to work with an uncle in the field of real estate. He had a talent for sales, became a licensed broker, and subsequently opened his own agency and made a success of it. Along the way he obtained a law degree with concentration in real estate law. His success led to an invitation to join the banking end of the field, an offer he eventually accepted. He is at the top of his field and continues to find his work challenging. He considers the most satisfying activities to be putting together financial arrangements for major corporate relocations.

Comment

This individual appears to be a late Foreclosure. There is no indication of serious consideration of career alternatives prior to or during the college years, although he undoubtedly held a variety of ideas at different times. Thus, when he joined his uncle's real estate firm he appears to have been Identity Diffuse. Then he discovered something of his talents and interests, forming a commitment to the real estate field. Because this choice represents a commitment to the first field seriously considered, scoring as Foreclosure is indicated. All the subsequent career changes are variations on a theme. Notice also that his high level of career success has no influence in identity status scoring.

Moratorium

Adults in the Moratorium status for vocation are currently engaged in active reconsideration of their career objectives. Perhaps the most frequent causes of such crises are job burnout and layoffs. In some instances a crisis may be triggered by the availability of an opportunity potentially more attractive than the respondent's current work. The activities of adults in moratorium will resemble those of college students engaged in career selection. Indeed, many adults will find it appropriate to resume their formal education in conjunction with a vocational identity crisis. Adults, however, may be expected to show a higher sense of urgency in looking to resolve their crises. Without a sense of urgency, it may be that career indecision represents avoidance of work responsibilities rather than an identity crisis.

Example

(Female, age 25) Marita is currently employed as a receptionist for a large corporation. She enjoys the work but does not consider it very challenging. The city in which she lives is actively recruiting women and minorities for admission to the police academy and she is considering applying. She anticipates that police work will be more interesting and demanding than her current employment. She is not put off by the danger associated with police work, but is concerned about the acceptance she might receive both from other officers and from the public. She reports being reluctant to give up her current position because it is in a very congenial setting. She does not know if she could get an equally attractive opportunity if for some reason she is not successful in police training. She must make her decision within the next several weeks, before the application deadline. She anticipates that she will apply, but also says that it is a big step to take.

Comment

This appears to be a classic example of a vocational identity conflict between a secure, generally attractive current career and a potentially more attractive but riskier alternative. The reasoning on both sides of the conflict is clearly delineated and the crisis is seen as time-bound, in this case because of external time pressures. The decision she has made is tentative, and the crisis will not be over just because an application is submitted. It is only when she feels secure in her new career choice, or has clearly rejected the prospect of a career change, that she will have emerged from the Moratorium status.

Identity Achievement

In discussing their feelings about their current work, individuals in the Identity Achievement status in the vocational domain will sound quite similar to respondents in the Foreclosure status. The difference is the developmental pathway by which they selected their career. For Identity Achievers, it is necessary to identify two or more distinctly different alternatives that had been considered at some time in their vocational development. Those alternatives may have either been simultaneously present or have emerged in sequence as the person changed from one field to another.

When a vocational identity crisis occurred during the high school years, or earlier in rare instances, memories of the alternatives considered and the emotions surrounding the decision-making process may have faded. When discussed in the interview, the process of choice may be described as less difficult and the choices themselves less seriously entertained than they actually were at the time. Careful questioning may help the respondent recover those memories clearly, but this will not always be possible. When coding interviews in which the seriousness with which early alternatives were considered will determine placement in either the Foreclosure or Identity Achievement status, some relaxation of the scoring criteria seems appropriate. However, scorers must also be cognizant of the opposite problem of projecting more concern into the respondent's decision-making process than was experienced at the time. It may be necessary in the field of identity research to become reconciled to the idea that the frequency of adult Identity Achievers in the vocational domain will be underestimated.

It is substantially easier to identify adult vocational Identity Achievers when the identity crisis has occurred more recently. The resumption of one's education or the making of a dramatic career change, whether in response to changing life circumstances, new interests, job burnout, or a mid-life crisis, are salient events in a person's life and memories of it will remain vivid. Though some respondents who have changed fields will express genuine commitment to their new careers somewhat more tentatively than they did to their past activities (if change was necessary once, it may be necessary again), most are likely to express commitment with comparable vigor.

Example

(Male, aged 46) Andrew has long been interested in the field of engineering. He obtained his B.S. degree in civil engineering and subsequently worked on the Alaska oil pipeline and other major construction projects. Approximately five years ago, he left a high-paying job in the private sector to join the Peace Corps. He is now working in Central Africa on water projects. He reports a major change in his thinking about his career. When he began, he was motivated primarily by the money to be made in engineering and he became highly successful. However, he found that money did not promote happiness and felt that most of the projects on which he worked were benefiting and enriching few people. He believed it necessary to make major changes in his life and find ways of more directly helping others. This decision motivated his desire to join the Peace Corps. Although he did not specify a desire to continue with engineering, the Peace Corps administrators saw his experience as a major asset to the program. Andrew reports his work now is highly satisfying and he will be continuing his participation for another tour of service.

Comment

Although engineering is a continuing focus to Andrew's work and does represent a Foreclosure theme, the major shift in his orientation to work represents a more important aspect of identity change. The engineering originally served as a means toward achieving personal success goals, but now serves as a means of contributing to the well-being of others. This shift in goals is discontinuous, in that it occurred in the context of reflective self-appraisal.

Religious Beliefs

As individuals enter the adult years, their religious beliefs will have been shaped by the religious views with which they were reared and any questioning of those ideas that may have occurred during adolescence and youth. Several issues about religious beliefs for adults may deeply influence how identity is judged for this age group. These issues include: (1) efforts to live in a manner consistent with one's religious and/or ethical beliefs, (2) conversions occurring at the time of marriage involving the adoption, formally or informally, of the spouse's religious orientation, (3) decisions about how one's children should be reared with respect to religion, and (4) the personal relevance of religion as one confronts the prospect of death.

The beliefs that many adolescents and youths hold about religion are somewhat abstract or intellectualized because in only a few areas are important life decisions seen as having a religious component. Among the decisions that do have such a component are whether or not to attend religious services, the extent and forms of sexual activity, and beliefs about abortion. For many adults many more life decisions may be viewed as bearing on the consistency with which one acts upon religious beliefs, including marital fidelity, divorce and remarriage, business ethics, charity and caring for the less fortunate, in addition to the issues of the younger age groups. As a consequence, adult interviewees may call attention to the discrepancies between their avowed religious or ethical beliefs and their actual behaviors. In considering the implications of this issue for identity status scoring, attention should be paid to the extent of the discrepancies, the frequency with which thought is given to them, the extent of the subjective discomfort experienced, and any active steps the person is taking to resolve the inconsistencies.

Because marriages by persons of differing religions often encounter social disapproval, pressures may be placed on one partner or the other to convert, thus creating at least the appearance of religious compatibility and resolving in advance questions as to how any children of the marriage will be reared with respect to religion. If the conversion appears to have been made *primarily* for family reasons or if the respondent reports strong continuity between past and present religious beliefs, then no identity crisis appears to exist. Where the decision to convert was a difficult one and considerable reflection was given to the change, a scoring involving crisis is indicated.

It is not unusual for individuals when they become parents, or as their children reach age 3 or 4, to resume religious observances that had been discontinued during the high school or college years. The respondents may report that what they are now doing is "for the children." If these activities are not personally expressive, they do not constitute evidence of a commitment. An active family debate and/or decision-making process about whether children should receive religious instruction can be considered evidence of an identity crisis only when the debate kicks up *personal*, unresolved issues about the role of religion in one's life.

One additional issue will be most applicable to individuals over age 50. As one begins to confront the prospect of one's own death, there may develop an increased concern with religion. Religious activity may increase along with thoughts about heaven, hell, and personal salvation. Alternatively, doubts about the existence of God may become accentuated. In trying to assess whether the changes in this area reflect an identity crisis, as opposed to one reflecting the age-related component of integrity versus despair, attention should be focused on the extent of differences between current beliefs and those of adolescence, youth, or the earlier adult years, the extent of reflective appraisal of alternatives, and the presence of efforts to reach an intellectual as well as an emotional resolution to the concerns, whether in the past or present.

Identity Diffusion

Adults in the Identity Diffusion status with respect to religious beliefs will either appear uninterested or express relatively superficial views that are not accompanied by personally expressive religious activity. When these individuals do attend religious services, it is either for the sake of appearances (e.g., it is expected of someone of the respondent's occupational standing), for the sake of the children, or in response to pressure from the spouse or other family members.

One pattern that may be found with some frequency is for an individual who was Foreclosed, or more rarely Identity Achieved, with respect to religion during adolescence or youth to gradually drift away from religious activity due to conflicting time pressures from work or from family. No conscious thought seems to have been given to the change, and when questioned the respondent may report continued identification with the religion. Still, the absence of current activity and the relative lack of continuing concern with religious ideas provide grounds for the scoring of Identity Diffusion.

Example

(Male, age 38) Doug reported that he is Roman Catholic, attending religious services only during Christmas and Easter. He describes his wife as more religious than himself and all their children as having been reared within the church. He believes in God, is opposed to abortion, and thinks artificial birth control acceptable. He has tried to persuade his wife about this last view. Because he is athletically inclined, he has coached soccer and baseball teams for the church in the Catholic Youth Organization (CYO) leagues. It gave him particular pleasure to coach his sons in these sports.

Comment

Scoring for Identity Diffusion, marginally involved type, is indicated. There is no evidence that religion has personal importance in his life. Yet he seems quite contented with his nominal affiliation and minimal activity. It provides an ideological label he can use when queried, but he shows no real interest in the substance of ideological issues. His involvement with CYO coaching is motivated by personal and family values, not religious concern.

Foreclosure

As adults, Foreclosures show continued allegiance to the religious views with which they were reared. Religion plays an important, though not necessarily central, role in their life. They present their idea clearly, often forcefully. They may convey the impression that theirs is the one true religion, though they may show tolerance for others with differing views. There are reports of accompanying religious activity, such as attending religious services regularly, prayer, and Bible reading.

Although there has been no active questioning of religious doctrines or values, Foreclosures will often describe a pattern of changes in their ideas as they matured. Belief in the literal truth of the Bible stories may give way to understanding the use of allegory and parable. At a later age, the person may give up a rigidly moralistic attitude about premarital sexuality in favor of greater flexibility and tolerance.

For individuals who are "born again," becoming increasingly concerned about religious values and more religiously active, scoring in the Foreclosure status is warranted if the person would have been categorized as

Foreclosed along compatible lines prior to the change. If the person would have been called Identity Diffuse before being "born again," arriving at a scoring is more problematic. Some identity researchers would be inclined to score the person Identity Achieved, focusing on the unconscious psychological dynamics that prepared the respondent for the evangelical conversion response. Other researchers prefer considering such changes as falling within the Foreclosure category because there is an absence of conscious reflection on alternatives, there is evidence of identification with a strong parental substitute figure, and the belief pattern that is adopted is taken over fully formed and is accepted in an unquestioning manner.

Example

(Female, age 25) Fran is an agnostic, having been raised in a family wherein both parents were agnostic. She presents reasoned arguments in support of an agnostic viewpoint. She has also developed secular justification for moral decision making, focused on trying to fulfil the legitimate needs of others, particularly those close to her. She plans to expose any children she may have to a variety of religions so that they can make their own decisions. She will, of course, discuss her own agnostic views and anticipates that her children will eventually come to adopt that position themselves. This is what her parents did with her.

Comment

One senses here that Fran is following a family script. It is true that she decided on agnosticism, but she did so without ever having held a belief in God or in any organized religion. On the other hand, her identification with her parents is clear, both in the content of her views and her style of childrearing in the area. Further, she shows no evidence of subjective discomfort or active questioning of religious or moral matters.

Moratorium

The issues that constitute the substance of an identity crisis in the religious area during the adult years are likely to be largely the same as those found among high school and college students, such as belief in God, value of religious services, and truth of conflicting religious claims. The primary difference between adult crises and those occurring earlier involves the precipitating events. Where the crises occurring in adolescence and youth are often initiated by questions arising from peers, teachers, or books, and thus are discussed somewhat abstractly, the crises occurring later may more often be triggered by some important real-life moral conflict, such as an abortion decision, the death of a child, or perceived immorality of church leaders. Because the level of emotionality in the interview will be higher under such circumstances, it becomes necessary to distinguish carefully between emotional crises and identity crises.

Example

(Male, age 48) The conflict for Mitchell began when his church council voted against establishing an emergency shelter for the homeless in the basement of the church building. For him, this refusal represented a rejection of Christian obligations for charity. He himself had been doing volunteer work one evening a week at the mission in a nearby town. He felt conflicted because he had been attending this church since childhood but now felt he could no longer support what it stood for. Having decided to disaffiliate, he felt cast adrift. He continued to believe in God, but there was no other church within the community he felt he could comfortably attend. He reported that more and more he was coming to the view of religion as a personal thing, between himself and God, that did not need the support or sanction of a formal organization. He did not, however, know where these changes might lead and would not speculate how he might be expressing his religious beliefs five years from now.

Comment

It is evident that Mitchell takes his religious beliefs seriously and is seeking a new format for their expression. Though he seems to have made substantial progress toward that goal, he is indicating he is still not comfortable with how things currently stand. For that reason he would be categorized as in the Moratorium status, though it might be anticipated that were another interview to be conducted in a year or two, he might well be an Identity Achiever.

Identity Achievement

As in the other content areas of the interview, adult Identity Achievers with respect to religion will express a coherent belief system that influences their day-to-day living. Because they have at some time questioned the ideas with which they were reared, and possibly considered a variety of alternative viewpoints, Identity Achievers are likely not to make absolutist religious claims. Rather, Achievers will describe the beliefs that they find personally expressive and are likely to show understanding about why others may adopt differing perspectives.

About the timing of an identity crisis: it could have occurred at any time from adolescence to the recent past. If the crisis did occur during adolescence and the resolution was in the direction of reaffirming religious beliefs, those ideas will be treated as a long-standing, stable aspect of the person's identity. As a consequence the respondent may at first impression sound Foreclosed. Further, given that adults often minimize the importance or significance of the questioning they did as adolescents (e.g., "I guess all teenagers have their doubts about God; it's just part of the stage"), it may be difficult to determine whether or not a genuine identity crisis did occur. Careful probing by the interviewer to assess whether the questioning was perceived as serious at the time it occurred will be most helpful here. However, when the record is not detailed but reference is made to questions during adolescence, this should be treated as evidence of a crisis unless there are overriding indications of the importance of identification figures in the area.

Recognition of Identity Achievers with respect to religion will be easier when the identity crisis occurred more recently. The freshness of the experience means that both the cognitive and the emotional components of the crisis will be conveyed in richer detail. The steps the person went through in resolving the crisis will be more fully described. Where the resolution of the crisis is in the direction of expressing a religious faith, religion may well play a central role in the person's life. This change will often occur after a religious conversion. Where the resolution is in the direction of loss of religious faith, the Identity Achieved respondent will usually discuss in detail the philosophical or moral beliefs that have been adopted to take the place of religion.

Example

(Female, age 30) Arlene described herself as only nominally religious prior to the birth of her first child. She was reared in the Jewish religion, believed in God, but seldom attended religious services. She felt herself to be largely ignorant of the Jewish religious tradition. However, upon becoming a parent she recognized that some decisions would have to be made about the children's religious education. Because her husband was largely indifferent to religion both personally and for the children, Arlene saw any decision as resting on her shoulders. She resolved to learn more about her religion and read extensively on both Jewish religious traditions and doctrines. After discovering numerous points that were incompatible with her strong feminist views, she decided not to rear her children within the religion. She reported that the experience had affected her thinking not only about Judaism, but also about the role of religion in her own life.

Comment

What apparently started as a task undertaken for the sake of the children became a far more personal experience. At the time she undertook the project she could best be characterized as Identity Diffuse. It is only when she finds incompatibility between different aspects of her belief system that she becomes ego involved in the decision-making process. In resolving the dissonance, she is at the same time working through her questions about religious identity. She emerges from the process as an Identity Achiever, holding a very different perspective on religion from the one with which she started.

Family/Career Priorities

The starting point for understanding the role of family/career priorities as an aspect of a person's sense of identity is with the four content possibilities in this domain: (1) family priority, (2) career priority, (3) dual priority, and (4) neither priority. A family priority is evident when personal decision making focuses on the best interests of the family—the spouse and children. A career priority can be said to exist when work is pursued for intrinsic motives (or when extrinsic rewards are sufficiently attractive) and when family arrangements are largely determined by work considerations. A dual priority is present when both family and career objectives appear to be given roughly comparable weight. Compromises on ideal arrangements should not be made exclusively in one direction. Neither priority would be indicated when moderate to intense dissatisfaction is expressed over both family and career roles or when priorities are confused.

Within the present cultural context, a family priority is more commonly found for women than for men and is often associated with the adoption of the homemaker career role. Among married women with children, the implementation of an exclusive homemaker role may be used as prima facie evidence of a family priority, provided the role appears to be self-chosen and is personally expressive. When a mother is working outside the home but the decision to work is the result of financial considerations and employment is deemed necessary for the optimal functioning of the family, then scoring for a family priority is still indicated. Also, a family priority may be said to exist when a woman works in some capacity to directly assist the husband's career. Where a woman is not married, or has not borne children, it is the desire to establish a family as the primary goal in her life that should be used as evidence for a family priority. Where a woman with children is separated or divorced, a primary concern on the making of decisions for the benefit of the children, accompanied by explicit or implied willingness to subordinate her own interests and needs, can be interpreted as reflecting a family priority. A desire to remarry may or may not be found among such women.

Although it is possible that adult men may also express a family priority by adopting the homemaker role, instances of such an association are not currently common. When a male is engaged in such activities, it should be determined whether the role is self-chosen and personally expressive or has been forced upon him by the exigencies of the job market. In the latter instance, commitment to a family priority cannot be said to exist. A more likely way for males to express a family priority is by placing family interests above those associated with career advancement. Thus, particular types of work may be desired because they will afford more time for family involvement. Correspondingly, a promotion may be declined because of its possible repercussions for family life. Again, where a man is not married or a father, it is the desire to establish a family as the primary goal in his life that should be used as evidence for a family priority.

A career priority implies that work activities are seen as expressive of the person's identity and that involvement with day-to-day family matters is viewed as of secondary importance. Responsibilities for child care are placed on the spouse, a grandparent, an in-law, an older child, or some agent outside of the family, such as a housekeeper-governess, babysitters, or nursery school. At present, males are more likely than females to be encouraged to place career considerations above family considerations.

A dual priority involves placing comparable emphasis on both career and family-life objectives. Because priorities in each area have a high social desirability association, there may be a tendency to verbalize a personal endorsement of both. It is important to ascertain whether or not the respondent's actions are consistent with a statement of a dual priority. Where compromises on ideal arrangements for reconciling family and career demands are consistently made in only one direction, a dual priority cannot be said to exist.

A dual priority may be expressed either by simultaneous pursuit of family and career objectives or by awareness of shifting priorities at different times in the individual's life. Among women, such a shift in priorities will most commonly involve temporary reduction or suspension of career activity during the children's preschool years followed by resumption (planned or implemented) of work activity when the youngest child enters school. There should be evidence of a genuine desire to pursue career objectives. If the woman is passively willing or prefers to remain home, even when she does work, a dual priority is not indicated. Among men, a shift in priorities may more often occur at a later age with a period of intense career involvement being followed by an increase in importance placed on family concerns and a corresponding reduction in the stress placed on career.

The lack of commitment implied in having neither a family nor career priority may be evidenced by expressed dissatisfaction with one's job, one's spouse, and one's children. The emotional tone may be one of hopelessness, helplessness, pervasive boredom, depression, unfocused anger, or pathological confusion. Alternatively, having neither priority may reflect the active reconsideration of identity alternatives, with some eventual commitment anticipated. Also included as having neither priority will be "free-spirit" types who wish to keep all their options open and experiment with many activities without committing themselves to any. Such individuals will usually express that they derive pleasure from their manner of living (and may well be committed to it).

Because potential identity crises over family and career priorities and the identity commitments formed may focus on either the parental aspects of family considerations or on the spousal aspects, or on both, it is appropriate to distinguish between these possibilities in the identity interview. When scoring an interview for identity status, the emphasis should be placed on whichever aspects involve the most extensive consideration of alternatives and/or whichever aspects involve the most important commitments.

Identity Diffusion

Where there is stable rejection of both family and career roles, scoring in the Identity Diffusion status is appropriate. The Diffusion status is also indicated where a preference for one or another pattern of priorities exists but where there is no intensity in the way in which the ideas are expressed. A similar conclusion is warranted if the person's actions do not correspond to the stated preference and little or nothing is being done to rectify that condition.

In this domain, the extent to which the respondent is being moved by circumstances outside his or her direction is particularly important. The person may be responding to implicit or explicit demands expressed by the spouse, employer, parents, or in some instances, children. It is about this domain that an Identity Diffusion may be most likely to express the feeling that his or her life is out of control. Other Identity Diffusions may show little or no distress, moving from day to day without trying to work out any long-range life direction. Such a casual attitude may be genuinely felt or may be a defense against underlying feelings of helplessness.

Example

(Female, age 24) Doris is married with three children, ages 4½, 3, and 1. She has been carrying out full-time parenting responsibilities, but reports a high level of frustration. She describes herself as not being a "natural mother," feels she is "too short" with the children, does not give them enough positive attention, and complains that her household is too disorganized. She reports that her husband tries to help out occasionally, but that it really does not improve the situation. When asked if she had thought about the possibility of her seeking outside employment and finding day-care arrangements for the children, she responded that anything that would get her out of the house would be a plus. However, she did not feel that this would be feasible because of her limited job skills, the cost of day care, and her husband's opposition to her working.

Comment

This is an example of a person whose life appears out of control. She started a family at an early age and may well feel trapped in her current situation. Doris feels frustrated with her parenting and would like to escape from at least some of that responsibility. However, she is taking no active steps to improve her situation. The list of reasons given to counter the suggestion that she might seek outside employment appears to be being used as a rationale for inaction. In the absence of clearly defined family and career goals, and without activity to alter an emotionally distressing situation, scoring in the Identity Diffusion status is indicated.

Foreclosure

Adult Foreclosures in the domain of family/career priorities may be committed to family, career, or dual priorities. Given the traditional nature of many Foreclosures, it is likely that women will typically be committed to a family priority and men will generally opt for a career priority. Exceptions to this pattern do occur, so that it is important to consider the correspondence between the priorities expressed by the respondent and the priorities reported to be held by the respondent's parents, particularly the same-sex parent. Where one or both parents hold dual priorities, it would not be unusual for a respondent to foreclose upon the same priorities in his or her life.

Whatever the priorities chosen, Foreclosures should appear comfortable with their decision and should be engaged in family and work activities that correspond to their stated preferences. When Foreclosures encounter problems in implementing their preferred alternative, they may experiment with a number of possibilities in an effort to find an arrangement that will work effectively. This condition should not be confused with an identity crisis, for the person's identity element is already established and is not in question. Rather, the concern is with finding a way to most effectively put the preferred priority into practice.

Example

(Male, age 44) Fulton is married with two children and is employed as a police officer. In addition to his regular shifts, he is obligated to put in specified amounts of overtime. Because his work schedule changes periodically, and often includes weekends, family routines are also variable. Fulton perceives no conflict between his family and work responsibilities. He reports that for him, the family is most important, with his primary responsibility to it being his role as the "breadwinner."

Comment

Although Fulton identifies himself as having a family priority, his priority seems more appropriately considered to be career. The role of breadwinner carries the implication that whatever is done to pursue or advance the career is done for the benefit of the family. Although this statement may sound like a dual priority, this description is not likely to be accurate. In practice, individuals holding the viewpoint expressed here often have limited involvement with family activities and there is often an assumption, as here, that the family must consistently accommodate to the job requirements of the respondent. It is clear that Fulton is committed to his value system in this domain and there is no suggestion that he has ever considered alternative priorities. Therefore, scoring in the Foreclosure status is warranted.

Moratorium

A Moratorium in the family/career priorities domain is indicated if active consideration is being given to any combination of family, career, and dual priorities. At present, it is likely that crises in this area for males will be between career and dual priorities, whereas for females the crises will be between family and dual priorities. However, the presence of a period of active decision making over whether or not to seek employment outside the home should *not* be considered a primary identity crisis *if* only family considerations are involved. Rather, such concerns seem best interpreted as a secondary crisis over the most appropriate means for implementing a family priority.

The level of distress experienced by a person in moratorium over family/career priorities will vary widely depending on the extent to which previously held ideas are associated with life dissatisfaction. Some people whose current activities are experienced as satisfying may be engaged in considering alternatives that may be several years in the future. For example, a woman with children may be contemplating whether or not to return to a paid career after the youngest child is of school age and, if so, how to balance the competing responsibilities of each role. At the other emotional extreme may be a woman who has found herself deeply frustrated by her experiences with full-time parenting, yet also concerned about the effect of a return to work on her children. Particularly distressing may be the discovery that adequate child care placements are either unavailable or beyond the financial capabilities of the family.

Example

(Female, age 32) Maxine has recently resumed her career after the younger of her children entered nursery school at age 3. She reported that she enjoys mothering but was distressed with being away from work as a graphic artist for the past five years. She is experiencing conflict over whether she should have delayed her return to work until both children were in public school. She considers herself lucky that she was able to find what appear to be suitable openings for her children but worries over the quality of child care her younger child will receive and about the after-school program for her older child. Her husband's work is described as precluding his being more actively involved in childrearing. There is an implication that she is frustrated with this relative lack of involvement and resents that the responsibilities have fallen entirely on her shoulders. She recognizes that in trying both to be primary parent and to pursue her career, she may be taking on more than she can handle. She talked about the "superwoman" role and is hoping it will work out for her. If it does not, she will have to reexamine her options, perhaps putting her career on hold for a while longer.

Comment

At present, Maxine is maintaining a dual priority to a family and career. She is not confident in her decision, however, so that her commitment cannot at present be described as firm. She worries whether she has made a good decision, whether the children will be well cared for, and whether she will be able to successfully juggle all her responsibilities. She is angry with her husband that he is not experiencing the same conflicts with which she has to deal. Though she knows what she would like to do, and in this sense her identity element is in place, she is still reviewing and repeating her decision, and thinking through alternative contingencies. Only when she becomes more relaxed and confident of her choice can her identity commitment be considered firm and can she be scored Identity Achieved. Until then, she appears to be in the later phases of Moratorium.

Identity Achievement

Respondents in the Identity Achievement status with respect to family and career priorities will have worked through the issues pertaining to how they wish to devote their energies in balancing competing demands on their time. Because they have consciously reflected on their options, they will be more aware than Foreclosures of the potential difficulties that could be encountered in implementing their priorities. Presenting a realistic appraisal of such problems does not imply any lack of commitment to their stated preference.

Many of the identity crises in this domain will have occurred during the adult years in response to the realities of parenting and career experiences. Though the person will have entered adulthood with particular expectations of the rewards and costs associated with family and career activities, actual experiences in these areas may produce outcomes very different from those anticipated. Specifically, attempts to juggle the competing demands arising from these sources may yield a reward/cost ratio that is far from satisfactory. As a consequence, there may be pressure to rethink the priorities that had been adopted.

Another circumstance that can lead to a change in family and career priorities may occur during the middle adult years when individuals have discovered the upward limits of their career potentials. It has frequently been observed that with increasing age, men experience a decrease in career concerns and an increase in family concerns. Whether a shift reflects an identity change in the respective priorities can be ascertained by assessing both the extent of the change made and the amount of conscious reflection given to working out the changes.

Corresponding to the shift in importance of career and family concerns evidenced by males, females are said to show decreasing involvement in family as their children approach the time of leaving home and commitment increase in career interests. Again, this may or may not reflect a change in priorities because, with the children now grown, there is less cause to implement a family priority. If a family priority were expressed if a subsequent need arose, such as a medical problem with a family member or an adult child returning to the household with children, then an identity change in priorities could not be said to have occurred. However, if a genuine reluctance were expressed to upset current plans to resume activities previously engaged in, then a change would have taken place in the identity elements pertaining to family and career priorities.

Example

(Male, age 52) Adrian has been married twice. He has four children from his first marriage and two from the second. His first marriage occurred at age 22, shortly following his college graduation. He played only a limited role in rearing the children in his first family, devoting his time to the pursuit of his career in business. At the time of his divorce, he had risen quite far in his company's hierarchy, and further advancement was doubtful. The youngest of his children was by that time in college. He remarried several years later, at age 47. His second wife was nearly twenty years younger than he, and he started a second family. He retired from his company and opened a small consulting firm, with which he has had gratifying success. He reported making the career move to reduce the pressure in his life and to give himself the time he feels he needs to enjoy his family. His involvement with the children in his second marriage is indeed far greater than with his first family. Though he reported occasionally missing the excitement of corporate decision making, he would not return to his former life-style if the opportunity were available.

Comment

There has been a clear change in Adrian's behavior with respect to parenting from his first to his second marriage, accompanied by reduced investment in career activities. It is unclear from the material provided what may have initiated the change: the lack of opening for further career movement, the pressures of work, his divorce, or the feeling that he had missed the experience of family during his first marriage. For whatever reason(s), he has shown a shift from a career priority to either a dual priority or a family priority, and is now committed to these new arrangements. The transition does not appear to have been particularly stressful, but the rationale offered for his shift suggests it was the product of reflective decision making. He seems more at peace with himself now than he was earlier in his life.

Part III
Epilogue

11 Epilogue

JAMES E. MARCIA

The purpose of this work is to provide a handbook useful for persons interested in conducting investigations into Erikson's psychosocial stages, especially identity and intimacy. As aids in this task, it furnishes a theoretical foundation, research reviews, interview schedules and scoring criteria, suggestions for interviewer training, and discussions of pertinent issues. There would be no point in assembling this material were there not questions still to be answered, issues still to be explored. Some of these are brought up in this final chapter.

The Meaning of the Identity Statuses in a Non-North American Context

The question of whether or not the identity statuses have the same significance in cultures other than North America, or even Western Europe, has been raised repeatedly, although not usually by identity researchers themselves. An a priori assumption is that the formation of an identity is, at this stage in human history, a developmental reality in the life of humankind. This identity may be an individual one (as in most Western cultures) or it may be a collective one—in which case it is still held individually, although its origin and contents are collective. Within the identity status paradigm, all collective identities would be Foreclosed. On the most manifest levels, one would expect Foreclosures, from any culture, to have characteristics in common. They would represent in their behaviors and values the most typical cultural beliefs. These would provide a context within which their life had an unquestioned meaning, and would give them a deserved reputation for reliability.[1] They would be seen as

[1] This passage is from *National Geographic*:

Surveying these comforts, I asked Tukkay if he would live in any other place. "Any other place?" he pondered. "Most likely not. I was born in the tundra, my parents and forefathers

the salt of whatever earth they inhabited. Their behavior should also be marked by an inflexibility that might never be displayed were they to remain in the culture on which they had foreclosed. The only context in which one can speak of the adaptive deficit of the Foreclosure status is one that calls for flexibility; that is, adjusting to a change in their own culture; adjusting to a new culture; creating new solutions to intransigent problems; and so on. Foreclosures have been depicted as having ascribed identities; for some, the identity seems inscribed. And the more inscribed it is, the less adaptive flexibility one would expect. In Western societies, particularly North America, where institutionalized moratoria exist, a Foreclosure identity can take on a somewhat more pejorative character than in a society whose struggles for survival preclude the luxury of a moratorium. In both contexts, however, the qualities of consistent cultural representation, dependability, and predictability should be manifested. What is written here is not intended to dilute the research findings for the Foreclosures, which are numerous, consistent, and speak for themselves. It is meant only to broaden the picture somewhat. As discussed previously (Marcia, 1980), each of the identity statuses—now, even Identity Achievement (Slugoski et al. 1984; Stephen et al., in press)—have their positive and negative aspects.

The empirical investigation of the differing meanings of the identity statuses in various cultural contexts is a fascinating research direction that awaits undertaking. For example, what could one discover about the developmental history of a Moratorium or Identity Achievement person who had grown up in a foreclosure context—assuming that such a person exists? Under what cultural conditions might it be adaptive to be an Identity Diffusion? When can and cannot a society afford to offer institutionalized moratoria? We now have sufficient assurance from the completed cross-cultural studies that the identity statuses are applicable in non-North American settings. But we do not know much about the characteristics of the statuses in those settings.

Research-Based Changes in Eriksonian Theory

Throughout this volume, the word "validate" has recurred. Its presence creates the impression that what has occurred is no more than the stamping of a preexisting truth with the imprimatur of much hard work. Had there not been changes to Erikson's theory as a result of our

---

were always reindeer herders. I studied at school, lived in the dormitory, then served in the army. Sometime the thought sprang up within me: Could I live in any other place but Arakachechen? To do that, I would be deprived of a certain part of my self. Here in the tundra, among the reindeer, although this is not the most comfortable and jovial existence, I feel the life I was created for."—Vladimir Tukkay, reindeer herder, Chukchi Peninsula, Soviet Arctic (Rytkheu, 1983, p. 215).

research, that impression might be accurate. It is particularly (and, perhaps, predictably) in the area of women's identity and intimacy development that the original psychosocial theory has had to be amended. Specifically, "inner space" and the kinds of interpersonal issues associated with it, are important to women—and are likely to be more important to women than men—but they are not the sole grounds upon which women found an identity, nor are they necessarily the most important domains for the majority of women. Both men and women consider occupation the most important identity-related area. Hence, based upon our research, Erikson was correct in identifying inner-space issues as salient for women, but not in the emphasis he placed on them, nor in his omission of men from this identity-relevant domain.

Another important change in theory following from our research has been the differing relationships between identity and intimacy for men and women. As Erikson suggested, identity does seem a necessary condition for intimacy for men; however, for women, identity and intimacy may codevelop. This statement has two implications. The first is that women's identity is more complex than men's. It seems to involve more a sense of balancing priorities and organizing different concerns into an organic (because it is always changing) whole. Men's identity, by contrast, seems more focused and more oriented toward resolving one issue at a time. The price women may pay for their complexity is lack of focus and goal orientation. The price men are likely to pay for their directedness is a truncation of experience. The second implication is that if sex-role prescriptions follow their current androgynous trajectory, men may begin to become less focused, more likely to combine intimacy with identity concerns (see Matteson's comments), and women may become more effectively competitive in the world of work. It is my impression that the latter is proceeding more quickly than the former.

Intrapsychic Dimensions

The specific nature of the intrapsychic dimensions, both psychodynamic and cognitive developmental, underlying the identity statuses and identity development in general, is not clear. Josselson (1988) has pursued both object relational and self-psychological issues, especially with respect to the development of women's identity. A major contribution of her work has been to emphasize the relational aspect of identity for women and to suggest that a woman's relationship with her mother may be a kind of marker against which to evaluate her continuing identity development. Kroger (1989) has suggested that ego-cognitive developmental processes described by Kegan (1982) and Noam (1988) may be a way of describing processes involved in identity formation. Blasi (1988), in a thoughtfully critical article, has pointed out that the identity status approach has overlooked some of the more existential-experiential aspects of Erikson's theory. All these views suggest an expanded theoretical network for the identity statuses and perhaps point to fundamental developmental principles underlying a number of theoretical perspectives (Marcia, 1988).

From the completely different perspective of social narrative, Slugoski and Ginsburg (1989) would find the "intrapsychic" issue meaningless, their position being that an identity interview yields only a story that an individual finds it advantageous to tell about himself or herself. Before this view can be taken as accurate it must provide its own alternative theoretical account for the considerable number and variety of significant findings already obtained for the identity statuses on dependent variables. Graafsma (1989) has spoken for that group of classical psychoanalysts who view identity as an epiphenomenon, reducible to constructs already in use. This may be a case where theoretical predilections determine how data are interpreted (see Greenberg & Mitchell's [1983] note in discussing Rangell's criticisms of Kohut and Fromm-Reichmann). Although it may be true that both those for whom identity is a valid phenomenon in its own right and those for whom it is an epiphenomenon see what their theoretical presuppositions lead them to see, the burden of proof rests with the orthodox psychoanalytic position that, if it is to establish its validity, must provide a theoretical accounting for the large body of research findings that have been accumulated based upon the proposition that identity is a valid construct. For this writer (Marcia) the identity statuses are only the tips of particular developmental icebergs, whose depths may go back to antecedents quite early in childhood. For example, I have sought to focus on the processes by which identity statuses are defined (exploration and commitment), and to ask what childrearing and social conditions might facilitate these processes (Marcia, 1988a,b; 1989b). Both variables are lifelong factors in personality development. At adolescence they give rise to identity; earlier, they may relate to individuation and cognitive/moral development; later, they may be important in a much more "internal" sense to the formation of Eriksonian Integrity.

Intra-Status Differentiation

The first time the issue of subtypes within an identity status arose was during the late 1960s when a group of persons, very much in the spirit of the times, adopted an ideology that precluded occupational commitment in the usual sense. They saw traditional occupational choice as complicity with a morally bankrupt society that was requiring their peers to participate in a war whose purpose and manner of pursuit was highly questionable to them. In the words of the time: "I ain't gonna work on Maggie's farm no more." The genuineness of at least some of these persons' commitments was clear and they could not be said to lack an identity because they were occupationally uncommitted. Hence, we called them "alienated Achievements" (Bob, 1968; Orlofsky et al., 1973), and they appeared very much like Identity Achievements on dependent variables. Since that time, "alienated Achievements" have disappeared; in fact, ideological commitment, in general, as would be attested by many in the university community, has declined appreciably. But some other intrastatus differences that have appeared are mentioned below.

For quite a while, Identity Achievements looked like a unitary group, except for the alienated Achievements. However, beginning with the Marcia follow-up study in 1976, which found former Achievements "becoming" Foreclosures after their college years, other researchers have reported that some Achievements are flexible but others may rigidify after their initial identity resolution and appear similar to Foreclosures in later life (Marcia, 1976; Stephen et al., in press; Slugoski et al., 1984). Among Moratoriums, some seem to experience the identity crisis with great emotional turmoil but others pass through equally genuine exploratory periods with considerably more equanimity (Ochberg, 1986; Offer & Offer, 1975). Also, some few Moratoriums, "characterological Moratoriums." stay in the exploratory mode all their life. Although this condition occurs more often in literature than in life, some characterological Moratoriums can be found on almost every university campus. An intrastatus distinction that is very important to make is that between a "developmental" and a "firm" Foreclosure. The former may be expected to go into a Moratorium at a later date and should appear more similar on dependent variables to Achievement than the latter, who is less likely to move developmentally. Some variables that may discriminate between these two and between flexible and rigid Achievements have been discussed by Bilsker and Marcia, (1991), Waterman (1982), and Stephen et al. (1992). They include engagement in creative activities such as poetry writing, the capacity for adaptive regression, dialectical reasoning, and an experiential, as contrasted with an instrumental, outlook. Archer and Waterman (1990) have discriminated an additional five varieties of Foreclosure, one of the most interesting of which is the "appropriated Foreclosure" who has adopted, totalistically, the outlook of a group. This may be a Diffusion who has undergone a "conversion experience."

The Identity Diffusion status presents the greatest variety of distinctions (see Marcia, 1989a and Archer & Waterman, 1990), ranging from the borderline personality (for whom identity diffusion is one of a number of symptoms and whose etiology lies earlier and elsewhere than adolescence) to the "adaptive Diffusion" whose uncommitted state is a realistic response to an environment offering a paucity of occupational and ideological alternatives, yet encouraging exploration. Because of the relatively great variety of ways of being diffuse, at least eight combining the categories in the two published articles, the greatest variability in ego strength is also likely to be present in this status. Almost no research has been done on these intrastatus distinctions.

Contexts of Identity Development

The necessary and sufficient social conditions for identity development have hardly been explored (exceptions being Costa & Campos, 1986, 1988; and Adams & Fitch, 1983). One clear advantage of Erikson's theory is that it acknowledges, and sometimes even specifies, connections between individual development on the one hand and relevant social institutions on the other. We now know some of the different forms identity can take and we have a fairly valid measure of these; it seems a logical next step to begin to specify what kinds of environments produce what kinds of identities. The taxonomy of environments that would be necessary for this task would have to transcend specific situations (e.g., college, workplace, armed forces) and instead consider transsituational commonalities (e.g., encouraging or discouraging of expression, skill-oriented). One clear implication of the Costa and Campos and Adams and Fitch studies is that the university is not a unitary experience, to the extent that it is not even, for all students, a psychosocial moratorium. For some in "crash" engineering and pre-med courses, it is more like educational boot camp. This taxonomy of environments has not been undertaken in part because of the individualistic appeal of the identity paradigm, which leads to its having been investigated more by psychologists than other social scientists (a valid point made by Côté & Levine [1988a,b]—see also Waterman [1988]). If we knew the relevant optimum environments for identity formation, we would be in a much stronger position to advocate specific social programs.

The Question of Intervention

When identity research began twenty-five years ago, it was hoped only that the most practical outcome would be good theory. Within the past few years, however, articles have begun to appear on interventional efforts stemming from the identity status research. For example, Markstrom-Adams et al. (unpublished ms.) have conducted some preliminary research on techniques for promoting identity development. A whole issue of the *Journal of Adolescence* (Archer, 1989) dealt with the topic of intervention and identity, and that is the theme of a forthcoming book by Archer (in preparation). The relationship between identity status research and intervention comes close to many psychologists' ideal of how interventions ought to be arrived at; viz., one begins with a theory, develops measures related to the theory, determines the theory's validity, and then proceeds to formulate ameliorative procedures based upon validated theory. Whether or not interventions following from this procedure are any more or less effective than those following from any other remains to be seen. At least, if they do not work, their failure should have some ramifications for changing theory.

Research on Other Psychosocial Stages

The current work was intended to be a handbook of psychosocial research, not just identity and intimacy research. It is hoped, then, that researchers seeking to validate other psychosocial stages will be heartened by our efforts. If nothing else, we have demonstrated that very complex concepts can be so defined and measured that one can proceed scientifically with them. Some initial efforts at developing measures of psychosocial stages other than identity and intimacy are currently under way. Bradley and Marcia (1990) have begun the development of a measure of Generativity; and Hearn (work in progress) is constructing a measure of Integrity. Both of these efforts employ a structured interview and scoring manual to determine statuses that have underlying process dimensions, similar to the approach taken with the identity and intimacy statuses. This method seems to capture best the complexity of adult resolutions of dialectical psychosocial issues. A measure of Industry has already been constructed and has undergone initial validational procedures (Kowaz & Marcia, 1991). Consistent with the less complex resolutions of the less dialectical earlier psychosocial stages, the Industry measure is a continuous-scale questionnaire-style measure. The general principle governing these efforts has been that the most useful and theoretically accurate way in which to validate a psychosocial stage issue is to construct an age-appropriate measure of that issue. Hence, if Autonomy, as a psychosocial developmental construct, is to be measured and validated, that measure should be one that is constructed for toddlers. Autonomy is an important concept at any chronological age, and its general construct validity might be determined at any age. But if one is speaking of establishing construct validity for Autonomy as a psychosocial developmental stage, then a measure of it constructed for, say, young adults is not adequate for assessing the overall validity of Erikson's psychosocial developmental scheme. What must be done first is to determine whether or not Autonomy is a valid way of describing the major personality developmental event of toddlerhood. If that is done successfully, then either an upward or downward extension of the measure can be constructed to assess Autonomy at other life-cycle stages, in the context of those stages' dominant issues. The point is that, in constructing a measure of Autonomy, one is not just constructing a measure of an isolated personality variable, but rather, one is attempting to determine the validity of a theory.

Life-Span Identity Development

The first identity resolution is achieved at late adolescence because that is the first time it can be; that is, when the necessary cognitive, physiological, social expectational, and experiential ingredients exist to make it possible. If this first resolution is an Achieved one, most persons will undergo further Moratorium-Achievement (MAMA) cycles throughout their life cycle. Based upon the longitudinal data that we have accumulated thus far, the prospects for life-span MAMA cycles for Foreclosures and Diffusions are weak. There are good psychosocial developmental reasons for this weakness: if one has not developed for oneself a clear sense of who one is then one's self-definition lies in the hands of others—either introjected others, for Foreclosures, or present others, for Diffusions. This extreme reliance upon external sources for one's identity necessarily detracts from the mutuality of a truly Intimate relationship, either because the partner is cast in terms of the introjects and not seen clearly for himself or herself (Foreclosure), or because of the identity-confirming burden laid upon the partner who is used for self-definition (Diffusion). The scope and depth of subsequent Generativity is then limited to "one's own kind" for Foreclosures, or, worse, to oneself for Diffusions. The disequilibration preceding a Moratorium is unlikely to occur for the Foreclosure who stays in a foreclosure setting and maintains foreclosure defenses intact because the potentially disequilibrating information is never perceived. For classic Diffusions, disequilibration is unlikely to occur because it presupposes a preexisting structure. And the only structure that is likely to exist is like an exoskeleton, present externally rather than internally, and more likely to be shattered than to undergo accommodation. However, although it seems not to be the norm, non-Identity Achievement persons do undergo identity crises after the optimal late adolescent period. This possibility is built into the form of Erikson's theory, which provides for the reemergence, and hence resolution, of every previous psychosocial stage at every succeeding one. But the task is not an easy one. Our society is willing to grant, and even encourage, a psychosocial moratorium for 18 year olds; but the applecarts overturned by a 40-year-old Foreclosure who begins to question occupational, marital, and parental roles are not applauded. This condition is especially true of Foreclosures just because of their particular strengths: reliability and predictability. The expectations that others have of them and that they have of themselves are more rigid than those established by Identity Achievements who expect, and to some extent are expected, to change. The Identity Achievement's identity crisis at 40 may also be painful, but not nearly as painful as the Foreclosure's.

Validation for the Structure of Psychosocial Developmental Theory

Although it is somewhat beyond the scope of this book, at least three sets of authors have proposed schemes whereby the underlying structure of Erikson's theory might be validated (van Geert, 1987; Logan, 1986; and Meacham & Santilli, 1982). Particularly interesting is van Geert's approach, suggesting a generative mathematical model, even though he acknowledges that "perhaps Erikson's theory is not a theory in the classical sense, but a heuristic framework, continuously changing, lacking a sufficient amount of logical-conceptual rigor. . . . Nevertheless, there is a definite advantage in applying a formal analytic tool to theories that are weakly structured. . . . The advantage is that formal analysis may provide explicitly formulated ways for making nontrivial extensions and specifications to the theory, leading to a real deepening of the understanding of what the theory amounts to, and to an extension of its empirical predictions and potential applications" (p. 254). If validity can be established for the measures of Generativity and Integrity currently under development, then we shall have those measures of the last five Eriksonian stages necessary to test some of the postulates of van Geert's model.

At the close of a book such as this, one usually makes an obligatory statement about there being much work yet to do and the importance of carrying out longitudinal studies. Both remarks are certainly valid here, but it is unlikely that anyone will do psychosocial developmental research because it is virtuous to do so. They may, however, do it for the reasons many of us have: it is conceptually challenging, intrinsically and personally interesting and involving, and potentially useful socially.

Part IV
Appendices

Appendix A
Identity Status Interview: Early and Middle Adolescent Form

SALLY L. ARCHER AND ALAN S. WATERMAN

General Opening

How old are you?

And you are in what grade?

Where are you from?

How do you feel about living in ______________________________?

Are both of your parents living?

[If not:] At what age were you when your (father) (mother) died?

Have your parents ever been separated or divorced?

[If yes:] At what age were you when your parents separated?

[If appropriate:] Whom have you lived with?

[If appropriate:] Has either of your parents remarried?

[If yes:] What age were you at that time?

Can you tell me something about your father's educational background?

And what type of work does he do?

And your mother, what was her educational background?

And has she been employed outside of the home?

[If appropriate:] Doing what?

Do you have any brothers or sisters? How many? Which are older and which are younger than you?

[If not already provided:] And your age is?

Vocational Plans—Opening

What grade are you in now?

[If High School:] What school program are you enrolled in here at ____________?

Do you have any ideas about what you'd like to do after graduation from high school in terms of work, school, and/or marriage?

[Proceed to the appropriate block(s) of questions: college or other education, work, and/or marriage.]

[If "don't know," ask: Do you think it is more likely that you will continue with your education after high school or that you will seek employment?

Proceed to the appropriate block(s) of questions.]

[If the answer is again "don't know," proceed to the closing block of questions on vocational plans.]

Vocational Plans—Further Education

[If appropriate:] Do you have any plans for a college major at this time?

What type of work would you like to do?

How did you come to decide on ____________? [Ask about future plans, if known; otherwise about major field].

If no definite interests are mentioned then omit this question and ask:] [What do you hope to gain by attending college? [Then skip to the closing block of questions on vocational plans.]

When did you first become interested in ____________?

What do you find attractive about ____________?

Is there anything not so attractive about this field?

[If several fields mentioned spontaneously, ask about each in turn.]

Have you ever considered any other fields besides ____________?

[List all the fields that were previously mentioned.]

[If yes, repeat questions about when interested and nature of attraction.]

How seriously were (are) you considering each of the fields you mentioned?

[For students who have specified a decision:] Did you ever feel that you were actively deciding between ____________ and ____________?

Was this a difficult decision to make?

What may have helped you make your choice here?

[For students who have not specified a decision:] Do you feel that choosing a career is something that you're trying to work out now, or do you feel that this is where you can let time take its course and just see what happens?

Do you have any ideas as to when you'd like to have this decision made?

How are you going about getting the information you'd like to have to make a decision?

Do you feel that this is an important decision for you to make now, or are you more concerned with other things right now?

[Proceed to the closing block of questions on vocational plans.]

Vocational Plans—Employment

What type of employment would you like to find?

How did you come to decide on ____________?

When did you first become interested in that type of work?

What do you find attractive about ____________?

What do you find not so attractive about this field?

[If several alternative possibilities are spontaneously mentioned, ask about each in turn.]

Have you ever considered any type of work besides ____________?

[List all the fields previously mentioned.]

Repeat cycle of questions above for each field mentioned that has not been previously discussed.]

How seriously were (are) you considering each of the plans you mentioned?

[For students who have specified a decision:] Do you feel that you were ever actively deciding between ____________ and ____________?

Was this a difficult decision for you to make?

What may have helped you to make your decision here?

[For students who have not specified a decision:] Do you feel that choosing a career is something that you're trying to work out now, or do you feel that this is something where you can let time take its course and just see what happens?

Do you have any idea as to when you'd like to have this decision made?

How are you going about getting the information you'd like to have to make a decision?

Do you feel that this is an important decision for you to make now or are you more concerned with other things right now?

Have you ever seriously considered continuing your education after high school?

[If yes:] Could you describe your thinking at that time?

[If appropriate:] Why did you decide not to go on with school?

[Proceed to the closing block of questions on vocational plans.]

Vocational Plans—Marriage

How did you come to decide on marriage as the best plan for you?

Do you plan to have children?

[If yes:] Do you plan to work or remain at home until you have children?

[If appropriate:] After you have children, would you continue to work?

When did you first become interested in these plans?

What do you find attractive about marriage (and work)?

What do you find unattractive about marriage (and work)?

Have you ever considered any other type of plan?

[If yes, repeat questions about when interested and nature of attraction.]

How seriously were you considering each of the plans you mentioned?

Have you ever seriously considered continuing your education (or going to work) after high school?

[If yes:] Could you describe your thinking at that time?

Why did you decide not to go on with school (work)?

Vocational Plans—Closing

Most parents have plans for their (sons) (daughters), things they'd like to see them go into, things they'd like to see them do. Did your folks have any plans like that for you?

Do you think your parents may have had a preference for one plan over another, although they would never have tried to pressure you about it?

[If yes:] Did you ever consider ____________?

[If appropriate:] How do your parents feel about your plans to go into ____________?

As you think about your activities in your coursework in school and any part-time work or hobbies you have had in the field(s) you might like to go into, what would you say is most satisfying or rewarding for you (for each of them)?

Is there anything about these activities that you would consider to be not so good?

How would you describe your feelings while you are engaged in these activities?

Why do you think you feel that way?

How willing do you think you'd be to change your plans from ____________ [the strongest one or two plans mentioned], if something better came along?

[If asked: "What do you mean by better? Respond: "Whatever might be better by your standards."]

[If Respondent indicates the possibility of change:]

What might you change to?

What might cause you to make such a change?

How likely do you think it is that you will make some change?

[Repeat for all the possibilities mentioned.]

On a 7-point scale, how important do you see your vocation as being to you in your life, where 7 means "extremely important" and 1 means "not at all important"?

Marriage and the Role of Spouse

[For those who were interviewed on the *Marriage—Vocational Plans*, use this beginning to the marriage domain:] I'd like to ask you more specific questions about marriage and parenting now. [Go first to "Why do you plan to marry," and so on within the marriage domain, and then on the parenting domain begin with, "Why do you plan to become a parent," and so on.]

[For all others, begin:] Do you plan to marry some day?

[If yes:] Why do you plan to marry?

When do you think would be a good time for you to marry?

Why then?

What kind of a person would you want to marry?

How do you picture what marriage might be like for you?

What do you see as your role as a (husband) (wife)?

[If no:] Have you ever thought about the idea of marriage?

Why do you think you would prefer not to marry?

What do you see as the advantages and disadvantages of being single versus being married? [If only one side is asked about, ask about the other position.]

Has your decision about (marrying) (not marrying) come easily to you or has it been a difficult decision to make?

Why ?

Who may have influenced your decision?

[If not already evident:] Have you ever gone through an important change in your thinking about marriage for yourself?

[If yes:] Please describe that change.

What started you thinking about these questions?

Who may have influenced your thinking?

How would you compare your ideas about marriage with those of your (father) (mother)? [Make comparison with the parent of the same gender as the Respondent.]

What is your parents' marriage like? How do you feel about the kind of marriage your parents (have) (had)?

Would you like your marriage to be similar to theirs?

How do your parents feel about your ideas on marriage? [If parents do not know:] How do you think they would feel about them if they did know?

Are you currently in a romantic relationship with someone?

[If yes:] How does your (boy) (girl) friend feel about your ideas about marriage?

How do your ideas about marriage compare with (his) (hers)?

What do you think are the best and worst things about marriage in terms of what you would be doing in the marriage in your role as a (husband) (wife)?

How willing would you be to change your plans about marriage?

[If appropriate:] What would it take to change your ideas about marriage?

Do you think you might think again about your decision at some time in the future?

[If yes:] When? Why then?

On a 7-point scale, how important do you see marriage and your having the role of (husband) (wife) as being to you in your life? Again, 7 means "extremely important" and 1 means "not at all important."

The Role of Parent

[Remember, for people who answered vocational plans in terms of marriage and parenting, to begin with "Why do you plan to become a parent."]

[For all others, begin:] Do you plan to become a parent some day?

[If yes:] Why do you plan to become a parent?

When do you think would be a good time in your life to start parenting?

How do you picture your role in parenting?

What type of behavior in your child would give you pleasure?

If you ever did become a parent, what role to you think your (husband) (wife) **should** have in parenting with you?

What role do you think your (husband) (wife) **will** have in parenting with you?

[If any difference is mentioned:] Why do you think that would be?

[If no:] Is this because you have never thought about the role of parent for you yourself or that you definitely do not want to be a parent?

How did you figure out that decision?

What do you see as the advantages and disadvantages of parenting?

[If only one side is presented, ask about the other.]

Has your decision about parenting come easily to you, or has it been a difficult decision to make?

Why?

Who or what has had a part in helping you to make your decision about this?

Have you ever gone thourgh an important change in your thinking about parenting?

[If yes:] When was that in your life?

Please describe the changes.

What started you thinking about these questions?

How did you go about working out your ideas?

Who may have influenced your decision about this?

How would you compare your ideas about parenting with those of your parents?

How would you describe your parents' thinking about parenting?

What do you think of the parenting you have had?

Would you like your parenting to be like theirs?

Would your parents like to see you be a parent some day?

How do you feel about that?

How do your parents feel about your ideas on parenting? [If parents don't know:] How do you think they would feel about them if they did know?

[If presently in a romantic relationship:] How does your (boy) (girl) friend feel about what you think about parenting?

How do your ideas about parenting compare with (his) (hers)?

Do you believe your ideas about parenting are now fairly well worked out, or do you feel that you are still working out your thinking about parenting?

[If still working out ideas:] What questions are you still thinking about?

What are you doing now to work out your thinking about these questions?

As you think about being a parent yourself, what would you like best and least about your role of parent?

How willing would you be to change your plans about parenting?

[If appropriate:] What would it take to change your ideas about parenting?

Do you think you might reconsider your decision at some time in the future?

[If yes:] When?

Why then?

What do you think might influence your decision about whether to be a parent or not?

On a 7-point scale, how important do you see the role of parent as being to you in your life? Again, 7 means "extremely important" and 1 means "not at all important."

Family and Career Priorities

Looking over the numbers you gave from 1 to 7 for each of the areas we have talked about so far, I notice that you rated career ____, in importance, marriage ____ and parenting ____, which seems to suggest that you value (____________ more) (each area about equally). How do you feel about that?

I would like you to share with me the types of problems you feel could develop because you have a career and a marriage, specifically with your being a (husband) (wife).

Now I would like you to tell me about possible problems you feel could happen because you have a career and are a parent.

I'd like you to give me a time line for how you plan to fit your education, employment, marriage, and parenting into your life relative to one another.

I'd like you to examine your time line about career and children more closely. If you were to have children, when would you want to fit them in with your education, career, and marriage?

How many children would you like to have?

How many years between them?

Would you plan to take time off from work to have children?

[If yes:] For how long?

Would you go back to work after having each child?

So the approximate total time off from work would amount to ____ years?

[If this is a considerable length of time:] Do you think it would be necessary for you to develop new or extra skills in your profession to get a similar job back?

What might some additional problems be for you that could arise about (marriage and career) (parenting and career) [in that order] as you look into your future?

How would you try to solve each of the problems you have mentioned?

How much have you thought about *marriage* and career conflicts before?

Have you ever gone through an important change in your thinking about marriage and career conflicts for yourself?

[If yes:] Please describe that change.

What started you thinking about such questions?

Who may have influenced your thinking about this question?

How are your thoughts about marriage and career problems like and not like those of your parents?

How do your parents handle such problems?

How does the way they do it make you think about how you would want to do it?

[If in a romantic relationship:] How does your (boy) (girl) friend feel about handling marriage and career conflicts?

How are your ideas similar and different?

How does your (friend) (partner) feel about your ideas on what the problems might be and how to handle them?

How much concern do you have now about this question? [If little or none:] Do you think it will become a serious question for you in the future?

[If yes:] At what time in your life?

[If no:] Why not?

[If not previously addressed concretely:] If you were confronted with a conflict between your work responsibilities and your responsibilities as a (husband) (wife), which would you give priority to? Why?

How much have you thought about *parenting* and career conflicts before?

Have you ever gone through an important change in your thinking about parenting and career conflicts for yourself?

[If yes:] Please describe that change.

What started you thinking about these questions?

Who or what helped you to make your decisions about this question?

How are your ideas like and not like those of your parents about how to handle problems or conflicts between doing things for your career and doing things for your children?

How do your parents handle such conflicts with you (and your brothers and sisters)?

Does the way they deal with it influence how you might deal with it? How so?

Would you like your handling of parenting and career conflicts to be like theirs?

[If in a romantic partnership:] How are your ideas about handling parenting and career conflicts like and not like those of your (boy) (girl) friend?

How does your (boy) (girl) friend feel about your ideas on the handling of parenting and career conflicts?

How much concern do you have now about this question?

[If little or none:] Do you think it may become a serious question for you in the future?

[If yes:] At what time in your life?

[If no:] Why not?

[If not previously addressed concretely:] If you were confronted with a conflict between your work responsibilities and your responsibilities as a parent, which would you give priority to? Why?

Religious Beliefs

Do you have any religious preference? [I.e., Do you belong to a religion?]

How about your parents: do they have any religious preference?

Were both of your parents reared ____________?

How important would you say religion is to your parents?

Have you ever been active in church or church groups? [Adapt for Jews and others.]

[If not already evident:] Do you go to religious services now?

[If yes:] What are your reasons for going?

How do you feel while you are doing things (in) (for) your (church) (temple)?

Why do you think you feel that way?

[If no:] Did you ever attend religious services fairly regularly?

[If appropriate:] What led to your attendance at services falling off?

Do you talk about religion with other people?

[If yes:] What kinds of things do you talk about? Do you get into arguments or discussions?

[If appropriate:] What do you argue for and against?

I'd like to find out something about your ideas in the area of religion, for example on such questions as the existence of God, and the importance of (organized religion) (having actual churches/temples to worship in and to go to school in to learn about your religion). What are your ideas?

[If Roman Catholic:] How about on the matter of the infallibility of the Pope? (I.e., Can the Pope ever make wrong decisions?)

[Ask about other religious questions as these appear appropriate.]

Was there ever a time when you came to question, to doubt, or perhaps to change your religious beliefs?

[If yes:] What types of things did you question or change?

What started you thinking about these questions?

[If not already in evidence:] How old were you at the time?

How serious were these questions for you?

Do you feel that you've solved these questions for yourself, or are you still working on them?

[If resolved:] What has helped you to answer these questions?

[If not resolved:] How are you going about trying to answer these questions?

How do your parents feel about your religious beliefs?

[If parents don't know:] How do you think they would feel about them if they did know?

Are there any important differences between your beliefs and those of your parents?

At this time, how well worked out do you think your ideas in the area of religion are?

Do you think your ideas in the area are likely to remain the same, or do you believe they may very well change in the future?

[If they may change:] In what direction do you think your beliefs might change?

What might bring about such a change?

How likely is it that such a change might occur?

[If you see evidence of continued thought being given to religious questions:] How important is it to you to work out your ideas in the area of religion?

Are you actively trying to work out your beliefs now, or are you more concerned with other things?

How would you like to see your own children reared with respect to religion?

On a 7-point scale, how important do you see your religious beliefs as being to you in your life? Again, 7 means "extremely important" and 1 means "not at all important."

[For agnostics and atheists, the last question in this domain should be phrased thus:]

On a 7-point scale, how important do you see your ideas about (agnosticism) (atheism) as being to you in your life? Again, 7 means "extremely important" and 1 means "not at all important."]

Political Beliefs

Do you have any political preference? [If asked "What do you mean by political preference?" Respond: Either party preference or a position on the liberal to conservative scale. For example, do you consider yourself a Democrat or a Republican? Do you consider youself as a liberal, moderate, or conservative?]

[If appropriate:] Have you heard of these terms before?

[If yes:] Can you tell me which terms you have heard about, and how?

Do your parents have any political preferences?

[If appropriate:] Do they belong to any political party?

[If appropriate:] Where would they fall on a scale from liberal through moderate to conservative?

[Ask the questions above separately for both father and mother.]

How important would you say political questions are to your parents?

Are there any political or social issues that you feel pretty strongly about?

[If asked, "Such as?" Respond: "Whatever might be important issues for you." If asked again, suggest such issues as the economy, how much weaponry is needed for defense, foreign policy, the environment, and so on.]

What would you like to see done about ____________________?

[Repeat for each issue raised.]

Are there other issues that you have views about?

What would you like to see done about ______________________?

[Repeat for each issue mentioned.]

Have you ever taken any political actions, like joining groups, participating in election campaigns, writing letters to government or other political leaders, signing petitions, participating in demonstrations?

[If yes, elicit a description of each if necessary.]

How did you get involved in these activities?

[Repeat for several of the activities mentioned.]

[If no issues or activities were discussed:] Do you feel that you are actively trying to arrive at a set of political beliefs, or do you feel that the area of politics isn't very important to you at present?

[If trying to work out ideas:] Can you tell me something about the types of things you are thinking about?

How are you going about getting the information you need to make a decision?

How important is it for you to work out these ideas?

Was there ever a time when you found your political ideas undergoing change, when you believed one thing on an issue and then, months or years later, you found you had very different ideas on the same issue?

[If yes:] Please describe the circumstances.

What led you to make that type of change?

Was there anyone or anything that may have influenced your thinking at the time?

How do you feel while you are engaged in activities related to your political beliefs?

Why do you think you feel that way?

How do your parents feel about your political ideas?

[If parents don't know:] How do you think they would feel about them if they did know?

Are there any important differences between your views and those of your parents?

At this time do you believe that your political beliefs are likely to remain the same for some time, or do you feel they may very well change in the future?

[If they may change:] In what direction do you think your beliefs might change?

What might bring about such a change?

How likely is it that such a change will occur?

[If appropriate:] Do you feel these changes would occur just on specific issues, or might there be a change in your general political attitude?

On a 7-point scale, how important do you see your political beliefs as being to you in your life? Again, 7 means "extremely important" and 1 means "not at all important."

Sex-Role Attitudes

Changing topics again, I'd like to talk with you about your ideas of men's (boys') and women's (girls') roles in society today.

What advantages and disadvantages do you see associated with the roles of men and women in today's society?

[Ask advantages **and** disadvantages for **both** genders.]

[Or for the younger ones, ask:] What do you think is good and bad about being a boy versus a girl in our society today?

How do you think things **should** be in terms of what women and girls are supposed to be like and what men and boys are supposed to be like?

If you could have chosen to be a man (boy) or a woman (girl) in today's society, which would you be?

Why?

[If appropriate:] What is best and worst for you yourself about being a (male/boy) (female/girl)?

How do you feel while you are doing things that go with your being a (male) (boy)/(female) (girl)?

Why do you think you feel that way?

How did you come to learn what it means to be a (man/boy) (woman/girl) in today's society?

Do you feel this is something that came rather naturally for you, or were there times when you were uncertain how you should act?

[If there were uncertainties:] Can you describe the circumstances for me?

How did you go about working out what you should do?

Who or what may have helped you with your thinking at the time?

Was there ever a time when you came to question, to doubt, or perhaps to change your ideas, your expectations, and/or how you acted in terms of your (male/boy) (female/girl) roles in this society?

[If yes:] What types of things did you question or change?

What started you thinking about these questions?

[If not already evident:] How old were you at the time?

How serious were these questions for you?

Do you feel you've solved these questions for yourself, or are you still working on them?

[If resolved:] What has helped you to answer these questions?

[If not resolved:] How are you going about trying to answer these questions?

How have your mother and father expressed their female and male roles, respectively?

How were your ideas, expectations, and behaviors in this area influenced by your parents?

Are there any important similarities and differences between the ideas, expectations, and behaviors you and your (father) (mother) have in expressing your role as a (male/boy) (female/girl) in today's society?

[If appropriate:] How about the effects your brothers or sisters may have had? [Adapt as appropriate for the gender of the sibs.]

Are there any important differences between their ideas, expectations, and behaviors and yours about men's and women's roles in society?

[If currently in a romantic relationship:] What are your dating partner's ideas, expectations, and behaviors about men's and women's roles in society today?

How are they similar to and different from yours?

How does (he) (she) feel about your ideas, expectations, and behaviors about your role as a (male/boy) (female/girl) in today's society?

How has (his)(her) perspective influenced yours?

How do your parents feel about your views on this area?

[If parents don't know:] How do you think they would feel about them if they did know?

Do you see your ideas about the roles of men and women in today's society remaining stable or do you see your ideas possibly changing in the future?

[If ideas may change:] In what direction might your ideas change?

What do you think might cause such a change?

How likely is it that such a change might occur?

[If you see evidence of continued thought being given to these questions:] How important is it to you to work out your ideas in this area?

Are you actively trying to work out your beliefs, expectations, and/or behaviors now, or are you more concerned with other things?

On a 7-point scale, how important do you see your role as a (male/boy) (female/girl) as being to you in your life? Again, 7 means "extremely important" and 1 means "not at all important."

Appendix B
Identity Status Interview: Late Adolescent College Form

James E. Marcia and Sally L. Archer

General Opening

How old are you?

Where are you from originally?

And where are you living now?

How do you feel about living in ______________________________?

Are both of your parents still living?

[If not:] At what age were you when your (father) (mother) died?

Have your parents ever been separated or divorced?

[If yes:] At what age were you when your parents separated?

[If appropriate:] Whom did you live with then?

[If appropriate:] Has either of your parents remarried?

[If yes:] What age were you at that time?

Can you tell me something about your father's educational background?

And what type of work does he do?

And your mother, what was her educational background?

And has she been employed outside the home?

[If appropriate:] What type of work does she do?

Do you have any brothers or sisters?

[If yes:] What are their ages?

What have you done about continued schooling, work, and marriage since you left high school?

[If married, inquire about the educational and employment background of the spouse, and the presence of children in the family.]

Vocational Plans[1]

How did you come to decide on attending ____________ (name of college or other postsecondary school)?

What year are you in now?

What is your major?

Do you have a minor? [If yes:] What is it?

How did you come to decide on ____________ as a major?

When did you first become interested in ____________?

What do you find attractive about this field?

What drawbacks do you see about the field?

What would you like to do with this major after you graduate from college?

How would you describe your feelings while you are engaged in activities related to your major?

Why do you think you feel that way?

Since you have been at college, have you thought about any other majors besides ____________?

[If yes:] What else have you considered?

When did you first become interested in ____________?

What did you find attractive about ____________?

What drawbacks did you see in this field?

Why did you decide not to pursue this field?

[1] If Respondent is currently employed, use the vocational activities section of the adult form.

Was this a difficult decision to make?

What do you think influenced your choice?

[Repeat for each possible major mentioned.]

How about when you were in high school—what was your thinking about your future vocational plans?

[Repeat cycle of questions above for each field mentioned that has not been previously discussed.]

[If not already evident:] Was there ever a time when you were trying to decide between two very different directions for your life, in terms of the work you wished to pursue?

[If yes:] What were your alternatives then?

Was that a difficult decision to make?

What influenced your decision here?

Most parents have plans for their (sons) (daughters), things they'd like to see them go into, things they'd like to see them do. Did your folks have any plans like that for you?

Do you think your parents may have had a preference for one field over another, although they would never have tried to pressure you about it?

[If necessary:] How do your parents feel about your plans to go into ______________ (Respondent's current career plans)?

How willing do you think you'd be to change your plans from ______________ [Respondent's current career plans], if something better came along?

[If asked: "What do you mean by better? Respond: "Whatever might be better by your standards."]

[If Respondent indicates the possibility of change:] What might you change to?

What might cause you to make such a change?

How likely do you think it is that you will make some change?

On a 7-point scale, how important do you see your vocation as being to you in your life, where 7 means "extremely important" and 1 means "not at all important"?

Marriage and the Role of Spouse

Do you plan to marry some day?

[If yes:] Why do you plan to marry?

When do you think would be a good time for you to marry?

Why then?

What kind of a person would you want to marry?

How do you picture what marriage might be like for you?

What do you see as your role as a (husband) (wife)?

[If no:] Have you ever thought about the idea of marriage?

Why do you think you prefer not to marry?

What do you see as the advantages and disadvantages of being single versus being married?

Has your decision about (marrying) (not marrying) come easily to you, or has it been a difficult decision to make?

Why do you think it has?

Who may have been a factor in your decision?

[If not already evident:] Have you ever gone through an important change in your thinking about marriage for yourself?

[If yes:] Please describe that change.

What started you thinking about these questions?

Who may have been a factor in your thinking?

How would you compare your ideas about marriage with those of your (father) (mother)? [Make comparison with the parent of the same gender as the Respondent.]

How would you describe your parents' marriage?

What do you think of the marriage your parents (have) (had)?

Would you like your marriage to be similar to theirs?

How do your parents feel about your ideas on marriage?

[If parents do not know:] How do you think they would feel about them if they did know?

Are you currently in a romantic relationship with someone?

[If yes:] How does the person you are presently involved with feel about your ideas on marriage?

How do your ideas about marriage compare with (his) (hers)?

As you think about the activities involved in marriage and your role as a (husband) (wife), what would you say you anticipate to be most satisfying or rewarding for you?

Is there anything about these activities that you anticipate will be a source of dissatisfaction for you?

How willing would you be to change your plans about marriage?

[If appropriate:] What would it take to change your ideas about marriage?

Do you anticipate that you might reexamine your decision at some time in the future?

[If yes:] When? Why then?

On a 7-point scale, how important do you see marriage and the role of a spouse as being to you in your life? Again, 7 means "extremely important" and 1 means "not at all important."

The Role of Parent

Do you plan to be a parent some day?

[If yes:] Why do you plan to be a parent?

When do you think would be a good time in your life to start parenting?

How do you picture your role in parenting?

What type of behavior in your child would give you pleasure?

If you ever did become a parent, what role do you think your spouse **should** have in parenting with you?

What role do you anticipate your spouse **would** have in parenting with you?

[If any difference is mentioned:] Why?

[If no:] Is this because you have never thought about the role of parent for you yourself, or that you definitely do not want to be a parent?

How have you arrived at that decision?

What do you see as the advantages and disadvantages of parenting?

[If only one side is presented, ask about the other.]

Has your decision about parenting come easily to you, or has it been a difficult decision to make?

Why do you think it has been?

What has influenced your decision?

Have you ever gone through an important change in your thinking about parenting?

[If yes:] When was that in your life?

Please describe the changes.

What started you thinking about these questions?

Who may have been a factor in your thinking?

How would you compare your ideas about parenting with those of your parents?

How would you describe your parents' thinking about parenting?

What do you think of the parenting you have had?

Would you like your parenting to be similar to theirs?

Would your parents like to see you be a parent some day?

How do you feel about that?

How do your parents feel about your ideas on parenting?

[If parents don't know:] How do you think they would feel about them if they did know?

[If presently in a romantic relationship:] How does the person you are presently involved with feel about your attitudes toward parenting?

How do your ideas about parenting compare with (his) (hers)?

Do you believe that your ideas about parenting are now fairly well worked out, or do you feel that you are still working out your thinking about parenting?

[If still working out ideas:] What questions are you still thinking about?

What are you doing now to work out your thinking about these questions?

How willing would you be to change your plans about parenting?

[If appropriate:] What would it take to change your ideas about parenting?

Do you anticipate that you might reexamine your decision at some time in the future?

[If yes:] When? Why then?

What do you think might influence your decision?

On a 7-point scale, how important do you see the role of parent as being to you in your life? Again, 7 means "extremely important" and 1 means "not at all important."

Family and Career Priorities

Looking over your previous responses, I notice that you rated career ____ in importance, marriage ____, and parenting ____, which seems to suggest that you value (____________ more) (each area about equally). How do you feel about that?

I would like you to share with me the types of conflicts you feel could develop as a result of your pursuit of a career and a marriage, specifically with your role as a (husband) (wife).

Now I would like you to elaborate on possible conflicts you feel could develop as a result of pursuing your career and parenting?

I'd like you to give me a time line for how you plan to fit your education, employment, marriage, and parenting into your life relative to one another.

I'd like you to examine your time line about career and children more closely. If you were to have children, at what time relative to your education, career, and marriage would you like to have them?

How many children would you like to have?

How many years apart?

Would you plan to take time off from work to have children?

[If yes:] For how long?

Would you reenter the work force between children?

So the approximate total time off from work would amount to ____ years?

[If this is a considerable length of time:] Do you think it would be necessary for you to develop reentry skills in your profession to gain employment comparable to the work you had before?

What might some additional conflicts be for you that could arise based on your projections of your future? [Ask first for marriage, then for parenting.]

How would you try to resolve each of the conflicts you have mentioned?

How much have you thought about **marriage** and career conflicts before?

Have you ever gone through an important change in your thinking about marriage and career conflicts for yourself?

[If yes:] Please describe that change.

What started you thinking about such questions?

Who may have been a factor in your thinking?

How would you compare your ideas about handling spouse/career conflicts with those of your parents?

How would you describe your parents' own behavior in their marriage over such potential conflicts?

Did their behavior and choices influence you? How?

Would you like to handle spouse and career conflicts in a way that would be similar to their handling of such conflicts?

[If in a romantic relationship:] What similarities and differences are there between your ideas about spouse and career conflicts and those of your romantic partner?

How does your romantic partner feel about your ideas on handling spouse and career conflicts?

How much concern do you have now about this question?

[If little or none:] Do you anticipate its becoming a serious question for you in the future?

[If yes:] At what time in your life?

[If no:] Why not?

[If not previously addressed concretely:] If you were confronted with a conflict between your work responsibilities and your responsibilities as a (husband) (wife), which would you give priority to? Why?

How much have you thought about **parenting** and career conflicts before?

Have you ever gone through an important change in your thinking about parenting and career conflicts for yourself?

[If yes:] Please describe that change.

What started you thinking about these questions?

Who may have been a factor in your thinking?

How would you compare your ideas about handling parenting and career conflicts with those of your parents?

How would you describe your parents' own behavior in parenting and career conflicts?

Did their way of handling such conflicts influence your decision about how to handle them? How?

Would you like your handling of parenting and career conflicts to be similar to theirs?

[If in a romantic partnership:] What similarities and differences are there between your ideas about parenting and career conflicts and those of your romantic partner?

How does your romantic partner feel about your ideas on handling parenting and career conflicts?

How much concern do you have now about this question?

[If little or none:] Do you anticipate its becoming a serious question for you in the future?

[If yes:] At what time in your life?

[If no:] Why not?

[If not previously addressed concretely:] If you were confronted with a conflict between your work responsibilities and your responsibilities as a parent, which would you give priority to? Why?

Religious Beliefs

Do you have any religious preference?

How about your parents—do they have any religious preference?

Were both of your parents reared ________?

How important would you say religion is to your parents?

Have you ever been active in church or church groups? [Adapt for Jews and others.]

Have you been active since (coming to college) (in the past several years)?

[If not already evident:] Do you currently attend religious services?

[If yes:] What are your reasons for attending services?

How do you feel while you are engaged in activities related to your religion?

Why do you think you feel that way?

[If no:] Did you ever attend religious services with any frequency?

[If appropriate:] What has led your attendance at services to fall off?

Do you find yourself getting into religious discussions?

[If yes:] What point of view do you express in these discussions?

I'd like to find out something about your ideas in the area of religion, for example on such questions as the existence of God, and the importance of organized religion. What are your ideas?

[If Roman Catholic:] How about the matter of the infallibility of the Pope?

[Ask other religious questions as these appear appropriate.]

Was there ever a time when you came to question, to doubt, or perhaps to change your religious beliefs?

[If yes:] What types of things did you question or change?

What started you thinking about these questions?

[If not already evident:] How old were you at the time?

How serious were these questions for you?

Do you feel that you've resolved these questions for yourself, or are you still working on them?

[If resolved:] What has helped you to answer these questions?

[If not resolved:] How are you going about trying to answer these questions?

How do your parents feel about your religious beliefs?

[If parents don't know:] How do you think they would feel about them if they did know?

Are there any important differences between your beliefs and those of your parents?

At this time, how well worked out do you think your ideas on religion are?

Do you think your ideas on religion are likely to remain stable, or do you believe they may very well change in the future?

[If they may change:] In what direction do you think your beliefs might change?

What might bring about such a change?

How likely is it that such a change might occur?

[If you see evidence of continued thought being given to religious questions:] How important is it to you to work out your ideas on religion?

Are you actively trying to work out your beliefs now, or are you more concerned with other things?

On a 7-point scale, how important do you see your religious beliefs as being to you in your life? Again, 7 means "extremely important" and 1 means "not at all important."

[For agnostics and atheists, the last question in this domain should be:] On a 7-point scale, how important do you see your ideas about (agnosticism) (atheism) as being to you in your life?

Again, 7 means "extremely important" and 1 means "not at all important."

Political Beliefs

Do you have any political preference?

Do you belong to, or do you see yourself as associated with, any political party?

Where would you describe yourself as falling on a scale from liberal through moderate to conservative?

Do your parents have any political preferences?

[If appropriate:] Do they belong to any political party?

[If appropriate:] Where would they fall on a scale from liberal through moderate to conservative? [If necessary, ask separately for both father and mother.]

How important would you say political matters are to your parents?

Are there any political or social issues that you feel pretty strongly about?

[If asked "Such as?" Respond: "Whatever might be important issues for you." If asked again, suggest such issues as the economy, how much weaponry is needed for defense, foreign policy, etc.]

What would you like to see done about ______________________________?

[Repeat for each issue raised.]

Are there other issues that you have views about?

What would you like to see done about ______________________________?

[Repeat for each issue mentioned.]

Have you ever taken any political actions, like joining groups, participating in election campaigns, writing letters to government or other political leaders, signing petitions, participating in demonstrations?

[If yes:] [If necessary, elicit a description of each.]

What were the circumstances of your becoming involved in these activities?

[Repeat for several of the activities mentioned.]

How do you feel while you are engaged in activities related to your political beliefs?

Why do you think you feel that way?

[If no issues or activities were discussed:] Do you feel that you are actively trying to arrive at a set of political beliefs, or do you feel that the area of politics isn't very important to you at present?

[If trying to work out ideas:] Can you tell me something about the types of things you are thinking about?

How are you going about getting the information you need to make a decision?

How important is it for you to work out these ideas?

Was there ever a time when you found your political ideas undergoing change, when you believed one thing on an issue and then, months or years later, you found you had very different ideas on the same issue?

[If yes:] Please describe the circumstances.

What led you to make that type of change?

Was there anyone who may have influenced your thinking at the time?

How do your parents feel about your political ideas?

[If parents don't know:] How do you think they would feel about them if they did know?

Are there any important differences between your views and those of your parents?

At this time do you believe your political beliefs are likely to remain stable for some time, or do you feel they may very well change in the future?

[If they may change:] In what direction do you think your beliefs might change?

What might bring about such a change?

How likely is it that such a change might occur?

[If appropriate:] Do you feel these changes would occur just on specific issues, or might there be a change in your general political philosophy?

On a 7-point scale, how important do you see your political beliefs as being to you in your life? Again, 7 means "extremely important" and 1 means "not at all important."

Sex-Role Attitudes

Changing topics again, I'd like to talk with you about your perceptions of men's and women's roles in society today.

What advantages and disadvantages do you see as associated with the roles of men and women in today's society?

[Make sure advantages **and** disadvantages are addressed for **both** genders.]

How do you think things **should** be in terms of what women are supposed to be like and what men are supposed to be like?

If you could have chosen to be a man or a woman in today's society, which would you be?

Why?

As you think about your activities as a (man) (woman) in today's society, what would you say is most satisfying or rewarding for you yourself?

Is there anything about these activities that you would consider a source of dissatisfaction?

How would you describe your feelings while you are engaged in these activities?

Why do you think you feel that way?

How did you come to learn what it means to be a (man) (woman) in today's society?

Do you feel this is something that came naturally for you, or were there times when you were uncertain how you should act?

[If there were uncertainties:] Can you describe the circumstances for me?

How did you go about working out what you should do?

Who may have been a factor in your thinking at the time?

Was there ever a time when you came to question, to doubt, or perhaps to change your ideas, expectations, and/or behavior about your roles as a (woman) (man) in this society?

[If yes:] What types of things did you question or change?

What started you thinking about these questions?

[If not already evident:] How old were you at the time?

How serious were these questions for you?

Do you feel that you've resolved these questions for yourself, or are you still working on them?

[If resolved:] What has helped you to answer these questions?

[If not resolved:] How are you going about trying to answer these questions?

How have your mother and father expressed their female and male roles, respectively?

How were your ideas, expectations, and behaviors in this area influenced by your parents?

Are there any important similarities and/or differences between the ideas, expectations, and behaviors with which you and your (father) (mother) express the role of a (man) (woman) in today's society?

[If appropriate:] How about the effects your brothers or sisters may have had on your ideas, expectations, and behaviors?

Are there any important differences between their ideas, expectations, and behaviors and yours on men's and women's roles in society?

[If currently in a romantic relationship:] What are your dating partner's ideas, expectations, and behaviors about men's and women's roles in society today?

How are they similar and different from yours?

How does (he) (she) feel about your ideas, expectations, and behaviors on your role as a (man) (woman) in today's society?

How has (his) (her) perspective influenced yours?

How do your parents feel about your ideas, expectations, and behaviors on your role as a (man) (woman) in today's society?

[If parents don't know:] How do you think they would feel about them if they did know?

Do you see your ideas about the roles of men and women in today's society remaining stable, or do you see your ideas possibly changing in the future?

[If ideas may change:] In what direction might your ideas change?

What do you think might cause such a change?

How likely is it that such a change might occur?

[If you see evidence of continued thought being given to these questions:] How important is it to you to work out your ideas in this area?

Are you actively trying to work out your beliefs, expectations, and/or behaviors now, or are you more concerned with other things?

On a 7-point scale, how important do you see your beliefs, expectations, and behaviors defined by your role as a (man) (woman) as being to you in your life? Again, 7 means "extremely important" and 1 means "not at all important."

Appendix C
Identity Status Interview: Adult Form

Sally L. Archer and Alan S. Waterman

General Opening

Where are you from originally?

And where are you living now?

How do you feel about living in ______________________________?

If I may ask, how old are you?

Are both of your parents still living?

[If not:] At what age were you when your (father) (mother) died?

Have your parents ever been separated or divorced?

[If yes:] At what age were you when your parents separated?

[If appropriate:] Whom did you live with then?

[If appropriate:] Has either of your parents remarried?

[If yes:] What age were you at that time?

Can you tell me something about your father's educational background?

And what type of work (does) (did) he do?

And your mother, what was her educational background?

And has (had) she been employed outside of the home?

[If appropriate:] What type of work does (did) she do?

Do you have any brothers or sisters?

[If yes:] What are their ages?

What have you done about continued schooling, work, and marriage since you left high school?

[If married, inquire into the educational and employment background of the spouse, and the presence of children in the family.]

Vocational Activities

How did you come to work for ____________ (name of company)?

And how did you come to choose to do ____________ (the type of work described)?

[If unemployed:] What type of work would you like to do?

How are you going about trying to obtain employment?

[For all Respondents:] When did you first become interested in ____________?

What do you find attractive about the work you are (doing) (seeking) now?

What drawbacks do you see about your (present) (sought) work?

How would you describe your feelings while you are engaged in these work activities?

Why do you think you feel that way?

Have there been other types of work that you have pursued?

[If yes:] What did they involve?

[As appropriate:] How long were you engaged in each of those types of work?

[As appropriate:] What did you see as attractive and as drawbacks to ____________? [Ask for each type of work.]

When you were deciding on employment, were there any other fields or types of work you were considering?

[If appropriate, ask "attractive" and "drawbacks" questions about each field mentioned.]

[If appropriate:] Why did you decide *not* to pursue that (those) careers?

[If Respondent attended college or other type of postsecondary school:] How did you come to decide on attending ____________?

What was your major?

Did you have a minor? [If yes:] What was it?

How did you come to decide on ____________ as a major?

When did you first become interested in ____________?

What did you find attractive about this field?

What drawbacks did you see about the field?

What did you plan to do with this major after you graduated from college?

While in college, did you think about any other majors besides____________?

[If yes:] What else did you consider?

When did you first become interested in ____________?

What did you find attractive about ____________?

What drawbacks did you see to this field?

Why did you decide not to pursue this field?

Was this a difficult decision to make?

What do you think influenced your choice?

[Repeat for each possible major mentioned.]

How about when you were in high school, what was your thinking about your future vocational plans?

[Repeat cycle of questions above for each field mentioned that has not been previously discussed.]

[If not already evident:] Was there ever a time when you were trying to decide between two very different directions for your life—the work you wished to pursue?

[If yes:] What were your alternatives then?

Was that a difficult decision to make?

What influenced your decision here?

Most parents have plans for their (sons) (daughters), things they'd like to see them go into, things they'd like to see them do. Did your folks have any plans like that for you?

Do you think your parents may have had a preference for one field over another, although they would never have tried to pressure you about it?

[If necessary:] How did your parents feel about your plans to go into ______________ [Respondent's current career activities]?

[If married:] How does your spouse feel about your current career activities?

How willing do you think you'd be to change your plans from ____________ [Respondent's current career activities], if something better came along?

[If asked: "What do you mean by better?" Respond: "Whatever might be better by your standards."]

[If Respondent indicates the possibility of change:] What might you change to?

What might cause you to make such a change?

How likely do you think it is that you will make some change?

On a 7-point scale, how important do you see your vocation as being to you in your life, where 7 means "extremely important" and 1 means "not at all important"?

Marriage and the Role of Spouse

Do you remember what your thoughts about marriage were like when you were a student in high school (and in college)?

[If necessary:] Can you describe your thinking?

[If married:] What were your thoughts about marriage leading up to the time when you married?

What did you think would be a good time for you to marry?

What kind of person did you want to marry?

How did you picture what marriage might be like for you?

What did you see as your role as a (husband) (wife)?

[If never married:] Have you ever thought about the idea of marriage?

[If not planning to marry:] Why do you think you preferred not to marry?

[If planning to marry:] Why do you think you would prefer to marry?

What do you see as the advantages and disadvantages of being single versus being married?

Has your decision about (marrying) (not marrying) come easily to you, or has it been a difficult decision to make?

Why?

Who may have been a factor in your decision?

[If divorced and not remarried:] Have you ever thought about the idea of marrying again?

[If not planning to remarry:] Why do you think you preferred not to remarry?

[If planning to remarry:] Why do you think you would prefer to remarry?

What do you see as the advantages and disadvantages of being single versus being married again? [If only one side is presented, ask about the other.]

Has your decision about (remarrying) (not remarrying) come easily to you, or has it been a difficult decision to make?

Why?

Who may have been a factor in your decision?

[For every Respondent:] Have you ever gone through an important change in your thinking about marriage for yourself?

[If yes:] Please describe that change.

What started you thinking about these questions?

Who may have been a factor in your thinking?

How would you compare your ideas about marriage with those of your (father) (mother)? [Make comparison with the parent of the same gender as the Respondent.]

How would you describe your parents' marriage?

What do you think of the marriage your parents (have) (had)?

Would you like your (marriage) (remarriage) to be similar to theirs?

How do your parents feel about your ideas on marriage?

[If parents do not know:] How do you think they would feel about them if they did know?

[If married or in a romantic relationship:] How does your (spouse) romantic partner) feel about your ideas on marriage?

How do your ideas about marriage compare with (his) (hers)?

As you think about the activities involved in marriage and your role as a (husband) (wife), what would you say (has been) (you anticipate to be) most satisfying or rewarding for you?

Is there anything about these activities that (has been) (you anticipate will be) a source of dissatisfaction to you?

How willing would you be to change your ideas about marriage?

[If appropriate:] What would it take to change your ideas about marriage?

Do you anticipate that you might reexamine your decision at some time in the future?

[If yes:] When? Why then?

On a 7-point scale, how important do you see marriage and the role of a spouse as being to you in your life? Again, 7 means "extremely important" and 1 means "not at all important."

The Role of Parent

Do you remember what your thoughts about parenting were like when you were a student in high school (and in college)? [If necessary:] Can you describe your thinking?

[If a parent:] What were your thoughts about parenting leading up to the time when you became a (father) (mother)?

What did you think would be a good time for you to start a family?

How did you picture what parenting might be like for you?

What (do) (did) you see as your role as a (father) (mother)?

What type of behavior in your child (gives) (gave) you pleasure?

What role do you think your spouse **should** have in parenting with you?

What role **does** your spouse have in parenting with you?

[If any difference is mentioned:] Why?

[If never a parent:] Have you ever thought seriously about the idea of parenting?

[If not planning to become a parent:] Why do you think you preferred not to be a parent?

[If planning to become a parent at some time in the future:] Why do you think you would like to be a parent?

When do you think would be a good time in your life to start parenting?

How do you picture your role in parenting?

What type of behavior in your child would give you pleasure?

If you do become a parent, what role do you think your spouse **should** have in parenting with you?

What role do you anticipate your spouse **will** have in parenting with you?

[If any difference is mentioned:] Why?

[For every Respondent:] What do you see as the advantages and disadvantages of being a parent?

[If only one side is presented, ask about the other.] Has your decision about (parenting) (not parenting) come easily to you, or has it been a difficult decision to make?

Why?

Who may have been a factor in your decision?

Have you ever gone through an important change in your thinking about parenting?

[If yes:] Please describe that change.

What started you thinking about these questions?

Who may have been a factor in your thinking?

How would you compare your ideas about parenting with those of your parents? [Ask for a comparison with the parent of the same gender as the Respondent, if not provided.]

How would you describe your parents' parenting?

What do you think of the parenting you had?

Would you like your parenting to be similar to theirs?

How do your parents feel about your ideas on parenting?

[If parents do not know:] How do you think they would feel about them if they did know?

[If married:] How does your spouse feel about your ideas on parenting?

How do your ideas about parenting compare with (his) (hers)?

[For all Respondents:] Do you believe your ideas about parenting are now fairly well worked out, or do you feel you are still working out your thinking about parenting?

[If still working out ideas:] What questions are you still thinking about?

What are you doing now to work out your thinking about these questions?

How willing would you be to change your ideas about parenting?

[If appropriate:] What would it take to change your ideas about parenting?

Do you anticipate that you might reexamine your decision at some time in the future?

[If yes:] When? Why then?

What do you think might influence your decision?

On a 7-point scale, how important do you see the role of parent as being to you in your life? Again, 7 means "extremely important" and 1 means "not at all important."

Family and Career Priorities

Looking over your previous responses, I notice that you rated career _____, in importance, marriage _____, and parenting _____, which seems to suggest that you value (_________ more) (each area about equally). How do you feel about that?

I would like you to share with me the types of conflicts you feel have developed or could develop as a result of your pursuit of a career and a marriage, specifically with your role as a (husband) (wife).

How much had you thought about **marriage** and career conflicts earlier in your life?

Have you ever gone through an important change in your thinking about marriage and career conflicts for yourself?

[If yes:] Please describe that change.

What started you thinking about such questions?

Who may have been a factor in your thinking?

How would you compare your ideas about handling spouse and career conflicts with those of your parents?

How would you describe your parents' own behavior in their marriage in such potential conflicts?

Did their position influence you? How?

Would you like your handling of spouse and career conflicts to be similar to theirs?

[If married:] What similarities and differences are there between your ideas about spouse and career conflicts and those of your spouse?

How does your spouse feel about your ideas on handling spouse and career conflicts?

How much do you worry now about conflicts between spouse and career roles?

[If little or none:] Do you anticipate its becoming a serious question for you in the future?

[If yes:] At what time in your life?

[If no:] Why not?

[If not previously addressed concretely:] If you were confronted with a conflict between your work responsibilities and your responsibilities as a (husband) (wife), which would you give priority to? Why?

Now I would like you to elaborate on possible conflicts you feel have developed or could develop as a result of pursuing your career and parenting.

How much had you thought about **parenting** and career conflicts earlier in your life?

Have you ever gone through an important change in your thinking about parenting and career conflicts for yourself?

[If yes:] Please describe that change.

What started you thinking about these questions?

Who may have been a factor in your thinking?

How would you compare your ideas about parenting and career conflicts with those of your parents?

How would you describe your parents' own handling of such conflicts?

Would you like your handling of parenting and career conflicts to be similar to theirs?

[If married:] What similarities and differences are there between your ideas about parenting and career conflicts and those of your spouse?

How does your spouse feel about your ideas on handling parenting and career conflicts?

How much do you worry now about parenting and career conflicts?

[If little or none:] Do you anticipate its becoming a serious question for you in the future?

[If yes:] At what time in your life?

[If no:] Why not?

[If not previously addressed concretely:] If you were confronted with a conflict between your work responsibilities and your responsibilities as a parent, which would you give priority to? Why?

What do you think are the likely consequences of making ______________ your priority?

Have you given much thought to (or experienced) such consequences?

What kind(s) of control(s) do you feel you have over such consequences?

Religious Beliefs

Do you have any religious preference?

How about your parents—do (did) they have any religious preference?

Were both of your parents reared ______________?

How important would you say religion (is) (was) to your parents?

Have you ever been active in church or church groups [Adapt for Jews and others.]

Since you were in (high school) (college), have your activities with respect to religion increased or decreased or remained about the same?

[If not already evident:] Do you currently attend religious services?

[If yes:] What are your reasons for attending services?

How do you feel while you are engaged in activities related to your religion?

Why do you think you feel that way?

[If no:] Did you ever attend religious services with any frequency?

[If appropriate:] What has led your attendance at services to fall off?

Do you find yourself getting into religious discussions?

[If yes:] What point of view do you express in these discussions?

I'd like to find out something about your ideas in the area of religion, for example on such questions as the existence of God, and the importance of organized religion. What are your ideas?

[If Roman Catholic:] How about the matter of the infallibility of the Pope?

[Ask about other religious questions as these appear appropriate.]

Was there ever a time when you came to question, to doubt, or perhaps to change your religious beliefs?

[If yes:] What types of things did you question or change?

What started you thinking about these questions?

[If not already evident:] How old were you at the time?

How serious were these questions for you?

Do you feel that you've resolved these questions for yourself, or are you still working on them?

[If resolved:] What has helped you to answer these questions?

[If not resolved:] How are you going about trying to answer these questions?

[If married:] Does your spouse have any religious preference?

Was your spouse reared ______?

How important would you say religion is to your spouse?

How does your spouse feel about your ideas on religion?

How (do) (did) your parents feel about your religious beliefs?

[If parents don't know:] How do you think they would feel about them if they did know?

Are there any important differences between your beliefs and those of your spouse and/or your parents?

[If yes:] How do you deal with them?

At this time, how well worked out do you think your ideas on religion are?

Do you think your ideas in this area are likely to remain stable, or do you believe they may very well change in the future?

[If they may change:] In what direction do you think your beliefs might change?

What might bring about such a change?

How likely is it that such a change might occur?

[If you see evidence of continued thought being given to religious questions:] How important is it to you to work out your ideas in the area of religion?

Are you actively trying to work out your beliefs now, or are you more concerned with other things?

On a 7-point scale, how important do you see your religious beliefs as being to you in your life? Again, 7 means "extremely important" and 1 means "not at all important."

[For agnostics and atheists, the last question in this domain should be phrased thus:] On a 7-point scale, how important do you see your ideas about (agnosticism) (atheism) as being to you in your life? Again, 7 means "extremely important" and 1 means "not at all important."

Political Beliefs

Do you have any political preference?

Do you belong to, or do you see yourself as associated with, any political party?

Where would you describe yourself as falling on a scale from liberal through moderate to conservative?

Do your parents have any political preferences?

[If appropriate:] Do they belong to any political party?

[If appropriate:] Where would you say they fall on a scale from liberal through moderate to conservative?

[If necessary, ask separately for both father and mother.] How important would you say political matters are to your parents?

Are there any political or social issues that you feel pretty strongly about?

[If asked "Such as?" Respond: "Whatever might be important issues for you." If asked again, suggest such issues as the economy, how much weaponry is needed for defense, foreign policy, etc.]

What would you like to see done about ______________________?

[Repeat for each issue raised.]

Are there other issues that you have views about?

What would you like to see done about ______________________?

[Repeat for each issue mentioned.]

Have you ever taken any political actions, like joining groups, participating in election campaigns, writing letters to government or other political leaders, signing petitions, participating in demonstrations?

[If yes, elicit a description of each, if necessary.]

What were the circumstances of your becoming involved in these activities?

[Repeat for several of the activities mentioned.]

How do you feel while you are engaged in activities related to your political beliefs?

Why do you think you feel that way?

[If no issues or activities were discussed:] Do you feel that you are actively trying to arrive at a set of political beliefs, or do you feel that the area of politics isn't very important to you at present?

[If trying to work out ideas:] Can you tell me something about the types of things you are thinking about?

How are you going about getting the information you need to make a decision?

How important is it for you to work out these ideas?

Was there ever a time when you found your political ideas undergoing change, when you believed one thing on an issue and then, months or years later, you found you had very different ideas on the same issue?

[If yes:] Please describe the circumstances.

What led you to make that type of change?

Was there anyone who may have been a factor in your thinking at the time?

[If married:] Does your spouse have any political preferences?

[If appropriate:] Does (he) (she) belong to any political party?

[If appropriate:] Where does (he) (she) fall on a scale from liberal through moderate to conservative?

How important would you say political questions are to your spouse?

How does your spouse feel about your ideas on politics?

How (do) (did) your parents feel about your political beliefs?

[If parents don't know:] How do you think they would feel about them if they did know?

Are there any important differences between your beliefs and those of your spouse and/or your parents?

How do you deal with them?

At this time do you believe your political beliefs are likely to remain stable for some time, or do you feel that they may very well change in the future?

[If they may change:] In what direction do you think your beliefs might change?

What might bring about such a change?

How likely is it that such a change might occur?

[If appropriate:] Do you feel these changes would occur just on specific issues, or might there be a change in your general political philosophy?

On a 7-point scale, how important do you see your political beliefs as being to you in your life? Again, 7 means "extremely important" and 1 means "not at all important."

Sex-Role Attitudes

Changing topics again, I'd like to talk with you about your perceptions of men's and women's roles in society today.

What advantages and disadvantages do you see associated with the roles of men and women in today's society?

[Make sure advantages **and** disadvantages are addressed for **both** genders.]

How do you think things **should** be in terms of what women are supposed to be like and what men are supposed to be like?

If you could have chosen to be a man or a woman in today's society, which would you be?

Why?

As you think about your activities as a (man) (woman) in today's society, what would you say is most satisfying or rewarding for you yourself?

Is there anything about these activities that you would consider a source of dissatisfaction?

How would you describe your feelings while you are engaged in activities related to your (masculinity) (femininity)?

Why do you think you feel that way?

How did you come to learn what it means to be a (man) (woman) in today's society?

Do you feel this is something that came naturally for you, or were there times when you were uncertain how you should act?

[If there were uncertainties:] Can you describe the circumstances for me?

How did you go about working out what you should do?

Who may have been a factor in your thinking at the time?

Was there ever a time when you came to question, to doubt, or perhaps to change your ideas, expectations, and/or behavior about your roles as a (woman) (man) in this society?

[If yes:] What types of things did you question or change?

What started you thinking about these questions?

[If not already evident:] How old were you at the time?

How serious were these questions for you?

Do you feel that you've resolved these questions for yourself, or are you still working on them?

[If resolved:] What has helped you to answer these questions?

[If not resolved:] How are you going about trying to answer these questions?

How (do) (had) your mother and father express(ed) their female and male roles, respectively?

How were your ideas, expectations, and behaviors in this area influenced by your parents?

Are there any important similarities and/or differences between the ideas, expectations, and behaviors with which you and your (father) (mother) express the role of a (man) (woman) in today's society?

[If appropriate:] How about the effects your brothers or sisters may have had on your ideas, expectations, and behaviors?

Are there any important differences between their ideas, expectations, and behaviors and yours on men's and women's roles in society?

[If married:] What are your spouse's ideas, expectations, and behaviors about men's and women's roles in society today?

How are they similar to and different from yours?

How does your spouse feel about your ideas, expectations, and behaviors on your role as a (man) (woman) in today's society?

How has your spouse's perspective influenced yours?

How (do) (did) your parents feel about your ideas, expectations, and behaviors on your role as a (man) (woman) in today's society?

[If parents don't know:] How do you think they would feel about them if they did know?

Do you see your ideas about the roles of men and women in today's society remaining stable, or do you see your ideas as possibly changing in the future?

[If ideas may change:] In what direction might your ideas change?

What do you think might cause such a change?

How likely is it that such a change might occur?

[If you see evidence of continued thought being given to these questions:] How important is it to you to work out your ideas in this area?

Are you actively trying to work out your beliefs, expectations, and/or behaviors now, or are you more concerned with other things?

On a 7-point scale, how important do you see your beliefs, expectations, and behaviors defined by your role as a (man) (woman) as being to you in your life? Again, 7 means "extremely important" and 1 means "not at all important."

Appendix D
Intimacy Status Interview and Rating Scales (1988 Version)

JACOB L. ORLOFSKY AND LAURIE A. ROADES*
University of Missouri—St. Louis

This is a list of recommended questions on subjects' relationship with friends and romantic partners, as well as general questions on friendship and love. The list is by no means exhaustive, nor should the interviewer feel constrained to use every question. It is important to ask open-ended questions whenever possible, moving to more specific questions as necessary.

Intimacy Interview

Instructions

"I'd like to ask you some questions about your relationships with other people and about attitudes you have toward these relationships. I'll be tape-recording our interview, but everything you say here will be kept completely confidential, and so I hope you'll feel comfortable expressing your feelings."

Part One: Friendships

I. General questions
   1. a. How do you usually like to spend your leisure time? (Activities you enjoy, and so on.)
      b. Do these usually involve spending time with others, or do you usually prefer to do them alone?
      c. What are you most likely to do with friends, and what do you usually do alone?
   2. Do you generally prefer to be with people or by yourself?
   3. Do you have any friends you're close to now?
      [If yes, go to Section II (Close Friendships).]
      [If no, ask the following: (Then begin Part Two—Dating and Love Relationships).]

* A graduate student.

a. Have you ever had any close friendships?
   i. When was this?
      Can you tell me about those friendships?
      Why do you think you're not friends any more?
   ii. How is that for you?
b. What do you think is preventing you from establishing friendships now?
c. Are there any changes you'd like to see in the way you relate to other people or the way they relate to you? [How might you accomplish this change?]
   [Go to Part Two: Dating and Love Relationships]

II. Close friendships

A. General questions about friendships

"I'd like to focus on one or two of your closest friendships."

1. Would you tell me about this (these) relationships?
2. [How did you meet? How long have you been close to (her) (him) (them)?]

B. Tasks and activities

1. How often do you get together or have contact with each other?
2. a. What kinds of things do you usually do together?
   b. Who usually plans your activities?
   c. Do you feel that these shared activities usually reflect (her) (his) interests or your interests?
3. a. Do you have much in common with your friends? (Tell me about it.)
   b. Have you had those interests long or did (she) (he) introduce you to them?

C. Closeness and emotional aspects

1. Tell me about some of the experiences you've had that contributed to your feeling close to each other. [Check for one-sided versus mutual experiences.]
2. What kinds of things do you talk about?
3. Are you the type of person who likes to talk about personal matters or problems with your friends, or do you prefer to keep them to yourself?
   [Give me an example of some things you might talk about.]
4. a. Do you share more of your personal concerns with (him) (her) or does (she) (he) share more with you?
   b. How do you feel about this balance?
5. a. Are there any matters that you wouldn't discuss with (him) (her) (them)?
   b. What would some of those be?
   c. What makes them difficult to share?
6. a. Do you do things for each other?
   b. Give me an example or two.

c. Do you go out of your way to help each other?
[Check for mutuality.]

D. Closest friends and friend spent most time with
"Now I'd like us to focus on your closest or best friend."
1. a. Tell me what this person is like.
   b. How would (she) (he) describe you?
   c. What do you like or admire most about (her) (him)?
   d. What do you dislike (or like least)?
2. a. Do you feel you can trust (her) (him)?
   b. How important is this trust to you?

"Even good friends sometimes have disagreements or conflicts and disagree or get angry with each other."
3. a. Has this ever happened between you and your friend?
   b. What happened?
   c. How did you deal with it?
   d. Has this happened with previous friends?
4. a. How important is this friendship to you?
   b. Will you still be friends in five years?
   c. How will you maintain the relationship that long?

III. Conclusion of friendship questions
1. How satisfied are you with your friendships?
   [Do you feel you're as close to friends as you'd like to be?]
2. What would you like to change about these relationships?
   [What are you doing or might you do to accomplish that?]
3. a. What kinds of conflicts or troubles have you experienced in your friendships?
   b. Do these keep you from enjoying your friendships as much as you might like?
4. Are there any changes you'd like to see in the way you relate to other people or the way they relate to you?
   [How might you accomplish this change?]
   [Go to Part Two Dating and Love Relationships.]

Part Two: Dating and Love Relationships

"I am going to be asking you some questions about your dating experiences now. Are you currently married, engaged, living with someone, or involved in a steady relationship?" [If no, ask: "Were you ever involved in an exclusive relationship with a (woman) (man) in the past?" If yes, ask: "When was that?"]

Interviewer: The three options are:

A. Subject is currently married or in a committed relationship. Use Section I.

B. Subject is not currently married or committed but previously was. Use Section I, asking questions in the past tense. Begin as follows: "I'd like to ask you some questions about that former relationship before we talk about any relationships or dating you are involved in now. Is that okay?"

C. Subject has not been involved in a committed relationship. Use Section II.

I. Married or committed

"I'd like to ask you a few questions about your relationship."

A. Description

1. Tell me about your (boyfriend) (girlfriend) (wife) (husband). What is (she) (he) like?
   [Follow up as necessary. Notice what seems important to the Respondent. Suggestions for follow-up are:
   a. What do you like or admire most about (her) (him)?
   b. What do you (dislike) (like) least?
   c. In what ways is (she) (he) special to you?
2. How would (she) (he) describe you? [and: What do you think (she) (he) likes most about you? What does (she) (he) dislike or like least?]

B. General question

1. Would you tell me about the relationship?
   [How did you meet?]
2. How long have you known (her) (him)?
   [How long have you been involved?]

C. Tasks and activities

1. How do you spend your time together?
2. Do you have mutual friends?
3. a. Do you have some interests or friendships that are separate from those of your partner?
   b. Tell me about some of these.
   c. What about your partner? What kinds of interests or activities does (she) (he) have separate from you?

D. Emotional closeness

1. a. How would you describe your feelings for (her) (him)?
   b. How much of this feeling have you told your partner about?
   c. Are you in love with (her) (him)?
2. a. How do you show (her) (him) that you care?
   b. How does (she) (he) show you that (she) (he) cares?
3. a. How close would you say the two of you are?
   b. Can you describe some of the experiences in which you've felt closest?
   c. How do you usually express your affection?
   d. Would you say you're a physically affectionate kind of person?
   e. What about your partner?

[How do you feel about this?]

4. a. What kinds of things do the two of you talk about?
   b. How comfortable are you discussing personal matters or problems with (her) (him)?
   c. What kinds of things couldn't you share with (her) (him) or would you find most difficult to talk about?
   d. How much does (she) (he) confide in you?
   e. Do you generally like your partner to discuss (her) (his) problems or concerns with you, or would you prefer sometimes that (she) (he) work them out (her) (himself)? Why?
5. a. What would you like from (her) (him) that (she) (he) doesn't give you as much of as you'd like?
   b. What do you think (she) (he) would like from you?
   c. Have you discussed these things with each other?
   d. What have you decided to do about this?
   e. What do you each do to try to get what you want from each other?

E. Conflict resolution

"People sometimes get on each other's nerves in one way or another and disagree or get angry with each other."
Has this ever happened with the two of you?
[If no:] Why do you think it is that the two of you never seem to argue or get on each other's nerves?
[If yes:]

   a. What kinds of issues have you had disagreements about?
      [About specific disagreements, ask the following:]
      1. What's your view about that?
      2. How do you think (she) (he) feels about that?
      3. Why do you think (she) (he) feels that way?
   b. How have you resolved things when you've had disagreements like these?
      [Does R take partner's feelings into account by modifying (her) (his) behavior, compromising, and so on?]
   c. Are there any other issues you would like to see resolved?
      [How might you accomplish that?]

F. Involvement and autonomy

1. a. How involved are you in this relationship?
   b. Your partner?
   c. Do you feel that one of you is more involved in the relationship or considers it more important than the other?
      [If yes:] How do you feel about it?
2. Some people feel concerned about becoming too dependent or too involved in a relationship.
   a. How much of a concern is this for you?
   b. How much for your partner?

c. Tell me more about it.
d. How do these issues affect your relationship?
Where do you see this problem going, or how do you see it getting resolved?

[Ask 3A or 3B depending on Respondent's answer to Question C3 above.]

3A. You mentioned earlier some separate interests and activities you each have.
a. How do you feel about (her) (his) separate interests and friends?
b. How does your partner feel about yours?
c. Does either of you ever feel left out or abandoned by the other?

3B. You mentioned earlier that you pretty much have the same interests and do most things together.
a. How do you feel about this arrangement?
b. Does either of you ever feel constrained [e.g., in personal growth] because of your relationship?
c. Do you think this condition will change?

4. a. Who makes most of the major decisions in your relationship [Major purchases, sexual activity, and so on.]
b. What about the minor ones? [activities, movies to see, and so on.]
c. How do you feel about this?

G. Sexuality

"Some people feel comfortable discussing sexual issues and others don't. Although I don't need to know specific details about your sexual life, I would like to ask some general questions about your attitude toward sexual involvement."

1. a. What are your feelings about sexual involvement before marriage?
b. How do you feel about expressing your feelings in physical or sexual ways?
c. How do you feel about other people doing this [expressing their feelings thus] with you?

2. a. What role does sex have in your relationship?
b. How important is this expression of sex to you?
c. Tell me about it.

3. How satisfied are you with the sexual component in your relationship?
[Do you usually feel satisfied by sexual involvement? What do you feel you get from it?]
[If not satisfied, Have you discussed it with (her) (him)?]

H. Satisfaction and commitment and future plans

1. a. How happy are you in this relationship?

b. How does this compare to other relationships you've had?

2. a. Where do you want this relationship to go in the future?
   b. Have you discussed future plans?
3. a. How critical is this relationship to your present and future happiness?
   b. What do you think life would be like if you were no longer involved with (her) (him)?
   c. How do you think your partner would handle it?
4. a. What would you like to change about this relationship?
   b. How satisfied are you with this relationship?
   c. Do you feel you're as close as you'd like to be with this person?
   d. Are there any conflicts or worries or difficulties that you experience in this relationship?
   [If yes:] Do these keep you from enjoying this relationship as much as you might like?
   [If Respondent has been discussing a past relationship, go to Appendix I; otherwise, conclude the interview with question 5.]
5. We've talked about a number of issues in the last half-hour. Are there any other problems or issues about your relationships that you think are important which we haven't discussed?

Appendix: For Respondent with a past committed relationship.

A. Conclusion of love relationship
   1. What do you think caused the relationship to end?
   2. Did you experience any specific conflicts or difficulties during the relationship? [Tell me some of these.]
   3. a. How did you experience the breakup?
      b. How do you feel about the relationship now?
   4. How has this experience affected the way you approach relationships now?
      [E.g.: More cautious now? Decided to improve some aspect of (her) (his) approach to relationships? Given up on romantic relationships?]
B. Current dating
   1. Are you dating now or have you dated since this relationship ended? [Tell me about this. How's this going?]

      [If no, go to section C.]
      [If yes, continue with next question.]

   2. What do you usually do on a date?
      [How do you usually spend your time together?]
   3. a. What kinds of things do you talk about with people you date?

b. How comfortable are you discussing personal matters or problems with (her) (him)?

4. a. What do you like about dating?
   b. Anything you particularly dislike?
5. Is the dating you've been doing now satisfying, or would you prefer to get involved in an exclusive relationship again? Why? [Go to Section D.]

C. Not currently dating
1. Is dating important to you?
2. Would you like to be dating someone? Tell me about it.

D. Future relationship preferences
1. How do you feel about not being involved in a committed relationship at this time?
2. Do you want to get married or have a relatively permanent relationship at some time (in the future) (again)?
   [If no:] Why do you think you're not interested in another committed relationship?
   [If yes:] How are you trying to become involved in a permanent relationship?
3. a. What makes up a meaningful or good love relationship as you see it?
   b. How much of this good relationship do you feel you've attained?
4. We've talked about a number of issues in the last half-hour. Are there any other concerns or issues about your relationships you think are important that we haven't discussed?

II. Dating (For subjects who have not been involved in a committed relationship.)

A. General
1. Do you date much?
   [If no:] a. Have you ever dated?
   [If yes, go to 2.]
   [If no, go to 1b.]
   b. How do you feel about that? How is that for you?
   c. Are there any reasons you don't date much? [What do you think has gotten in the way?]
   [Go to Section III—Never Dated.]
   [If yes:] a. Some people like to find one person to have a steady relationship with, whereas others prefer to date more than one person. What do you prefer? [Tell me something about that.]
   b. Have you ever dated one person exclusively for a time?
   [If yes, go back to Section I and Section I—Appendix.]
   [If no, continue with this dating section.]

2. How often do you date?
3. Is there a usual length of time that you see someone? [What's the longest you've ever dated someone?]

B. Description
1. a. Describe for me one or two of the people you've dated. [What were they like? What did you like about them?]
   b. How would (she) (he) describe you?
2. What are your dating relationships usually like? [Encourage spontaneous description and follow up with these questions as needed.]

C. Tasks and activities
1. What do you usually do on a date?
2. How do you usually spend time together?

D. Emotional closeness
1. a. What kinds of things do you like to talk about with people you date? [School, work, personal matters, problems, and so on?]
   b. How comfortable are you discussing personal matters or problems with these (women) (men)?
   c. What kinds of things couldn't you share with (her) (him) (them) or would be most difficult to talk about?
2. a. How do you show someone you're dating that you care for (her) (him)?
   b. How do your dates show you that they care?
   c. How do you feel about this?
3. a. What do you like about dating?
   b. Anything you especially dislike?
4. Is dating important to you? [Tell me about it.]
5. Some people worry about becoming too dependent or too involved in a relationship.
   a. How much of a worry is this for you?
   b. How about for the people you date?
   c. How do these issues affect your relationship(s)? [How do you feel about this dependence?]
6. People sometimes get on each other's nerves in one way or another and disagree or get angry with each other. Has this ever happened with you and someone you were dating?
   [If no:] Why do you think this never seems to happen?
   [If yes:] i. Tell me about it.
   ii. What kinds of issues have you had disagreements about?
   iii. Are there any specific conflicts or difficulties that seem to come up pretty often?

E. Sexuality
"Some people feel comfortable discussing sexual issues and others don't. Although I don't need to know specific details about your

sexual life, I would like to ask some general questions about your attitudes toward sexual involvement.

1. What are your feelings about sexual involvement before marriage?
2. a. What role does sex have in your relationship with (men) (women)?
   b. How important is this expression of sex to you?
3. a. How do you feel about expressing your feelings in physical or sexual ways?
   b. How do you feel about other people doing this [expressing their feelings thus] with you?
4. Do you feel satisfied with the sexual component in your relationship(s)? [Do you usually feel satisfied by sexual involvement?] [If no:] Are you able to discuss this with (her) (him)?

F. Conclusion

1. What kinds of things about a (woman) (man) would prompt you to go out with (her) (him) again?
2. In your dating, have you ever met someone with whom you would like to have an enduring relationship?
   [If yes:] What happened? Tell me about it.
   [If no:] Why do you think that is? [Or:] What keeps you from wanting a longer relationship with the (men) (women) you date?
3. What makes up a meaningful or good love relationship as you see it?
4. How much of this relationship do you feel you've attained?
5. How do you feel about not being involved in a relationship with one person now?
6. Do you think you want to get married or have a relatively permanent relationship at some time in the future?
   [If no:] Why do you think you're not interested in an exclusive relationship?
   [If yes:] How are you trying to become involved in a permanent relationship?
7. We've talked about a number of issues in the last half-hour. Are there any other concerns or issues about your relationships that you think are important?

III. Never dated

"I'd like to ask you a few questions about your attitudes about dating."

1. What makes up a meaningful or good love relationship, as you see it? [What would you like in a relationship?]
2. How much of this relationship do you feel you've attained so far?
3. How do you feel about not being involved in a dating relationship at this time?
   [If not interested:] Why do you think you're not interested in a relationship?

[If subject prefers to be dating:] How are you trying to become involved in a dating relationship? [What do you think has been getting in your way up to now?]

4. What kind of social life or relationship would you like for yourself in the future?
5. We've talked about a number of issues in the last half-hour. Are there any other problems or issues about your relationships that you think are important which we haven't discussed?

Interview Rating Scales

(Make separate ratings for the section on Friendships and the section on Dating and Love Relationships)

1. Commitment

a. Duration

1	2	3	4	5
Dates around		Involved, but ambivalent about future plans		Currently involved and has definite plans for future

b. Quality

1	2	3	4	5
Thinks relationship should take care of itself				Invested in enhancing and maintaining quality of their interactions (wants to meet Partner's needs as well as own)

2. Communication

a. Intrapersonal self-disclosure (confiding about worries, problems, and other personal matters)

1	2	3	4	5
Low level of sharing. May be mistrustful		Some confiding, or confides but feels uncomfortable doing so		High level—feels comfortable sharing

b. Interpersonal

1	2	3	4	5
Closed, distant, or dishonest				Shares angry and affectionate feelings openly

3. Caring and affection

1	2	3	4	5
Dislikes or devalues Partner or utilitarian attitude toward Partner		Some caring or ambivalent feelings toward Partner		Genuine caring for Partner

4. Knowledge of Partner's traits

1	2	3	4	5
Superficial description, or describes Partner in terms of own needs				Rich description of Partner as unique and special

5. Perspective-taking

1	2	3	4	5
Unable to see Partner's point of view, or is highly judgmental		Can see, but doesn't have sympathetic understanding of Partner's feelings and concerns	Can see Partner's point of view and is somewhat accepting of it	Can see Partner's point of view and values it

6. Power and decision making

1	2	3	4	5
Controlling or self-subordinating (circle one)		Slightly controlling or self-subordinating (circle one)		Values mutuality

7. Maintains Own Interests

1	2	3	4	5
Gives up own interests		Maintains own interests without regard for Partner		Maintains own interests (while caring for Partner's needs and wishes)

8. Acceptance of Partner's Separateness

1	2	3	4	5
Is very needy, clinging, or struggles against Partner's autonomy; is manipulative	Resigned to Partner's separate interests	Accepts Partner's autonomy		Encourages and prizes Partner's autonomy

9. Dependency or Detachment

1	2	3	4	5
Needy, dependent		Mutually interdependent		Detached

Rules for Distinguishing the Nonisolate Intimacy Statuses (Intimate and Preintimate vs. Pseudointimate and Stereotype vs. Merger Committed and Uncommitted)

	Intimate	Pseudointimate	Merger
1. Commitment			
a. Duration*	Medium–high	Medium–high	Medium–high
b. Quality	High	Low–medium	Medium–high
2. Communication			
a. Intrapersonal self-disclosure	High	Low–medium	Medium–high
b. Interpersonal	High	Low–medium	Medium–high
3. Caring and affection	High	Low–medium	Medium–high
4. Knowledge of partner's traits	High	Low	Low–medium
5. Perspective-taking	High	Low–medium	Low–medium
6. Power and decision making	High	Low–medium (control)	Low–medium (submissive)
7. Maintains own interests	Medium–high	Medium–high	Low–medium
8. Acceptance of partner's separateness	Medium–high	Medium	Low–medium
9. Dependency and detachment	Medium	Medium–high	Low

* Low levels of commitment or involvement indicate the noncommitted version of the statuses: preintimate, stereotyped, and merger-uncommitted, respectively.

Appendix E
Intimacy Status Rating Manual (1989 Version)

Jacob L. Orlofsky
University of Missouri—St. Louis

Intimacy Status Rating Manual

The main objective in rating each interview is to locate the individual in one of the seven "intimacy statuses," each status being a mode for coping with the intimacy–isolation crisis of young adulthood. The four major statuses are Intimate, Merger (committed), Stereotype, and Isolate. Additional categories are Preintimate, a subdivision of Intimate; Merger (uncommitted), a subdivision of Merger (committed); and Pseudointimate, a subdivision of Stereotyped Relationships. The Intimate and Preintimate, the Merger (committed) and Merger (uncommitted), and the Pseudointimate and Stereotyped Relationship statuses are differentiated by whether the subject has established an enduring, committed relationship.

The following is a list of the dimensions along which individuals are rated for intimacy status. Generally, individuals whose relationships are characterized by a high degree of communication and closeness are rated high in intimacy (Intimate and Preintimate). Those who appear overly and intensely involved, dependent, and needful in relationships are rated Merger. Those who shun involvement with others are rated Isolated. Those who are not isolated but whose relationships are characterized by minimal emotional closeness, openness, mutual respect, and so on are rated low in intimacy (Pseudointimate and Stereotyped Relationships).

Criteria for rating intimacy status in relationships

1. Presence of close relationships with friends and/or boyfriend or girlfriend or spouse.
2. Degree of closeness
   - Do they maintain close contact with their friends?
   - Do they share interests?
   - What does closeness mean to them? friendship? Does it mean having a good time together, knowing each other deeply, and so on?

- How close do they feel in their relationships?
- Is there a bond of mutual trust and care?
- Do they really know their friends, understand their needs or is their understanding of them limited or superficial?
- Can they describe close experiences they have had together?
- Can they say what it is they like or dislike about their friend?
- Can they communicate something about what the other person is like?

3. Degree of respect for individuality
   - Can they see their friends as unique and separate individuals with both strengths and vulnerabilities? Do they idealize or devalue the other?
   - Can they see both similarities and differences between themselves and their friends, or is the other "just like" them?
   - Can they maintain their independence within close relationships, or are they overly dependent on and needful of others? Can their relationships survive distance, or is there a need to maintain close contact? Can they pursue interests and activities comfortably apart from their relationships?
   - Can they maintain more than one close friend and accept this independence of their friends as well—or are they overly possessive and jealous of their friends' other involvements?
   - Is there continual bickering or arguing with friends?
   - Do they feel they could eventually cope with life without the relationship? Or do they feel they would fall apart, be unable to live without the friend?
4. Degree of openness and communication
   - Do they share personal problems and worries with the other? (Why do they do so in the first place?—to feel better, to gather other viewpoints, to share aspects of themselves with them?) Are there things they cannot share with their friend (what kinds of things?)?
   - Is it easier or more difficult to be open with a friend rather than a boyfriend or girlfriend or spouse? (Why?)
   - Are they open to the other's feelings?
   - Can they express affection, anger, accept and resolve differences?
5. Degree of responsibility
   - Are they responsible for being themselves? Are they straight with others, really themselves? Do they accept responsibility for their feelings, or do they tend to overdramatize or manipulate?
   - Do they go out of their way to help out the other, listen when the other needs to talk, or are they mostly on the receiving end?
6. Mutuality
   - Is the relationship two-sided?
   - Do both have approximately equal investment in the relationship?
   - Are both open and responsible?

7. Commitment
   - Is the relationship enduring: do they switch friends or partners often?
   - Are they there when the other needs them?
   - Is there discussion of future plans, such as marriage, living together?
   - Is there a commitment to discussing and resolving problems in the relationship (as opposed to keeping differences to oneself or pretending they don't exist)?
   - Is the relationship strong, surviving distances, differences of opinion?
8. Sexuality
   - Are they physically affectionate?
   - Is the relationship mutually satisfying and meaningful?
   - Do they treat sexual partners as people (or as caretakers or objects of sexual conquest)?

Instructions for Rating

The following is a description of the way in which these criteria are combined to yield an intimacy status. (Note: When the two ratings are different, the "relationships with boyfriends/girlfriends" is weighted more heavily. Otherwise, the overall feeling of the interview is used.)

1. *Isolates*

   a. These individals have no close relationships with peers; their acquaintances tend to be formal and stereotyped.

These individuals may see some peers at school, work, or church, but rarely do they talk with them at length or attempt to initiate social contacts. Isolates rarely date and it is unlikely that they will date the same person more than a few times. Isolate individuals may rationalize their lack of dating as a desire to avoid being tied down or as a result of their being too busy. Otherwise, they may want to date more but are too uncomfortable on dates or see themselves as too unattractive or otherwise unacceptable for others to be interested in them.

Isolates tend to be withdrawn and lacking in social skills. They may appear insecure and self-deprecating; or smug, self-satisfied, and defensive, living in a world of "splendid isolation" and denying any need or desire to be close to others.

1. She has no close friends now and never had a close friend. Sometimes she wants one—like when she's lonely—but mostly she's satisfied with working and studying all the time. She is quiet and lacks confidence in herself. She was once betrayed by a playmate when she was little. She doesn't date and doesn't want to, although she has a guy she could be dating if she wanted to. Has difficulties with this guy but won't say what they are.

2. She has friends but doesn't feel close to any of them. Feels afraid of and threatened by people. She is always wearing a mask—is never herself because she has to pretend she's perfect to be accepted. Closeness is bad for her. Can't accept that no one is perfect and till she does she shouldn't be close. Feels constant pain and loneliness but doesn't miss the closeness because "you can't miss what you've never had."

3. Lives with his parents. Stays home a lot, watches television. His school work keeps him pretty busy; he doesn't have too much time to see people. Actually, lately he has been thinking of working nights.

4. Dated a girl in high school for a while. Since he's come to college, though, he hasn't dated; maybe a few dates a year. He doesn't want to "get tied down, get married too early like some people" he knows. He's going to wait until he's well set up financially before he thinks about dating.

5. Gets pretty lonely. He wants to talk to people, but is afraid he'll "talk their ears off." And so he stays away from people for the most part, won't initiate contacts. Doesn't date much; concentrates on his work. Very uncomfortable with girls.

6. Lives in a rented room; some other guys have rooms in the same house. They talk occasionally, but he stays by himself for the most part. Never dated. He's too "horrible." A girl "could never like" him.

2. *Stereotyped Relationships*

a. These individuals have friends and dating relationships but have not established a long-term heterosexual commitment.

b. Their relationships lack openness or deep involvement and communication is at a low level.

These individuals may have several friends whom they see frequently and enjoy being with. They may describe these relationships as close. There appears to be little real closeness between them, however. They rarely discuss personal matters or problems with friends; that would be overstepping the implicit bounds of the relationship. To the limited extent that they do share problems with others, it is only to "gather other viewpoints" or "feel better." They generally prefer to keep conversations on a superficial, impersonal level. Friendships typically mean having a good time or partying with the crowd.

Stereotyped individuals may date frequently, but rarely do they see the same person for more than a few months. They may prefer to play the field, not get too involved, and date several people at the same time. Dates are often formal—parties, movies, sporting events. Seldom are dates spent talking and getting to know each other. Stereotyped individuals may be sexually inhibited and immature or promiscuous, going from one partner to the other and experiencing sexuality as conquest or excitement. The emphasis in their relationships is on what can be obtained from others rather than on mutuality. The idea of genuine closeness and mutuality appears foreign to them.

In general, stereotyped individuals are characterized by constriction, shallowness, and paucity of self-awareness.

1. She used to party all the time in high school with two groups of friends but didn't feel close to any group or individual in the group. Her goal was just to have fun. These girls still party, but she claims that now that she's started college she has matured and no longer wants to get drunk and party. However, she hasn't shared this with them and just makes up excuses when they call. She guesses "they'll eventually get the message." She's been dating a guy for a few months. They don't really talk and she doesn't share problems with him because she thinks "a guy would rather have a happy girl around." She's disappointed that he's not romantic and that she no longer feels that excited feeling when he calls.

2. She has one friend with whom she's not completely open. Just dropped another friend because she got on her nerves. She never discussed it with her. The longest she ever dated a guy was two or three months. He was "nice" and "outgoing." "Nothing in particular" caused the relationship to end.

3. Her close friend is "nice" and "fun to be with." There is nothing she dislikes about her and no conflicts in the relationship. Her boyfriend of three months is also "nice" and "fun." She'll share everything with him "if it's not too secretive."

4. Dated one guy four or five months. They didn't share personal problems. She broke it off because "he just turned me off after a while." She once met a man she might have liked to marry. He was a "good-looking, athletic type" and they had some things in common.

5. Has many friends with whom she tries to spread her time evenly. Wouldn't like to spend too much time with any one friend because "I get bored easily." She never wants to get married. She doesn't like commitment or feeling she has to answer to anyone.

6. He lived in the dorm for a while, then moved into an apartment with a guy he knew and a couple of other guys. They didn't get along too well. Since then he's moved in with some other people. They get along okay, but don't talk to each other too much.

7. Has some friends with whom he goes drinking and enjoys being with. People are generally pretty open with him, tell him about their problems. He's a good listener. But he doesn't like to discuss his problems with others. He lets them do the talking.

8. Dated a girl in high school for a while. Since being in college he's dated around for a couple of years. Nothing serious. Liked one girl but she wasn't interested in him.

9. Dates several girls. Goes to parties and to movies and likes to do these things with a date. None of the relationships have been enduring. He generally dates on the weekends; sees each girl maybe once a week for a couple of months. Then the relationship usually fizzles out.

3. *Pseudointimate*
   a. These individuals have established a long-term heterosexual relationship.
   b. This and other relationships lack open communication and deep emotional involvement.

Like the stereotyped individuals, pseudointimates form relationships that tend to be superficial. Rarely do they share their personal problems or innermost feelings with others. Their sense of responsibility to friends and partner are limited. Generally they tell others only what is convenient and are available to hear the other's concerns, feelings, and problems only when it is convenient for them. These individuals approach relationships as conveniences in which others are treated as objects who provide status, respectability, and material or other external gains. When asked why they married or became engaged they may not know or they may reply that others expected it or "it was about time." They appear to live their life in parallel to others, never really meeting or experiencing them. They are limited in their ability to perceive their friends or partner as unique individuals. When asked to describe their partner, they may be able to say very little about them or else mention external characteristics or degree of fun the partner provides. They may or may not have a satisfactory sexual relationship.

Pseudointimates are generally characterized by constriction, shallowness, and lack of self-awareness. They do not appear to value open, honest relationships or are unaware of such a possibility.

1. She feels pretty close to a few friends but they're away at school so she's not that close any more. She's planning to marry a guy she's been dating for six months. He's "nice, considerate, and fun to be with." She's never thought about what she admires about him. They never fight, have no conflicts, and there's nothing she'd like changed about the relationship.

2. She became engaged to her boyfriend after knowing him eight months. This is the second engagement for both of them. She was engaged two years ago when she was 16. They never discuss this with each other. They are jealous of each other's other relationships, but "we just keep it quiet—we don't talk it out." She feels she should have more time for herself—he disagrees but she sees talking about this as "just leading to an argument," and so she drops it. She's not involved in the relationship as much as he is and she's kind of concerned that maybe she's too young to be married. She doesn't think there are any emotional conflicts in the relationship—just that they're short on time and money.

3. Has lots of friends. He sees them often and has a lot of fun with them, lots of laughs, etc. Has a girlfriend from back home. She's a few years younger than he and just finished high school. He sees her on vacations and sometimes on weekends. He goes out with several girls; his girlfriend back home is waiting for him. Plans to go back and marry her when he's through with school.

4. Been seeing a girl for a while. She'll do anything for him. He stays with her, alternately impressed with and turned off by how much she cares for him. Knows this other girl. He really wants her; she is his ideal, but she does not want to get involved with him.

5. Used to be in a fraternity. Since he met his girlfriend he has dropped out of it pretty much, although he still goes to the parties sometimes. Been seeing her for several months. She's pretty and fun-loving. Sometimes he thinks about marrying her.

4. *Merger (Committed)*

a. These individuals have established a long-term heterosexual relationship.

b. Their relationships are characterized by high involvement to the point of enmeshment, dependency, and unrealistic perceptions of others.

Committed mergers are intensely involved with a partner. Some are similarly involved with one or two close friends; others have abandoned such relationships for exclusive involvement with a partner. Individuals in this status differ from intimates in that they attempt to gain a sense of self through these relationships. They have difficulty discussing themselves or pursuing interests and activities separate from their partner or friends. They are highly dependent on their partner emotionally as well as practically. They tend to look to their partner to make decisions for themselves as well as for both of them. Some are the more dominant one and attain their sense of self by dominating their partner. Either way, individuals in this status lack respect for the autonomy and integrity of the self and others. Satisfaction from the relationship is mainly derived by achieving a sense of security, wholeness, or direction, feeling taken care of, and avoiding feeling alone and empty. Jealousy and possessiveness are typically major issues in the relationships formed by the individuals in this status. Though not necessarily happy in the relationship or in love with their partner, they would find its termination intolerable or fear that leaving would cause their partner intolerable pain.

Committed mergers may unrealistically idealize their partner, whom they are eager to please. Or else they may devalue them as weak, passive, dependent, possessive, insecure, insensitive, and so on. Alternation between these two positions may also appear. Committed mergers have difficulty absorbing frustrations in the relationship and working out conflicts in an equitable way.

Individuals in this status appear quite needful and may have low self-esteem. For some, the sense of self depends on fulfilling the partner's excessive need for security. They may be somewhat self-aware and eager to communicate their internal world, but they have trouble seeing others as separate from themselves or letting others take care of themselves.

1. Has one close friend who is a year younger and still in high school. Her friend is her "look-alike" and likes everything the same as she. She feels jealous of her friend's other friends in high school because they get to see her in school and she gets mad at her friend when she talks about these friends. She is seriously involved with a guy and spends her afternoons hanging around where he works. He's extremely jealous and it's hard for her to be without him . . . "I cling."

2. She's seriously involved with a 16-year-old guy. She idealizes him. "He's fantastic . . . he's the substance that holds me together." She's also especially close to a woman twice her age who is like a mother. Closeness means "having someone to take a problem to."

3. She lost her best friend of many years because of her boyfriend. "She was jealous . . . and it was hard to please both." Now she has no really close friends because her best friend is her boyfriend. Closeness to him is like a "journal or

diary." She dislikes his temper and that he gets mad at little things. "He's jealous and lacks trust." She doesn't know if it's that he's immature or what.

4. Feels very close to and is planning to marry her boyfriend. Jealousy and possessiveness is a problem in the relationship. It was such a big problem last year that she felt "all closed in . . . like there was a leash on me," and so she tried to break it off. However, he was miserable and threatened suicide. He told her that "he was going to play dirty . . . not let me get out of this so easily . . . bribe me . . . make me feel guilty." She felt guilty and didn't want to "cause a tragedy" and so they got back together.

5. Is extremely attached to a guy who cooled their relationship. She is hoping he will change his mind and is waiting for him. She won't date anyone else. She speaks to him on the phone two or three times a day but doesn't get to see him much. When on the phone with him she'll often hear other women in the background. She has never been able to tell her friends about the intensity of her attachment and can't understand it herself.

6. He had been engaged to his girlfriend for six months until she was killed in a car accident. He says they talked about everything and that she was the one and only person he ever totally opened up to. "She made it easier—I didn't have to keep everything bottled up." He can't remember ever arguing or needing to make decisions because they were so much alike. "We seemed to know what the other was thinking." When she went out with friends, he describes that he felt left behind and "lonely."

7. His best friend became jealous when he wanted to hang around with another group of guys and "would get mad because I would go out with my girlfriend when before we used to always go out together." When he's with his girlfriend, he makes most of the decisions. "Sometimes we fight about that because I say 'Why don't you make a decision?'" He says he's shared so much with her he feels "she's like a part of me." He shows he cares by doing what she asks of him. He's beginning to think he wants more freedom and that "I don't want to rely on her or become too dependent. I don't want her to become totally hurt." He thinks they will move apart for a while and then back together before they marry.

8. He likes how his girlfriend cares so much about him and says "I never cared so much about me." They don't have separate friends and interests and that "bothers me a little" because he doesn't get to see any of his friends. When he does have friends over, his girlfriend gets upset and so the next weekend he tries to spend more time with her. On the other hand, he says he doesn't have any friends since his grade-school friend was "the only person I ever hung around with." He thinks "he doesn't care because he doesn't call me."

5. *Merger (Uncommitted)*

a. These individuals have not established a long-term heterosexual relationship.

b. Their relationships are characterized by high involvement to the point of enmeshment, dependency, and unrealistic perceptions of others or in fostering this sense of neediness in others.

Uncommitted mergers experience their relationships as extensions of themselves. They continually seek intensely close encounters through which they can define and experience themselves. Their friends may be unrealistically idealized when they meet their expectations and devalued when they disappoint them. For this reason their relationships may be transient—quickly formed and abandoned—and they often lack insight into the dynamics of being "left behind."

These individuals may dwell on such issues or conflicts pertaining to dependency, security, autonomy, entrapment, bickering, domination, jealousy, possessiveness, and loyalty when discussing their relationships. They may have difficulty with a third party (e.g., a friend's boyfriend or girlfriend) "intruding" on their closeness with their friend. At times they may feel pressured to choose between two conflicting loyalties.

Any loss of a close or needed relationship is also described with a great deal of intensity. A friend moving out of town or a breakup with a boyfriend or girlfriend, for example, is extremely painful for uncommitted mergers because they have few internal resources to deal with the loss. Mergers tend to view relationships as permanent and do not easily tolerate change in a friend or in the friend's interests. Mergers are typically satisfied with the status quo, and anything that could change the relationship is perceived as a threat. Uncommitted mergers have trouble enjoying themselves or pursuing interests apart from close friends.

Individuals in this status may use their sexuality freely as a means to obtain affection and gratify their need to be held and cared for. Or else they are fearful of their sexuality and threatened by others who arouse such feelings in them. Mergers are still most comfortable in relationships that parallel mother–child mirroring or early adolescent closeness.

Like the committed mergers, individuals in this status appear quite needful. They are generally sensitive, communicative, and somewhat insightful, yet have trouble differentiating themselves from others.

1. Feels satisfied with her close friends except when her "inferiority complex" takes over. Then she doesn't feel a strong bond and gets depressed. She's known her boyfriend for seven years. They were engaged but not now. She feels ambiguous about the relationship. Very fearful of making a commitment. She'd hate to part but has a problem with commitment and a fear of getting very seriously hurt. She will go out with others for evaluation. Feels she will struggle with dependency problems all her life.

2. Has two very close friends who have helped her become less shy and less serious. She is extremely shy and reserved with people unless she knows them very well. She won't get involved in groups because she's fearful of others' reactions. She is fearful of guys and has never dated or been asked out. She fears there's something wrong with her.

3. Her best friend and she are so much alike. They can read each other's minds. Her friend is egotistical and needs a lot of ego boosting and she knows how to feed her ego. She sometimes manipulates her in this way. She could never tell her friend anything that would hurt her because "I'd be hurt too."

4. Her best friend went away to school. They used to argue a lot but now she misses her so much that she calls her every night to share her day and visits her friend's family regularly "just to be in her surroundings." She can always feel

when something is changing in her life and calls her . . . Likewise, her friend knows her moods and knows what she will be like. Any guy who tries to date either of them knows he has to win the friend's approval as well. One of her problems with relationships is that "my personality changes for whomever I am with."

5. She was extremely close to her boyfriend. She was very surprised when he asked her to marry him. It frightened her and made her furious. She felt "he was trying to trap me." She decided she could never see him again after that day.

6. He had a girlfriend over the summer and another for a couple of months after that and both times he thought he was in love. "But not seeing each other gets in the way. I trust her but I wonder if she's doing something. . . . Those relationships started out good and ended terrible, so right now I'm not looking for anything unless I meet the right girl. . . . Maybe I shouldn't let them play with my emotions and believe every word they say."

7. He describes his best friend as being just like him: "We both said the same things at exactly the same time and we thought about things in exactly the same way and in the same situations." But he says that since his friend began dating, he's not the same as he used to be. Now that he doesn't see him as much any more, he's a lot closer to two other friends.

6. *Preintimate*

a. These individuals have one or more close friends, but have not established an enduring heterosexual relationship.

b. Their relationships are characterized by open communication, affection, caring, and respect.

Preintimates have close friends whom they enjoy being with and see regularly. They discuss personal problems with them and are open and sympathetic to their concerns. They value openness and generally want to know others and be known by them on a deep emotional level.

Preintimates may or may not date much. Generally their dating relationships are characterized by the same kind of openness and honesty as their friendships are. They are generally somewhat experienced sexually but have some conflicts in this area. However, their sexual encounters are not primarily conquest or approval seeking. Preintimates are generally somewhat conflicted about commitment, desiring a close sexual relationship yet feeling not quite ready to form such an attachment. Preintimates have deep respect for the integrity of others, perceive them in a realistic manner, and are on guard against using them for their own gain.

Preintimate individuals have a good deal of self-awareness and genuine interest in others. They give the impression of being capable of engaging in an enduring love relationship and being likely to do so at some future time.

1. She has three close girlfriends with whom she can share personal things. Doesn't really have many acquaintances. Closeness is very special to her . . . "like a bond, you really know the person." She's been dating a guy for three months who is very sensitive and caring. They are really good friends. She can share with him as much as she shares with her closest girlfriend. However, he has dated

more and wants to become more serious than she does. This scares her and she shares it with him. She tries to take one day at a time. Though she wants an enduring relationship in a few years, she doesn't feel ready or mature enough for it now.

2. She feels very close to her friends. Friendship is very important to her—"I don't like a lot of material things—I hold on to special relationships." She feels close to her coworkers as well—"I like people—I'm not prejudiced—people I work with are mostly white but I'm not hung up on color." She's just begun dating a guy whom she can easily talk to and respects. He is a serious, open, and sincere person.

3. She has one very close friend whom she's known since grade school. Her friend is engaged and she gave her a bridal shower. She used to get "bugged" because her friend is very attractive and "could always get the guys," but she looks at it differently now because she feels good about herself. She can understand her friend's attachment to her fiance and knows they'll remain good friends. She falls in love easily and has been hurt but it doesn't keep her from being open to relationships with guys. She dated a guy exclusively for a while but was able to break it off when she realized that he was forever indulging in self-pity and didn't want to change. Also, their values were too different to make for a compatible marriage or family life. She is now dating a guy who is more open and feels good about himself.

4. Has made some good friends here. Feels very close to them. They do lots of talking and philosophizing together. He got a lot of support from his two closest friends recently when he was having problems with his family.

5. Believes in "pure" relationships: relationships without dependency or possessiveness, between friends who become lovers without tying each other down.

6. Has some girlfriends whom he can talk to pretty easily. But usually with girls he's a little shy. Recently he was seeing one girl for about a month; they started sleeping with each other. After a while, though, he wasn't sure about his feelings for her. She started falling in love with him. He didn't feel he could give her all that she needed and didn't want to lead her on, and so he "put the brakes on." They've remained good friends, but they've stopped having sex. He really likes her, and for a while considered trying it again, but then she started to go out with someone else, so. . . .

7. *Intimate*

a. These individuals have established a long-term heterosexual relationship and made a commitment to continuing the relationship.
b. This relationship and the intimate's relationships with friends are characterized by openness of communication, mutual affection and caring, sharing of responsibility, and respect for the integrity of the self and others.

Intimate individuals work at developing mutual personal relationships. They share private worries and problems with their partner and friends and are able to express both angry and affectionate feelings with them. They are open to others' feelings and problems as well. They have a strong commitment to their partner and work to overcome problems and resolve differences in an equitable way. They perceive their partner and friends as unique individuals and view their limitations and strengths in a realistic way. They enjoy interests and activities with others; however, they also have interests and activities apart from them and respect their individual needs as well. They are not overly dependent on, or jealous or manipulative of others.

Intimate individuals are characterized by a good deal of self-awareness, genuine interest in others, and absence of significant defensiveness.

1. Has known her closest friend since grade school. In junior high they were inseparable but since then they've grown a lot. They now have separate friends but can still be close. She's both similar and different from her friend. She's been involved with a guy for a year and a half. They started dating as friends. "It's like a friendship that's grown." She now loves and cares for him very much. She admires how aware he is of how a person feels.

2. She's been dating her boyfriend exclusively for a year and a half and they plan to marry. She maintains close relationships with her girlfriends. She and her boyfriend have similar values and goals. One major priority in life they share is to "make each other and the family we're going to have happy." They are really good friends and help each other through personal problems. She dislikes that he has some fixed ideas in his head, particularly about roles husbands amd wives should take. However, she talks this out with him and he has become open to altering his ideas.

3. Has made some close friends, kind of a tight-knit group with common intellectual interests. One or two of them are moving out of the circle, living with their girlfriends. But he's still pretty close with them and with their girlfriends as well.

4. Been going with a girl for about a year. She has a "good head" and is an intellectual companion as well as lover. They care a great deal about each other, been sleeping with each other for about ten months. Recently they have tried living together, and though they've had some problems, it has generally been working out pretty well. He's going to travel during the summer, but when he comes back they plan to live together again.

5. Is finishing up school this year. Had some very close friends but many of them graduated last year. He's living with one guy; they've gotten close and can discuss most anything with each other. His girlfriend has been in another city for the past year. He sees her about every other weekend. Loves her and recently they've decided to get married and both go to graduate school. The separation hasn't been easy, but he feels they've grown a great deal and become less dependent on each other than they were in their first year together. They have been able to make it okay alone and feel ready to be with each other in a more mature way than before.

References

Abraham, K.G. (1986). Ego-identity differences among Anglo-American and Mexican-American adolescents. *Journal of Adolescence*, *9*, 151–166.

Adams, G.R. (1985). Family correlates of female adolescents' ego-identity development. *Journal of Adolescence*, *8*, 69–82.

Adams, G.R., Abraham, K.G., & Markstrom, C.A. (1987). The relations among identity development, self-consciousness, and self-focusing during middle and late adolescence. *Developmental Psychology*, *23*, 292–297.

Adams, G.R., Bennion, L., & Huh, K. (1987). *Objective Measure of Ego Identity Status: A reference manual.* Unpublished manuscript. Department of Family Relations, Utah State University, Logan, UT.

Adams, G.R. & Fitch, S.A. (1981). Ego stage and identity status development: A cross-lag analysis. *Journal of Adolescence*, *4*, 163–171.

Adams, G.R. & Fitch, S.A. (1982). Ego stage and identity status development: A cross-sequential analysis. *Journal of Personality and Social Psychology*, *43*, 574–583.

Adams, G.R. & Fitch, S.A. (1983). Psychological environments at university departments: Effects on college students' identity status and ego stage development. *Journal of Personality and Social Psychology*, *44*, 1266–1275.

Adams, G.R. & Gulotta, T. (1983). *Adolescent life experiences.* Monterey, CA: Brooks/Cole.

Adams, G.R. & Jones, R.M. (1983). Female adolescents' identity development: Age comparisons and perceived child-rearing experience. *Developmental Psychology*, *19*, 249–256.

Adams, G.R., Ryan, J.H., Hoffman, J.J., Dobson, W.R., & Nielsen, E.C. (1984). Ego identity status, conformity behavior, and personality in late adolescence. *Journal of Personality and Social Psychology*, *47*, 1091–1104.

Adams, G.R. & Shea, J.A. (1979). The relationship between identity status, focus of control, and ego development. *Journal of Youth and Adolescence*, *8*, 81–89.

Adams, G.R., Shea, J., & Fitch, S.A. (1979). Toward the development of an objective assessment of ego identity status. *Journal of Youth and Adolescence*, *8*, 223–228.

Adorno, T.W., Frenkel-Brunswik, E., Levinson, D.J., & Sanford, R.N. (1950). *The authoritarian personality*. New York: Harper.

Afrifah, A. (1980). *The relationship between logical cognition and ego identity: An investigation of Piagetian and Eriksonian hypotheses about adolescence*. Unpublished doctoral dissertation, Columbia University, New York, NY.

Amstey, F.H. (1977). *The relationship between continuing education and identity in adult women*. Unpublished doctoral dissertation, University of Rochester, Rochester, NY.

Anderson, D.C. & Borkowski, J.G. (1972). *Experimental psychology: Research tactics and their applications*. Glenview, IL: Scott, Foresman.

Anderson, S.A. & Fleming, W.M. (1986a). Late adolescents' home-leaving strategies: Predicting ego identity and college adjustment. *Adolescence*, *21*, 453–459.

Anderson, S.A & Fleming, W.M. (1986b). Late adolescents' identity formation: Individuation from the family of origin. *Adolescence*, *21*, 785–796.

Andrews, J. (1973). The relationship of values to identity achievement status. *Journal of Youth and Adolescence*, *2*, 133–138.

Archer, S.L. (1981a, April). Ego identity development among early and mid-adolescents. Paper presented at the meeting of the Eastern Psychological Association, New York.

Archer, S.L. (1981b). *Identity interview schedule for working women*. Unpublished mansucript. Trenton State College, Trenton, NJ.

Archer, S.L. (1982). The lower age boundaries of identity development. *Child Development*, *53*, 1551–1556.

Archer, S.L. (1985a). Career and family: The identity process for adolescent girls. *Youth and Society*, *16*, 289–314.

Archer, S.L. (1985b). Identity and social roles. In A.S. Waterman (Ed.), *Identity in adolescence: Processes and contents*. New Directions for Child Development. Sourcebook #30. San Francisco, CA: Jossey-Bass.

Archer, S.L. (1985c, April). Reflections on earlier life decisions: Implications for adult functioning. In G.R. Adams (Chair), *Identity development from adolescence to adulthood: Advances in conceptualization and methodology*. Symposium conducted at the meetings of the Society for Research in Child Development, Toronto, Canada.

Archer, S.L. (Ed.). (1989a). Adolescent identity: An appraisal of health and intervention [Special issue]. *Journal of Adolescence*, *12*(4).

Archer, S.L. (1989b). The status of identity: Reflections on the need for intervention. *Journal of Adolescence*, *12*, 345–359.

Archer, S.L. (1989c). Gender differences in identity development: Issues of process, domain, and timing. *Journal of Adolescence*, *12*, 117–138.

Archer, S.L. (1992). A feminist's approach to identity research. In G.R. Adams, R. Montemayor, & T.P. Gullota (Eds.), *Adolescent identity formation. Advances in Adolescent Development*, Vol. 4. (pp. 25–49.) Newbury Park, CA: Sage Publications.

Archer, S.L. (Ed.). (In preparation). *Interventions for adolescent identity development*. Newbury Park, CA: Sage Publications.

Archer, S.L. & Waterman, A.S. (1983). Identity in early adolescence: A developmental perspective. *Journal of Early Adolescence*, *7*, 223–251.

Archer, S.L. & Waterman, A.S. (1988). Psychological individualism: Gender differences or gender neutrality? *Human Development*, *31*, 65–81.

Archer, S.L. & Waterman, A.S. (1990). Varieties of identity diffusions and foreclosures: An exploration of subcategories of the identity statuses. *Journal of Adolescent Research*, *5*, 96–111.

Archer, S.L., Waterman, A.S., & Owens, P.O. (1988, March). Women's identity: Comparison among three patterns of life activities. Paper presented at the meeting of the Association for Women in Psychology, Bethesda.

Arora, U. (1981). *Ego identity status of marital dyads: Their sense of intimacy and interpersonal perception of relationship*. Unpublished doctoral dissertation, Indian Institute of Technology, Ranpur, India.

Arora, U. & Marcia, J.E. (1987). *A multi-cultural study of ego identity status, perceptions of culture, cultural identification, and family permissiveness*. Unpublished manuscript. Simon Fraser University, Burnaby, British Columbia, Canada.

Ausubel, D.P. & Sullivan, E.V. (1970). *Theory and problems of child development* (2nd ed.). New York: Grune and Stratton.

Bakan, D. (1966). *The duality of human existence*. Chicago: Rand-McNally.

Barath, A. & Cannell, C. (1976). Effect of interviewer's voice intonation. *Public Opinion Quarterly*, *40*, 370–373.

Bary, B. (1978). *Impact of parents in their adolescent son's identity crisis*. Unpublished doctoral dissertation, Temple University, Philadelphia, PA.

Baumeister, R.F. (1986). *Identity: Cultural change and the struggle for self*. New York: Oxford University Press.

Baumeister, R.F., Shapiro, J.P., & Tice, D.M. (1985). Two kinds of identity crisis. *Journal of Personality*, *53*, 407–424.

Bayley, N. (1974). Research in child development: A longitudinal perspective. *Developmental psychology*. Englewood Cliffs, NJ: Prentice-Hall.

Behar, B.A. (1983). *The relationship between androgyny and identity during adolescence*. Unpublished doctoral dissertation, California School of Professional Psychology, Berkeley, CA.

Bellew-Smith, M. & Korn, J.H. (1986). Merger intimacy status in adult women. *Journal of Personality and Social Psychology*, *50*, 1186–1191.

Bem, S.L. (1974). The measurement of psychological androgyny. *Journal of Consulting and Clinical Psychology*, *42*, 155–162.

Bem, S.L. (1975). Sex-role adaptability: One consequence of psychological androgyny. *Journal of Personality and Social Psychology*, *31*, 634–643.

Bem, S.L. (1977). On the utility of alternative procedures for assessing psychological androgyny. *Journal of Consulting and Clinical Psychology*, *45*, 196–205.

Bem, S.L., Martyna, W., & Watson, C. (1976). Sex typing and androgyny: Further explorations of the expressive domain. *Journal of Personality and Social Psychology*, *34*, 1016–1023.

Bennion, L. & Adams, G.R. (1986). A revision of the extended version of the Objective Measure of Ego Identity Status: An identity instrument for use with late adolescents. *Journal of Adolescent Research*, *1*, 183–198.

Benny, M., Riesman, D., & Star, S.A. (1956). Age and sex in interview. *American Journal of Sociology*, *82*, 143–152.

Berzonsky, M.D. (1985). Diffusion within Marcia's identity status paradigm: Does it foreshadow academic problems? *Journal of Youth and Adolescence*, *14*, 527–538.

Berzonsky, M.D. (1989a). Identity style: Conceptualization and measurement. *Journal of Adolescent Research, 4*, 267–281.
Berzonsky, M.D. (1989b). Self-theorists, identity status, and social cognition. In D.K. Lapsley & F.C. Power (Eds.). *Self, ego, and identity: Integrative approaches* (pp. 243–262). New York: Springer-Verlag.
Berzonsky, M.D. (1990). Self-construction over the life-span: A process perspective on identity formation. In G.J. Neimeyer & R.A. Neimeyer (Eds.). *Advances in personal construct theory*. Vol. 1. (pp. 155–186). Greenwich, CT: JAI.
Berzonsky, M.D. & Barclay, C.T. (1981). Formal reasoning and identity formation: A reconceptualization. In J.A. Meacham & N.F. Santilli (Eds.), *Social development in youth: Structure and content*. Basel: Karger.
Berzonsky, M.D. & Niemeyer, G.J. (1988). Identity status and personal construct systems. *Journal of Adolescence, 11*, 195–204.
Berzonsky, M.D., Rice, K.G., & Neimeyer, G.J. (1990). Identity status and self-construct systems: Process x structure interactions. *Journal of Adolescence, 13*, 251–263.
Berzonsky, M.D. & Sullivan, C. (1992). Social-cognitive aspects of identity style: Need for cognition, experiential openness, and introspection. *Journal of Adolescent Research, 7*, 140–155.
Berzonsky, M.D., Weiner, A.S., & Raphael, D. (1975). Interdependence of formal reasoning. *Developmental Psychology, 11*, 258.
Bilsker, D. & Marcia, J.E. (1991). Adaptive regression and ego identity. *Journal of Adolescence, 14*, 75–84.
Bilsker, D., Schiedel, D., & Marcia, J. (1988). Sex differences in identity status. *Sex Roles, 18*, 231–236.
Blasi, A. (1988). Identity and the development of the self. In D.K. Lapsley & F.C. Power (Eds.), *Self, ego, and identity: Integrative approaches*. New York: Springer-Verlag.
Blasi, A. & Hoeffel, J. (1974). Adolescence and formal operations. *Human Development, 17*, 344–363.
Block, J. (1961). Ego identity, role variability, and adjustment. *Journal of Consulting Psychology, 25*, 392–397.
Block, J. (1971). *Lives through time*. Berkeley, CA: Bancroft Books.
Block, J. (1973). Conceptions of sex roles: Some cross-cultural and longitudinal perspectives. *American Psychologist, 28*, 512–526.
Block, J. (1978). *The Q-Sort method in personality assessment and psychiatric research*. Palo Alto, CA: Consulting Psychologists Press.
Blos, P. (1962). *On adolescence: A psychoanalytic interpretation*. New York: Free Press.
Blos, P. (1974). The genealogy of the ego ideal. *Psychoanalytic Study of the Child, 29*, 43–89.
Blustein, D.L. & Phillips, S.D. (1990). Relation between ego identity statuses and decision-making styles. *Journal of Counseling Psychology, 37*, 160–168.
Bob, S. (1966). *Ego identity and two cognitive styles*. Unpublished master's thesis, State University of New York at Buffalo, Buffalo, NY.
Bob, S. (1968). *An investigation of the relationship between identity status, cognitive style, and stress*. Unpublished doctoral dissertation, State University of New York at Buffalo, Buffalo, NY.

Bosma, H.A. (1985). *Identity development in adolescents: Coping with commitments*. Groningen, The Netherlands: University of Groningen Press.

Bosma, H.A. & Gerrits, R.S. (1985). Family functioning and identity status in adolescence. *Journal of Early Adolescence, 5*, 69–80.

Bosma, H.A. & Graafsma, T.L.G. (Eds.). (1982). *The development of identity in adolescents*. Nijmegen: Dekker and van de Vegt.

Bourne, E. (1978a). The state of research on ego identity: A review and appraisal. Part 1. *Journal of Youth and Adolescence, 7*, 223–251.

Bourne, E. (1978b). The state of research on ego identity: A review and appraisal. Part 2. *Journal of Youth and Adolescence, 7*, 371–392.

Bowlby, J. (1969). *Attachment and loss: I. Attachment.* New York: Basic Books.

Boyes, M.C. & Chandler, M. (1992). Cognitive development epistemic doubt, and identity formation in adolescence. *Journal of Youth and Adolescence, 21*, 3, 277–304.

Bradley, C. & Marcia, J.E. (1990). *Towards construct validity of generativity-stagnation: A status approach*. Unpublished manuscript. Simon Fraser University, Burnaby, British Columbia, Canada.

Bronson, G.W. (1959). Identity diffusion in late adolescents. *Journal of Abnormal and Social Psychology, 59*, 414–417.

Bruner, J.S., Goodnow, I.J., & Austin, G.A. (1956). *A study of thinking*. New York: Wiley.

Bukowski, W.M. & Newcomb, A.F. (1983). The association between peer experiences and identity formation in early adolescence. *Journal of Early Adolescence, 3*, 265–274.

Bunt, M. (1968). Ego identity: Its relationship to the discrepancy between how an adolescent views himself and how he perceives that others view him. *Psychology, 5*, 14–25.

Caldwell, R.A., Bogat, G.A., & Cruise, K. (1989). The relationship of ego identity to social network structure and function in young men and women. *Journal of Adolescence, 12*, 309–313.

Campbell, E., Adams, G.R., & Dobson, W.R. (1984). Familial correlates of identity formation in late adolescence: A study of the predicted utility of connectedness and individuality in family relations. *Journal of Adolescence, 6*, 509–525.

Cannell, C.F. & Kahn, R.L. (1953). The collection of data by interviewing. In L. Festinger & D. Katz (Eds.), *Research methods in the behavioral sciences*. New York: Holt, Rinehart & Winston.

Caracelli, V.J. (1988, March). Reentry women students: Identity status stability and change during an "off-time" transition. Paper presented at the meeting of the Society for Research on Adolescence, Alexandria, VA.

Carkhuff, R.R. (1972). *The art of helping*. Amherst, MA: Human Resource Development Press.

Cauble, M.A. (1976). Formal operations, ego identity, and principled morality: Are they related? *Developmental Psychology, 12*, 362–364.

Cella, D.F., DeWolfe, A.S., & Fitzgibbon, M. (1987). Ego identity status, identification, and decision-making style in late adolescents. *Adolescence, 22*, 849–861.

Chandler, M. (1987). The Othello effect: An essay on the emergence and eclipse of skeptical doubt. *Human Development, 30*, 137–159.

Chapman, J.W. & Nicholls, J.G. (1976). Occupational identity status, occupational preference, and field dependence in Maori and Pakena boys. *Journal of Cross-Cultural Psychology*, *7*, 61–72.

Ciaccio, N.V. (1971). A test of Erikson's theory of ego epigenesis. *Developmental Psychology*, *4*, 306–311.

Constantinople, A. (1969). An Eriksonian measure of personality development in college students. *Developmental Psychology*, *1*, 357–372.

Constantinople, A. (1970). Some correlates of average level of happiness among college students. *Developmental Psychology*, *2*, 447.

Constantinople, A. (1973). Masculinity-femininity: An exception to a famous dictum? *Psychological Bulletin*, *80*, 389–407.

Cooke, T.P., Apolloni, T., & Cooke, S.A. (1977). Normal preschool children as behavioral models for retarded peers. *Journal of Exceptional Children*, *43*, 531–532.

Cooper, C.R., Grotevant, H.D., & Condin, S.M. (1983). Individuality and connectedness in the family as a context for adolescent identity formation and role-taking skill. In H.D. Grotevant & C.R. Cooper (Eds.), *Adolescent development in the family*. San Francisco, CA: Jossey-Bass.

Costa, M.E. & Campos, B.P. (1986). Identity in university students: Differences in course of study and gender. *Cadernos de Consulta Psicologica*, *2*, 5–13.

Costa, M.E. & Campos, B.P. (1988, July). A longitudinal study of identity development in university students. Paper presented at the First International Conference on Counseling Psychology and Human Development, Porto, Portugal.

Costa, M.E. & Campos, B.P. (1989, July). University area of study and identity development: A longitudinal study. Paper presented at the meeting of the International Society for the Study of Behavioural Development, Jyväskylä, Finland.

Côté, J.E. (1986). Identity crisis modality: A technique for assessing the structure of the identity crisis. *Journal of Adolescence*, *9*, 321–335.

Côté, J.E. & Levine, C. (1988a). A critical examination of the ego identity status paradigm. *Developmental Review*, *8*, 147–184.

Côté, J.E. & Levine, C. (1988b). On critiquing the identity status paradigm. *Developmental Review*, *8*, 209–218.

Côté, J.E. & Reker, G.T. (1979). Cognitive complexity and ego identity formation: A synthesis of cognitive and ego psychology. *Social Behavior and Personality*, *7*, 107–112.

Craig-Bray, L. & Adams, G.R. (1986). Different methodologies in the assessment of identity: Congruence between self-report and interview techniques? *Journal of Youth and Adolescence*, *15*, 191–204.

Craig-Bray, L., Adams, G.R., & Dobson, W.R. (1988). Identity formation and social relations during late adolescence. *Journal of Youth and Adolescence*, *17*, 173–187.

Cronbach, L. & Meehl, P. (1955). Construct validity in psychological tests. *Psychological Bulletin*, *52*, 281–302.

Cross, H. & Allen, J. (1970). Ego identity status, adjustment, and academic achievement. *Journal of Consulting and Clinical Psychology*, *34*, 288.

Crown, P.A. (1985). *Ego identity, intimacy, and sex role orientation of young adults*. Unpublished doctoral dissertation, University of Denver, Denver, CO.

Deldin, L.S. (1977). *Sex role development and identity achievement.* Unpublished doctoral dissertation, University of Florida, Gainesville, FL.
Della Selva, P.D. & Dusek, J.B. (1984). Sex role orientation and resolution of Eriksonian crises during the late adolescent years. *Journal of Personality and Social Psychology, 47,* 204–212.
Dellas, M. & Jernigan, L.P. (1987). Occupational identity status development, gender comparisons, and internal-external control in first-year Air Force cadets. *Journal of Youth and Adolescence, 16,* 587–600.
Dellas, M. & Jernigan, L.P. (1990). Affective personality characteristics associated with undergraduate ego identity formation. *Journal of Adolescent Research, 3,* 306–324.
Dignan, M.H. (1965). Ego identity and maternal identification. *Journal of Personality and Social Psychology, 1,* 476–483.
Donovan, J.M. (1970). *A study of ego identity formation.* Unpublished doctoral dissertation, University of Michigan, Ann Arbor, MI.
Donovan, J.M. (1975a). Identity status and interpersonal style. *Journal of Youth and Adolescence, 4,* 37–55.
Donovan, J.M. (1975b). Identity status: Its relationship to Rorschach performance and to daily life pattern. *Adolescence, 10,* 29–44.
Douglas, J.E. (1985). *Creative interviewing.* Beverly Hills, CA: Sage Publications.
Douvan, E. & Adelson, J. (1966). *The adolescent experience.* New York: Wiley.
Dufresne, J. & Cross, J.H. (1972). *Personality variables in student drug use.* Unpublished master's thesis, University of Connecticut, Storrs, CT.
Dunivant, N., Jr. & Bieri, J. (1973, April). A multi-method comparison of various measures of Erikson's concept of ego identity. Paper presented at the meeting of the Southwestern Psychological Association, Dallas, TX.
Dye, R., Marquess, J., & LaVoie, J.D. (1975). *Ego identity in normal and socially maladjusted adolescent females.* Unpublished manuscript. University of Nebraska at Omaha, Omaha, NE.
Egan, G. (1975). *The skilled helper: A model for systematic helping and interpersonal relating.* Monterey, CA: Brooks-Cole.
Egan, G. (1990). *The skilled helper* (3rd ed.). Monterey, CA: Brooks/Cole.
Enright, R.D., Lapsley, D.U., & Cullen, J. (1982). A psychometric examination of Rasmussen's ego identity scale. *International Journal of Behavioral Development, 6,* 89–103.
Enright, R.D., Lapsley, D.U., Drivas, A.E., & Fehr, L.A. (1980). Parental influences on the development of adolescent autonomy and identity. *Journal of Youth and Adolescence, 9,* 526–545.
Erikson, E.H. (1952, September). Remarks made at an interagency conference at Princeton, NJ. *Healthy personality development in children: As related to programs of the federal government.* New York: Josiah Macy Jr. Foundation.
Erikson, E.H. (1959). Identity and the life cycle. *Psychological Issues.* Monograph No. 1.
Erikson, E.H. (1963). *Childhood and Society,* 2nd ed. New York: Norton.
Erikson, E.H. (1968). *Identity: Youth and crisis.* New York: Norton.
Erikson, E.H. (1975). *Life history and the historical moment.* New York: Norton.
Erikson, E.H. (1980). *Identity and the life cycle: A reissue.* New York: Norton.

Erikson, E.H. (1982). *The life cycle completed: A review*. New York: Norton.

Erikson, E.H. (1987). Remarks on the "wider identity." In S. Schlein (Ed.), *A way of looking at things*. New York: Norton.

Erwin, T.D. & Schmidt, M.R. (1981). Convergent validity of the Erwin Identity Scale. *Educational and Psychological Measurement*, *41*, 1307–1310.

Evans, D., Hearne, M.T., Uhlemann, M.R., & Ivey, A.E. (1979). *Essential interviewing: A programmed approach to effective communication*. Monterey, CA: Brooks-Cole.

Fannin, P.N. (1979). The relation between ego identity status and sex role attitude, work role salience, atypicality of major, and self-esteem in college women. *Journal of Vocational Behavior*, *14*, 12–22.

Fitch, S.A. & Adams, G.R. (1983). Ego identity and intimacy status: Replication and extension. *Developmental Psychology*, *19*, 839–845.

Flum, H. (1990, March). What is the evolutive style of identity formation? Paper presented at the meeting of the Society for Research in Adolescence, Atlanta, GA.

Freilino, M.K. & Hummel, R. (1985). Achievement and identity in college age vs. adult women students. *Journal of Youth and Adolescence*, *14*, 1–11.

Freud, A. (1936). *The ego and the mechanisms of defense*. New York: International Universities Press.

Freud, S. (1923/1961). *The ego and the id*. In Vol. XIX of *The Standard Edition*. London: Hogarth.

Frieze, I.H., Parsons, J.E., Johnson, P.B., Ruble, D.N., & Zellman, G.L. (1978). *Women and sex roles: A social psychological perspective*. New York: Norton.

Fromm, E. (1956). *The art of loving*. New York: Harper and Row.

Fry, P.S. (1974). Developmental changes in identity status of university students from rural and urban backgrounds. *Journal of College Student Personnel*, *15*, 183–190.

Geert, P. van (1987). The structure of Erikson's model of the eight stages: A generative approach. *Human Development*, *30*, 236–254.

Genthner, R.W. & Neuber, K.A. (1975). Identity achievers and their rated levels of facilitation. *Psychological Reports*, *36*, 754.

Gerber, L. (1968). *Openness to experience, environmental conditions and classroom participation*. Unpublished doctoral dissertation, University of Chicago, Chicago, IL.

Gilligan, C. (1982). *In a different voice: Psychological theory and women's development*. Cambridge, MA: Harvard University Press.

Ginsburg, S.D. & Orlofsky, J.L. (1981). Ego identity status, ego development, and locus of control in college women. *Journal of Youth and Adolescence*, *10*, 297–307.

Gold, D.W. (1980). *Disadvantaged women's ego identity status as related to achievement, self-esteem, and demographic information*. Unpublished doctoral dissertation, University of Pittsburgh, Pittsburgh, PA.

Goldman, J.A., Rosenzweig, M., & Lutter, A.D. (1980). Effect of ego identity statuses on interpersonal attraction. *Journal of Youth and Adolescence*, *9*, 153–162.

Gombosi, P.G. (1972). *Regression in the service of the ego as a function of identity status*. Unpublished doctoral dissertation, Boston University, Boston, MA.

Gordon, R.L. (1954). *An interaction analysis of the depth-interview*. Unpublished doctoral dissertation, University of Chicago, Chicago, IL.

Gordon, T. (1970). *P.E.T.: Parent Effectiveness Training*. New York: Peter H. Wyden.

Gottman, J.M. (1979). *Marital interaction: Experimental investigations* (pp. 120–123). New York: Academic Press.

Graafsma, T.L.G. (1989, July). Working paper on psychoanalytic views of identity. Paper presented at the meeting of the International Society for the Study of Behavioural Development, Jyväskylä, Finland.

Greenberg, J.R. & Mitchell, S.A. (1983). *Object relations in psychoanalytic theory*. Cambridge, MA: Harvard University Press.

Greenhouse, E.M. (1975). *The relationship between identity status and several aspects of heterosexual relationships in college women*. Unpublished doctoral dissertation, Columbia University, New York, NY.

Grossman, S.M., Shea, J.A., & Adams, G.R. (1980). Effects of parental divorce during early childhood on ego development and identity formation of college students. *Journal of Divorce*, *3*, 263–272.

Grotevant, H.D. & Adams, G.R. (1984). Development of an objective measure to assess ego identity in adolescence: Validation and replication. *Journal of Youth and Adolescence*, *13*, 419–438.

Grotevant, H.D. & Cooper, C.R. (1983). The role of family communication patterns in adolescent identity and role-taking. Paper presented at the meeting of the Society for Research in Child Development, Detroit, MI.

Grotevant, H.D. & Cooper, C.R. (1985). Patterns of interaction in family relationships and the development of identity exploration in adolescence. *Child Development*, *56*, 415–428.

Grotevant, H.D. & Cooper, C.R. (1986). Individuation in family relationships: A perspective on individual differences in the development of identity and role-taking skill in adolescence. *Human Development*, *29*, 82–100.

Grotevant, H.D. & Thorbecke, W.L. (1982). Sex differences in styles of occupational identity formation in late adolescence. *Developmental Psychology*, *18*, 396–405.

Grotevant, H.D., Thorbecke, W.L., & Meyer, M.L. (1982). An extension of Marcia's identity status interview into the interpersonal domain. *Journal of Youth and Adolescence*, *11*, 33–47.

Gruen, W. (1960). Rejection of false information about oneself as an indication of ego identity. *Journal of Consulting Psychology*, *24*, 231–233.

Hansburg, H.G. (1980). *Adolescent separation anxiety: A method for the study of adolescent separation problems*. Huntington, N.Y.: Robert E. Krieger.

Hartmann, H. (1964). *Essays on ego psychology*. New York: International Universities Press.

Hartmann, H., Kris, E., & Lowenstein, R.M. (1946). *Papers on psychoanalytic psychology. Psychological Issues*, Monograph No. 14. New York: International Universities Press.

Hauser, S.T. (1971). *Black and white identity formation*. New York: Wiley.

Hauser, S.T. (1972). Black and white identity development: Aspects and perspectives. *Journal of Youth and Adolescence*, *1*, 113–130.

Hauser, S.T. (1976). Loevinger's model of ego development: A critical review. *Psychological Bulletin*, *83*, 928–957.

Hearn, S. (In progress). Development and construct validation of a measure of Eriksonian integrity. Work in progress. Simon Fraser University, Burnaby, British Columbia, Canada.

Hefner, R., Rebecca, M., & Olshansky, B. (1975). Development of sex-role transcendence. *Human Development*, *18*, 143–158.

Henson, R., Roth, A., & Cannell, C.F. (1977). Personal versus telephone interviews: The effects of telephone reinterviews on reporting of psychiatric symptomatology. In *NCHSR*.

Heyduk, C. (1983). *The relationship of identity status and intimacy status: An overlapping stage resolution perspective*. Unpublished doctoral dissertation, Bryn Mawr College, Bryn Mawr, PA.

Hildum, D. & Brown, R.W. (1956). Verbal reinforcement and interviewer bias. *Journal of Early Adolescence*, *4*, 47–52.

Himelstein, P. & Lubin, B. (1965). Attempted validation of the self-disclosure inventory by the peer nomination technique. *Journal of Consulting and Clinical Psychology*, *53*, 108–111.

Hodgson, J.W. & Fischer, J.L. (1979). Sex differences in identity and intimacy development in college youth. *Journal of Youth and Adolescence*, *8*, 37–50.

Hoffman, L.W. (1974). Fear of success in males and females. *Journal of Consulting and Clinical Psychology*, *42*, 353–358.

Hogan, R. (1973). Moral conduct and moral character: A psychological perspective. *Psychological Bulletin*, *79*, 217–232.

Hood, T.C. & Black, K.W. (1971). Self-disclosure and the volunteer: A source of bias in laboratory experiments. *Journal of Personality and Social Psychology*, *17*, 130–136.

Hooker, E. (1965). An empirical study of some relationships between sexual patterns and gender identity in male homosexuals. In J. Money (Ed.), *Sex research: New developments*. New York: Holt, Rinehart & Winston.

Hopkins, L.B. (1980). Inner space and outerspace identity in contemporary females. *Psychiatry*, *43*, 1–12.

Hopkins, L.B. (1982). Assessment of identity status in college women using outer space and inner space interviews. *Sex Roles*, *8*, 557–566.

Horner, M.S. (1972). Toward an understanding of achievement-related conflicts in women. *Journal of Social Issues*, *28*, 157–175.

Howard, L.P. (1960). Identity conflict in adolescent girls. *Smith College Studies in Social Work*, *31*, 1–21.

Howard, M.R. (1975). *Ego identity status in women, fear of success, and performance in a competitive situation*. Unpublished doctoral dissertation, State University of New York at Buffalo, Buffalo, NY.

Huh, K.S. (1984). *A study on the relationship between the college student's ego identity status and their personality traits*. Unpublished master's thesis, Graduate School of Seoul Women's University, Seoul, Korea.

Hult, R.E. (1979). The relationship between ego identity status and moral reasoning in university women. *Journal of Psychology*, *103*, 203–207.

Hummel, R. & Roselli, L.L. (1983). Identity status and academic achievement in female adolescents. *Adolescence*, *17*, 17–27.

Imberman, E. (1983). *The relationship of intimacy, ego identity and marital adjustment in married and cohabiting young adults: A comparative study of norma-*

tive adult development. Unpublished doctoral dissertation, Boston University, Boston, MA.
Inhelder, B. & Piaget, J. (1958). *The growth of logical thinking from childhood to adolescence*. New York: Basic Books.
Institute for Social Research (1969). *Interviewer's manual: Survey Research Center*. Ann Arbor: University of Michigan.
Ivey, A.E., Normington, C.J., Miller, C.D., Morill, W.H., & Haase, R.F. (1968). Microcounseling and attending behavior. *Journal of Counseling Psychology*, *15*, 1–12 (Monograph).
Janis, I.L. & Mann, L. (1977). *Decision-making: A psychological analysis of conflict, choice and commitment*. New York: Free Press.
Jegede, R.D. (1976). The identity status of Nigerian University students. *Journal of Social Psychology*, *100*, 175–179.
Johnson, R.W., Holborn, S.W., & Turcotte, C. (1979). Perceived attractiveness as a function of active vs. passive support for the feminist movement. *Personality and Social Psychology Bulletin*, *5*, 227–230.
Jones, M.C. (1957). The later careers of boys who were early or late maturing. *Child Development*, *28*, 113–128.
Jones, M.C. (1965). Psychological correlates of somatic development. *Child Development*, *36*, 899–911.
Jones, R.M. & Hartmann, B.R. (1988). Ego identity: Developmental differences and experimental substance use among adolescents. *Journal of Adolescence*, *11*, 347–360.
Jones, R.M. & Streitmatter, J.L. (1987). Validity and reliability of the EOM-EIS for early adolescents. *Adolescence*, *22*, 647–659.
Jones, W.H., Chernovetz, O.C., & Hansson, R.O. (1978). The enigma of androgyny: Differential implications for males and females. *Journal of Consulting and Clinical Psychology*, *46*, 298–313.
Jordan, D. (1970). *Parental antecedents of ego identity formation*. Unpublished master's thesis, State University of New York at Buffalo, Buffalo, NY.
Jordan, D. (1971). *Parental antecedents and personality characteristics of ego identity statuses*. Unpublished doctoral dissertation, State University of New York at Buffalo, Buffalo, NY.
Josselson, R.L. (1972). *Identity formation in college women*. Unpublished doctoral dissertation, University of Michigan, Ann Arbor, MI.
Josselson, R.L. (1973). Psychodynamic aspects of identity formation in college women. *Journal of Youth and Adolescence*, *2*, 3–51.
Josselson, R.L. (1980). Ego development in adolescence. In J. Adelson (Ed.), *Handbook of adolescent psychology*. New York: Wiley.
Josselson, R.L. (1982). Personality structure and identity status in women viewed through early memories. *Journal of Youth and Adolescence*, *11*, 293–299.
Josselson, R.L. (1987). Identity diffusion: A long-term follow-up. *Adolescent Psychiatry*, Vol. XIV. Chicago: University of Chicago Press.
Josselson, R.L. (1988). *Finding herself: Pathways of identity development in women*. New York: Jossey-Bass.
Josselson, R.L., Greenberger, E., & McConochie, D. (1977a). Phenomenological aspects of psychosocial maturity in adolescence. Part I. Boys. *Journal of Youth and Adolescence*, *6*, 25–55.

Josselson, R.L., Greenberger, E., & McConochie, D. (1977b). Phenomenological aspects of psychosocial maturity in adolescence. Part II. Girls. *Journal of Youth and Adolescence*, *6*, 145–167.

Jourard, S.M. (1971). *Self-disclosure: An experimental analysis of the transparent self*. New York: Wiley Interscience.

Jourard, S.M. & Landsman, M.J. (1960). Cognition, catharsis, and the "dyadic effect" in men's self-disclosing behavior. *Merrill-Palmer Quarterly*, *6*, 178–186.

Jourard, S.M. & Lasakow, P. (1958). Some factors in self-disclosure. *Journal of Abnormal and Social Psychology*, *56*, 91–98.

Jourard, S.M. & Richman, P. (1963). Disclosure output and input in college students. *Merrill-Palmer Quarterly*, *9*, 141–148.

Kacerguis, M.A. & Adams, G.R. (1980). Erikson stage resolution: The relationship between identity and intimacy. *Journal of Youth and Adolescence*, *9*, 117–126.

Kahn, S., Zimmerman, G., Csikszentmihalyi, M., & Getzels, J.W. (1985). Relations between identity in young adulthood and intimacy at midlife. *Journal of Personality and Social Psychology*, *49*, 1316–1322.

Kamptner, N.L. (1988). Identity development in late adolescence: Causal modeling of social and familial influences. *Journal of Youth and Adolescence*, *17*, 493–514.

Kato, A. (1983). A study of identity statuses and their structure in university students. *Japanese Journal of Educational Psychology*, *31*, 292–302.

Kegan, R. (1982). *The evolving self: Problem and process in human development*. Cambridge, MA: Harvard University Press.

Kelly, G. (1955). *The psychology of personal constructs*. (2 vols.) New York: Norton.

Kendis, R.J. & Tan, A.L. (1978). Ego identity perception of parents among female college students. *Perceptual and Motor Skills*, *47*, 1201–1202.

Kinsler, P. (1972). *Ego identity status and intimacy*. Unpublished doctoral dissertation, State University of New York at Buffalo, Buffalo, NY.

Kirby, C.S. (1977). *Complexity-simplicity as a dimension of identity formation*. Unpublished doctoral dissertation, Michigan State University, East Lansing, MI.

Kohlberg, L. (1973). Continuities in childhood and adult moral development revisited. In P.B. Baltes & K.W. Schaie (Eds.), *Life-span developmental psychology: Personality and socialization*. New York: Academic Press.

Kohlberg, L. (1976). Moral stages and moralization: The cognitive developmental approach. In T. Lickona (Ed.), *Moral development and moral behavior*. New York: Holt, Rinehart & Winston.

Kohlberg, L. & Gilligan, C. (1972). The adolescent as a philosopher: The discovery of the self in a post-conventional world. In J. Kagan & R. Coles (Eds.), *12 to 16: Early adolescence* (pp. 144–180). New York: Norton.

Kohut, H. (1971). *The analysis of the self: A systematic approach to the treatment of narcissistic personality disorders*. New York: International University Press.

Kowaz, A.M. & Marcia, J.E. (1991). Development and validation of a measure of Eriksonian industry. *Journal of Personality and Social Psychology*, *60*, 390–397.

Kroger, J. (1983). A developmental study of identity formation among late adolescent and adult women. *Psychological Documents*, *13* (Ms. No. 2537).

Kroger, J. (1985). Separation-individuation and ego identity status in New Zealand university students. *Journal of Youth and Adolescence, 14*, 133–147.
Kroger, J. (1986). The relative importance of identity status interview components: Replication and extension. *Journal of Adolescence, 9*, 337–354.
Kroger, J. (1987). *Sex differences in the relative importance of ego identity status content areas*. Unpublished manuscript. Victoria University of Wellington, Wellington, New Zealand.
Kroger, J. (1988a). A longitudinal study of ego identity status interview domains. *Journal of Adolescence, 11*, 49–64.
Kroger, J. (1988b). Separation-individuation and ego identity status in late adolescence: A two-year longitudinal study. *Journal of Youth and Adolescence, 17*, 59–79.
Kroger, J. (1989). *Identity in adolescence: The balance between self and other.* London and New York: Routledge.
Kroger, J. (1990a). Ego structuralization in late adolescence as seen through early memories and ego identity status. *Jouranl of Adolescence, 13*, 65–77.
Kroger, J. (1990b). *Intrapsychic dimensions of identity during late adolescence.* Unpublished manuscript. Victoria University of Wellington, Wellington, New Zealand.
Kroger, J. & Haslett, S.J. (1987). A retrospective study of ego identity status change by mid-life adults. *Social and Behavioral Sciences Documents, 17* (Ms. No. 2797).
Kroger, J. & Haslett, S.J. (1991). *A comparison of ego identity status transition pathways and change rates across five identity domains*. Unpublished manuscript. Victoria University of Wellington, Wellington, New Zealand.
Kumar, U., Nandkishore, M., Balasubramarian, R., Mathur, S., & Sheikh, S. (1980). Identity status and preference for managerial styles. *Journal of Social Psychology, 110*, 295–296.
Kurfiss, J. (1981). Cognitive development: *Sine qua non* of identity achievement? Paper presented at the meeting of the Rocky Mountain Psychological Association, Denver, CO.
Lamke, L.K. & Peyton, K.G. (1988). Adolescent sex-role orientation and ego identity. *Journal of Adolescence, 11*, 205–215.
LaVoie, J.C. (1976). Ego identity formation in middle adolescence. *Journal of Youth and Adolescence, 5*, 371–385.
LaVoie, J.C. & Adams, G.R. (1981). *Eriksonian developmental stage resolution and attachment behavior in young adulthood.* Unpublished manuscript. University of Nebraska at Omaha, Omaha, NE.
Leadbetter, B.J. & Dionne, J.P. (1981). The adolescent's use of formal operational thinking in solving problems related to identity resolution. *Adolescence, 16*, 111–121.
Leiper, R.N. (1981). *The relationship of cognitive developmental structures to the formation of identity in young men.* Unpublished doctoral dissertation, Simon Fraser University, Burnaby, British Columbia, Canada.
Levinson, D.J. (1978). *The seasons of a man's life*. New York: Knopf.
Levitz-Jones, E.M. & Orlofsky, J.L. (1985). Separation-individuation and intimacy capacity in college women. *Journal of Personality and Social Psychology, 49*, 156–169.
Lifshitz, M. (1978). Girls' identity formation as related to perception of parents. *Social Behavior and Personality, 6*, 81–87.

Loevinger, J. (1976). *Ego development: Conceptions and theories*. San Francisco, CA: Jossey-Bass.

Loevinger, J. & Wessler, R. (1970). *Measuring ego development*. (2 vols.) San Francisco, CA: Jossey-Bass.

Logan, R.D. (1986). A re-conceptualization of Erikson's theory as the repetition in adulthood of existential and instrumental themes from childhood. *Human Development*, *29*, 125–136.

Luria, E.S. (1980). *Housewives who begin professional school and housewives who do not: Identity and intimacy issues*. Unpublished doctoral dissertation, University of Cincinnati, Cincinnati, OH.

Lutes, C. (1981). Early marriage and identity foreclosure. *Adolescence*, *16*, 809–816.

Mahler, M.S., Pine, F., & Bergman, A. (1975). *The psychological birth of the human infant*. New York: Basic Books.

Mallory, M.E. (1983). *Longitudinal analysis of ego identity status*. Unpublished doctoral dissertation, University of California at Davis, Davis, CA.

Mallory, M.E. (1989). Q-sort definitions of ego identity status. *Journal of Youth and Adolescence*, *18*, 399–412.

Marcia, J.E. (1964). *Determination and construct validity of ego identity status*. Unpublished doctoral dissertation, The Ohio State University, Columbus, OH.

Marcia, J.E. (1966). Development and validation of ego identity status. *Journal of Personality and Social Psychology*, *3*, 551–558.

Marcia, J.E. (1967). Ego identity status: Relationship to change in self-esteem, "general maladjustment," and authoritarianism. *Journal of Personality*, *35*, 119–133.

Marcia, J.E. (1976a). Identity six years after: A follow-up study. *Journal of Youth and Adolescence*, *5*, 145–160.

Marcia, J.E. (1976b). *Studies in ego identity*. Unpublished research monograph. Simon Fraser University, Burnaby, British Columbia, Canada.

Marcia, J.E. (1980). Identity in adolescence. In J. Adelson (Ed.), *Handbook of adolescent psychology*. New York: Wiley.

Marcia, J.E. (1983). Some directions for the investigation of ego identity development in early adolescence. *Journal of Early Adolescence*, *3*, 215–223.

Marcia, J.E. (1986a). Clinical implications of the identity status approach within psychosocial developmental theory. *Cadernos de Consulta Psicologica*, *2*, 23–35.

Marcia, J.E. (1986b). Doubt and "distancing": Developmental perspectives on identity formation. Paper presented at the meeting of the Canadian Psychological Association, Toronto, Canada.

Marcia, J.E. (1988a). Common process underlying ego identity, cognitive/moral development, and individuation. In E. Lapsley & C. Power (Eds.), *Integrative approaches to self, ego, and identity*. New York: Springer-Verlag.

Marcia, J.E. (1988b). Counseling and psychotherapy from a developmental perspective. Paper presented at the First International Conference on Counseling Psychology and Human Development, Porto, Portugal.

Marcia, J.E. (1989a). Identity and intervention. *Journal of Adolescence*, *12*, 401–410.

Marcia, J.E. (1989b). Identity diffusion differentiated. In M.A. Luszcz & T. Nettelbeck (Eds.), *Psychological development: Perspectives across the life-span*. North Holland: Elsevier Science Publishers.

Marcia, J.E. (1989c, July). Implications of methodologies for identity theory: The Identity Status Interview. Paper presented at the meeting of the International Society for the Study of Behavioural Development, Jväskylä, Finland.

Marcia, J.E. & Friedman, M. (1970). Ego identity status in college women. *Journal of Personality*, *38*, 249–262.

Marcia, J.E. & Miller, E.C. (1980). Ego identity in mature women. Paper presented at the meeting of the Eastern Psychological Association, Hartford, CT.

Markstrom, C.A. (1987, February). Ego identity, sex-role orientation, and locus of control in four middle adolescent ethnic groups. Paper presented at the Fourth Biennial Conference on Adolescent Research, Tucson, AZ.

Markstrom-Adams, C.A., Ascione, F.R., Braegger, D., & Adams, G.R. (in press). The effects of two forms of perspective-taking training on ego-identity formation in late adolescence. *Journal of Adolescence*.

Marquis, K.H. & Cannell, C.F. (1969). *A study of interviewer–respondent interaction in the Urban Employment Survey*. (Research Report). Survey Research Center, University of Michigan, Ann Arbor, MI.

Maslow, A.H. (1954). *Motivation and personality*. New York: Harper and Row.

Matteson, D.R. (1974). *Alienation vs. exploration and commitment: Personality and family correlaries of adolescent identity statuses*. Report for the Project for Youth Research. Copenhagen Royal Danish School of Educational Studies. Copenhagen, Denmark.

Matteson, D.R. (1975). *Adolescence today: Sex roles and the search for identity*. Homewood, IL: Dorsey.

Matteson, D.R. (1977a). Exploration and commitment: Sex differences and methodological problems in the use of the identity status categories. *Journal of Youth and Adolescence*, *6*, 353–379.

Matteson, D.R. (1977b). *Peer support for adolescent identity formation*. Unpublished manuscript. Governors State University, Park Forest South, IL.

Matteson, D.R. (1977c). Two transitions and two crises in youth: A response to P.S. Fry's "Changes in youth's attitudes toward authority." *Journal of Counseling Psychology*, *24*, 79–80.

Matteson, D.R. (1978). Communication and identity formation in Danish and American adolescents. Paper presented at the meeting of the International Communications Conference, Chicago, IL.

Matteson, D.R. (1979). Training in identity formation: A practical proposal for bridging the worlds of school and adulthood. Paper presented at the meeting of the International Society for the Study of Behavioural Development, Lund, Sweden.

Matteson, D.R. (1980). *Teenagers' attitudes toward sex roles*. Unpublished manuscript. Governors State University, Park Forest South, IL.

Mayseless, O. (1990). Identity formation and emotional maturity of released soldiers in Israel. Research in progress.

McClain, E.W. (1975). An Eriksonian cross-cultural study of adolescent development. *Adolescence*, *10*, 527–541.

Meacham, J.A. & Santilli, N.R. (1982). Interstage relationships in Erikson's theory: Identity and intimacy. *Child Development*, *53*, 1461–1467.

Meilman, P.W. (1979). Cross-sectional age changes in ego identity status during adolescence. *Developmental Psychology*, *15*, 230–231.

Melgosa, J. (1987). Development and validation of the occupational identity status. *Journal of Adolescence*, *10*, 385–397.

Mellor, S. (1989). Gender differences in identity formation as a function of self–other relationships. *Journal of Youth and Adolescence*, *18*, 361–375.

Meyers, L.S. & Grossen, N.E. (1974). *Behavioral research: Theory, procedure and design*. San Francisco, CA: W.H. Freeman.

Minuchin, S. (1974). *Families and family therapy*. Cambridge, MA: Harvard University Press.

Mohammed, A.A. (1990). Using Marcia's ego identity status interview to study identity statuses in university students. *Journal of the Faculty of Education*, Zagazig University, Egypt, *5*(11) (Supplementary), 198–234.

Morash, M.A. (1980). Working class membership and the adolescent identity crisis. *Adolescence*, *15*, 313–320.

Moreland, J.R., Harren, V.A., Krimsky, M.E., & Tinsley, M.E.A. (1979). Sex-role self-concept and career decision-making. *Journal of Counseling Psychology*, *26*, 329–336.

Morgan, E. & Farber, B.A. (1982). Toward a reformulation of the Eriksonian model of female identity development. *Adolescence*, *17*, 199–211.

Munro, G. & Adams, G.R. (1977). Ego identity formation in college students and working youth. *Developmental Psychology*, *13*, 523–524.

Murray, H.A. (1943). *Thematic Apperception Test*. Cambridge, MA: Harvard University Press.

Mussen, P.H. (1962). Long-term consequences of masculinity of interests in adolescence. *Journal of Consulting Psychology*, *26*, 435–440.

Mussen, P.H. & Jones, M.C. (1957). Self-conceptions, motivations, and interpersonal attitudes of late- and early-maturing boys. *Child Development*, *28*, 243–256.

Muto, K. (1979). Modification and development of EISI and ego identity of Japanese university students. *Japanese Journal of Educational Psychology*, *27*, 178–187.

Neimeyer, G.J., & Rareshide, M.B. (1991). Personal memories and personal identity: The impact of ego identity development on autobiographical memory recall. *Journal of Personality and Social Psychology*, *60*, 562–569.

Neuber, K.A. & Genthner, R.W. (1977). The relationship between ego identity, personal responsibility, and facilitative communication. *Journal of Psychology*, *95*, 45–49.

Newman, F. (1986). *Ego development in women in an urban hostel*. Unpublished doctoral dissertation, Simon Fraser University, Burnaby, British Columbia, Canada.

Noam, G. (1988). A constructivist approach to developmental psychopathology. In E.D. Nannis & P.A. Cowan (Eds.), *Developmental psychopathology and its treatment*. New Directions for Child Development, No. 39. San Francisco, CA: Jossey-Bass.

Norris, L. & Katz, M. (1970). *The measure of academic interests. Part I. Characteristics of the Academic Interest Measure*. (ETS RB 70-67). Princeton, NJ: Educational Testing Service.

Norris, L., Katz, M.R., & Chapman, W. (1978). Sex differences in the career decision-making process. Final report. Princeton, NJ: Educational Testing Service.

Ochberg R.L. (1986). College dropouts: The developmental logic of psychosocial moratoria. *Journal of Youth and Adolescence, 15*, 287–302.
Ochse, R. & Plug, C. (1986). Cross-cultural investigation of the validity of Erikson's theory of personality development. *Journal of Personality and Social Psychology, 50*, 1240–1252.
O'Connell, A.N. (1976). The relationship between life style and identity synthesis and re-synthesis in traditional, neo-traditional, and non-traditional women. *Journal of Personality, 44*, 675–688.
Offer, D. & Offer, J.B. (1975). *From teenage to young manhood: A psychological study*. New York: Basic Books.
Offer, D., Ostrov, E., & Howard, K.I. (1981). *The adolescent: A psychological self-portrait*. New York: Basic Books.
Orlofsky, J.L. (1974). *Intimacy status, partner perception and resolution of previous developmental crises*. Unpublished doctoral dissertation, State University of New York at Buffalo, Buffalo, NY.
Orlofsky, J.L. (1976). Intimacy status: Relationship to interpersonal perception. *Journal of Youth and Adolescence, 5*, 73–88.
Orlofsky, J.L. (1977). Sex role orientation, identity formation, and self-esteem in college men and women. *Sex Roles, 3*, 561–574.
Orlofsky, J.L. (1978a). Identity formation, nAchievement, and fear of success in college men and women. *Journal of Youth and Adolescence, 7*, 49–62.
Orlofsky, J.L. (1978b). The relationship between intimacy status and antecedent personality components. *Adolescence, 8*, 419–441.
Orlofsky, J.L. & Frank, M. (1986). Personality structure as viewed through early memories and identity status in college men and women. *Journal of Personality and Social Psychology, 50*, 580–586.
Orlofsky, J.L. & Ginsburg, S.D. (1981). Intimacy status: Relationship to affect cognition. *Adolescence, 16*, 91–100.
Orlofsky, J.L., Marcia, J.E., & Lesser, I.M. (1973). Ego identity status and the intimacy versus isolation crisis of young adulthood. *Journal of Personality and Social Psychology, 27*, 211–219.
Orlofsky, J.L. & Windle, M.T. (1978). Sex role orientation, behavioral adaptability, and personal adjustment. *Sex Roles, 4*, 801–811.
Orne, M.T. (1962). On the social psychology of the psychological experiment: With particular reference to demand characteristics and their implications. *American Psychologist, 17*, 776–783.
Oshman, H.P. & Manosevitz, M. (1974). The impact of the identity crisis on the adjustment of late adolescent males. *Journal of Youth and Adolescence, 3*, 207–216.
Oshman, H.P. & Manosevitz, M. (1976). Father absence: Effects of stepfathers upon psychosocial development in males. *Developmental Psychology, 12*, 479–480.
Owen, R.G. (1984). *Cultural influences on ego identity status distributions and associated levels of psychological adjustment and development*. Unpublished doctoral dissertation, University of Miami, Miami, FL.
Owens, P.A., Archer, S.L., & Waterman, A.S. (1987). *Women's identity and work orientation: Comparisons among four life styles*. Unpublished manuscript. Trenton State College, Trenton, NJ.
Pack, A.T., Brill, N.Q., & Christie, R.L. (1976). Quitting marijuana. *Diseases of the Nervous System, 37*, 205–209.

Papini, D.R., Sebby, R.A., & Clark, S. (1989). Affective quality of family relations and adolescent identity exploration. *Adolescence*, *26*, 457–466.

Park, Y.S. (1984). *The relationship between ego identity status and religiosity in college students*. Unpublished master's thesis, Department of Education, Graduate School of Sook-Myung Women's University, Korea.

Parsons, T. & Bales, R.F. (1955). *Family socialization and interaction process*. New York: Free Press.

Passons, W.R. (1975). *Gestalt approaches in counseling*. New York: Holt, Rinehart and Winston.

Pederson, D.M. & Breglio, V.J. (1968). Personality correlates of actual self-disclosure. *Psychological Reports*, *22*, 495–501.

Pederson, D.M. & Higbee, K.L. (1969). Personality correlates of self-disclosure. *Journal of Social Psychology*, *78*, 81–89.

Perls, F., Hefferline, R.F., & Goodman, P. (1951). *Gestalt therapy: Excitement and growth in the human personality*. New York: Julian Press.

Peterson, R.E. (1965). *Technical manual: College Student Questionnaires*. Princeton, NJ: Educational Testing Service.

Phinney, J.S. (1990). Ethnic identity in adolescence and adulthood: A review of research. *Psychological Bulletin*, *108*, 499–514.

Phinney, J.S. (1992). The Multigroup Ethnic Identity Measure: A new scale for use with diverse groups. *Journal of Adolescent Research*, *7*, 156–176.

Phinney, J.S. & Alipuria, L.L. (1990). Ethnic identity in college students from four ethnic groups. *Journal of Adolescence*, *13*, 171–183.

Phinney, J.S. & Tarver, S. (1988). Ethnic identity search and commitment in Black and White eighth graders. *Journal of Early Adolescence*, *8*, 265–277.

Phye, G.D. & Sola, J.L. (1984). Stability of expressive and instrumental traits in an adolescent female population. *Journal of Genetic Psychology*, *145*, 179–184.

Piaget, J. (1965). *The moral judgement of the child*. (M. Gabain, Trans.). New York: Free Press.

Podd, M.H. (1972). Ego identity status and morality: The relationship between two developmental constructs. *Developmental Psychology*, *6*, 497–507.

Podd, M.H., Marcia, J.E., & Rubin, B.M. (1970). The effects of ego identity and partner perception on a prisoner's dilemma game. *Journal of Social Psychology*, *82*, 117–126.

Pomerantz, S.C. (1979). Sex differences in the relative importance of self-esteem, physical self-satisfaction, and identity in predicting adolescent satisfaction. *Journal of Youth and Adolescence*, *8*, 51–61.

Poppen, P.J. (1974). *The development of sex differences in moral judgment for college males and females*. Unpublished doctoral dissertation, Cornell University, Ithaca, NY.

Prager, K.J. (1977). The relationship between identity status, intimacy status, self-esteem, and psychological androgyny in college women. *Dissertation Abstracts International*, *38*, 2347–2348B. (University Microfilms No. 7723020).

Prager, K.J. (1982). Identity development and self-esteem in young women. *Journal of Genetic Psychology*, *141*, 177–182.

Prager, K.J. (1985). Intimacy status and couple communication. *Journal of Social and Personal Relationships*, *6*, 435–449.

Prager, K.J. (1986). Identity development, age, and college experience in women. *Journal of Genetic Psychology*, *147*, 31–36.

Prince-Embury, S. & Deutchman, I.E. (1981). The identity status of politically active pro- and anti-ERA women. *Journal of Mind and Behavior*, *2*, 309–321.
Protinsky, H.O. (1975). Eriksonian ego identity in adolescents. *Adolescence, 10*, 428–432.
Rachman, A. (1965). *Changes in cognitive dimensions of affective responses as a result of psychotherapy. Unpublished doctoral dissertation, University of Chicago, Chicago, IL.*
Rall, W.J. (1984). *A comparison of married and living together couples*. Unpublished master's thesis, University of South Africa.
Rapaport, D. (1959). The structure of psychoanalytic theory: A systematizing attempt. *Psychological Issues*, Monograph No. 6. New York: International Universities Press.
Raphael, D. (1975). *An investigation into aspects of identity status of high school females*. Unpublished doctoral dissertation, University of Toronto, Toronto, Ontario, Canada.
Raphael, D. (1977). Identity status in university women: A methodological note. *Journal of Youth and Adolescence*, *6*, 57–62.
Rasmussen, J.E. (1964). Relationship of ego identity to psychosocial effectiveness. *Psychological Reports*, *15*, 815–825.
Read, D., Adams, G.R., & Dobson, W.R. (1984). Ego identity status, personality and social influence style. *Journal of Personality and Social Psychology*, *46*, 169–177.
Richardson, S.A., Dohrenwend, B.S., & Klein, D. (1965). *Interviewing: Its form and functions*. New York: Basic Books.
Rogers, C. R. (1972). *Becoming partners: Marriage and its alternatives*. New York: Delacorte Press.
Rogow, A.M., Marcia, J.E., & Slugoski, B.R. (1983). The relative importance of identity status interview components. *Journal of Youth and Adolescence*, *9*, 87–99.
Romano, N.C. (1975). *Relationship among identity confusion and resolution, self-esteem, and sex role perceptions in freshman women at Rutgers University*. Unpublished doctoral dissertation, Rutgers University, New Brunswick, NJ.
Romer, N. (1977). Sex-related differences in the development of the motive to avoid success, sex role identity, and performance in competitive and non-competitive conditions. *Psychology of Women Quarterly*, *1*, 260–272.
Rosenthal, D.A., Gurney, R.M., & Moore, S.M. (1984). From trust to intimacy: A new inventory for examining Erikson's stages of psychosocial development. *Journal of Youth and Adolescence*, *10*, 525–537.
Rosenthal, R. & Jacobson, L. (1966). Teachers' expectancies: Determinants of pupils' I.Q. gains. *Psychological Reports*, *19*, 115–118.
Rotheram-Borus, M.J. (1989). Ethnic differences in adolescents' identity status and associated behavior problems. *Journal of Adolescence*, *12*, 361–374.
Rothman, K.M. (1978). Multivariate analysis of the relationship of psychosocial crisis variables to ego identity status. *Journal of Youth and Adolescence*, *7*, 93–105.
Rothman, K.M. (1984). Multivariate analysis of the relationship of personal concerns to adolescent ego identity status. *Adolescence*, *19*, 713–727.
Rotter, J.B. (1966). Generalized expectancies for internal versus external control of reinforcement. *Psychological Monographs*, *80*(1): Whole No. 609.

Rowe, I. & Marcia, J.E. (1980). Ego identity status, formal operations, and moral development. *Journal of Youth and Adolescence*, *9*, 87–99.

St. Clair, S. & Day, H.P. (1979). Ego identity status and values among young females. *Journal of Youth and Adolescence*, *8*, 317–326.

Saslow, G., Matarazzo, J.D., Phillips, J.S., & Matarazzo, R.G. (1957). Test-retest stability of interaction patterns during interviews conducted one week apart. *Journal of Abnormal and Social Psychology*, *54*, 295–302.

Saulnier, G. (1990). Differences in identity status and perceived social support in homosexual and heterosexual males. Unpublished master's thesis. Simon Fraser University, Burnaby, British Columbia, Canada.

Schaie, K.W. & Baltes, P.B. (1975). On sequential strategies in developmental research. *Human Development*, *18*, 384–390.

Schenkel, S. (1975). Relationship among ego identity status, field-independence, and traditional femininity. *Journal of Youth and Adolescence*, *4*, 73–82.

Schenkel, S. & Marcia, J.E. (1972). Attitudes toward premarital intercourse in determining ego identity status in college women. *Journal of Personality*, *3*, 472–482.

Schiedel, D.G. & Marcia, J.E. (1985). Ego identity, intimacy, sex role orientation, and gender. *Developmental Psychology*, *18*, 149–160.

Schuster, A.L. (1982). *Ego and sexual identity status and marital adjustment*. Unpublished doctoral dissertation, California School of Professional Psychology, Fresno, CA.

Selltiz, C., Wrightsman, L.S., & Cook, S.W. (1976). *Research methods in social relationships* (3rd ed.). New York: Holt, Rinehart and Winston.

Shain, L. & Farber, B.K. (1989). Female identity development and self-reflection in late adolescence. *Adolescence*, *24*, 381–392.

Shanken, L.C. (1984). Identity and intimacy formation in young adults. *Dissertation Abstracts International*, *45*, 1000B. (University Microfilms No. 84–13029).

Siegel, S. (1956). *Non-parametric statistics*, New York: McGraw-Hill.

Simmons, D. (1970). Development of an objective measure of identity achievement status. *Journal of Projective Techniques and Personality Assessment*, *34*, 241–244.

Simmons, D. (1985). Identity achievement and axiological maturity. *Social Behavior and Personality*, *11*, 101–104.

Simon, J.A. (1976). *Administrative behavior: A study of decision-making process in administrative organization* (2nd ed.). New York: Free Press.

Skoe, E.E. & Marcia, J.E. (1991). The development and partial validation of a care-based measure of moral development. *Merrill-Palmer Quarterly*, *37*, 289–304.

Slugoski, B.R. & Ginsburg, S. (1989). Ego identity and explanatory speech. In J. Shotter & K.J. Gergen (Eds.), *Texts of identity*. (pp. 240–245) London: Sage.

Slugoski, B.R., Marcia, J.E., & Koopman, R.F. (1984). Cognitive and social interactional characteristics of ego identity statuses in college males. *Journal of Personality and Social Psychology*, *47*, 646–661.

Smith, J.M. (1972). *Interviewing in market and social research*. Boston, MA: Routledge and Kegan Paul.

Sola, J.L. (1976). *Effects of presentation mode, instructions, grade, and cognitive style on a concept formation task*. Unpublished doctoral dissertation, Iowa State University, Ames, IA.

Sola, J.L. (1980). Vocational maturity and decision-making and their relationship to sex role orientation in adolescent and late adolescent women. Paper presented at the Conference on Psychology of Adolescence, Michael Reese Hospital, Chicago, IL.

Spence, J.T. & Helmreich, R.L. (1978). *Masculinity and femininity*. Austin, TX: University of Texas Press.

Spence, J.T., Helmreich, R.L., & Stapp, J. (1973). A short version of the Attitudes toward Women Scale (AWS). *Bulletin of the Psychonomic Society*, *2*, 219–220.

Spence, J.T., Helmreich, R.L., & Stapp, J. (1975). Ratings of self and peers on sex-role attributes and their relation to self-esteem and conceptions of masculinity and femininity. *Journal of Personality and Social Psychology*, *32*, 29–39.

Stark, P.A. & Traxler, A.J. (1974). Empirical validation of Erikson's theory of identity crises in late adolescence. *Journal of Psychology*, *86*, 25–33.

Stein, S.L. & Weston, L.C. (1982). College women's attitudes toward women and identity achievement. *Adolescence*, *17*, 895–899.

Stephen, J., Fraser, E., & Marcia, J.E. (1992). Moratorium-achievement (MAMA) cycles in lifespan identity development: Value orientations and reasoning system. *Journal of Adolescence*, *15*, 283–300.

Sterling, C.M. & Van Horn, K.R. (1989). Identity and death anxiety. *Adolescence*, *24*, 321–326.

Stolesen, S.N. (1981). Identity and intimacy development in working women. *Dissertation Abstracts International*, 42, 2087B. (University Microfilms No. 81-21940).

Streitmatter, J.L. (1987). The effect of gender and family status on ego identity development among early adolescents. *Journal of Early Adolescence*, *7*, 179–189.

Streitmatter, J.L. (1988). Ethnicity as a mediating variable of early adolescent identity development. *Journal of Adolescence*, *11*, 335–346.

Streitmatter, J.L. (1989). Identity development and academic achievement in early adolescence. *Journal of Early Adolescence*, *9*, 99–116.

Streitmatter, J.L. & Pate, G. (1989). Identity status development and cognitive prejudice in early adolescents. *Journal of Early Adolescence*, *9*, 142–152.

Sullivan, H.S. (1953). *The interpersonal theory of psychiatry*. New York: Norton.

Tan, A.L., Kendis, R.J., Fine, J.T., & Porac, J. (1977). A short measure of Eriksonian ego identity. *Journal of Personality Assessment*, *41*, 279–284.

Tesch, S.A. (1980). *Intimacy and identity development in early adulthood*. Unpublished doctoral dissertation, University of Rochester, Rochester, NY.

Tesch, S.A. (1984). Sex-role orientation and intimacy status in men and women. *Sex Roles*, *11*, 451–465.

Tesch, S.A. (1985). Psychosocial development and subjective well-being in an age cross-section of adults. *International Journal of Aging and Human Development*, *21*, 109–120.

Tesch, S.A. & Cameron, K.A. (1987). Openness to experience and development of adult identity. *Journal of Personality*, *55*, 615–630.

Tesch, S.A. & Whitbourne, S.K. (1982). Intimacy and identity status in young adults. *Journal of Personality and Social Psychology*, *43*, 1041–1051.

Thompson, M.St.G. (1963). *Modifications in identity. A study of socialization process during a sister formation program*. Unpublished doctoral dissertation, University of Chicago, Chicago, IL.

Thorbecke, W. & Grotevant, H.D. (1982). Gender differences in interpersonal identity formation. *Journal of Youth and Adolescence*, *11*, 479–492.

Toder, N.L. & Marcia, J.E. (1973). Ego identity status and response to conformity pressure in college women. *Journal of Personality and Social Psychology*, *26*, 287–294.

Tresemer, D.W. (1977). *Fear of success*. New York: Plenum Press.

Tzuriel, D. (1984). Sex role typing and ego identity in Israeli, Oriental, and Western adolescents. *Journal of Personality and Social Psychology*, *46*, 440–457.

Tzuriel, D. & Klien, M.M. (1977). Ego identity: Effects of ethnocentrism, ethnic identification, and cognitive complexity in Israeli, Oriental, and Western ethnic groups. *Psychological Reports*, *40*, 1099–1110.

Vaillant, G. (1977). *Adaptation to life*. Boston: Little, Brown.

Valdez, R., Jr. (1984). *An examination of patterns of ego identity and intimacy development in college women of differing sex role identities*. Unpublished doctoral dissertation, Michigan State University, East Lansing, MI.

Vinokur, A., Oksenberg, L., & Cannell, C.F. (1977). Effects of feedback and reinforcement on the report of health information. In *NCHSR*.

Vreeland, A.P. (1982). *A study of ego identity status categories and personality in college men and women*. Unpublished master's thesis, Northeast Louisiana State University, Monroe, LA.

Wagner, J.A. (1987). Formal operations and ego identity in adolescence. *Adolescence*, *22*, 23–35.

Waterman, A.S. (1980, April). Ego identity status among married, adult women. Paper presented at the meeting of the Eastern Psychological Association, Hartford, CT.

Waterman, A.S. (1982). Identity development from adolescence to adulthood: An extension of theory and a review of research. *Developmental Psychology*, *18*, 342–358.

Waterman, A.S. (1984). Identity formation: Discovery or creation? *Journal of Early Adolescence*, *4*, 329–341.

Waterman, A.S. (1985). Identity in the context of adolescent psychology. In A.S. Waterman (Ed.), *Identity in adolescence: Processes and contents*. San Francisco, CA: Jossey-Bass.

Waterman, A.S. (1988). Identity status theory and Erikson's theory: Communalities and differences. *Developmental Review*, *8*, 185–208.

Waterman, A.S. & Archer, S.L. (1979). Ego identity status and expressive writing among high school and college students. *Journal of Youth and Adolescence*, *8*, 327–341.

Waterman, A.S. & Archer, S.L. (1990). A life-span perspective on identity formation: Developments in form, function, and process. In P.B. Baltes, D.L. Featherman, & R.M. Lerner (Eds.), *Life-span development and behavior*, Vol. 10. Hillsdale, NJ: Erlbaum.

Waterman, A.S., Geary, P.S., & Waterman, C.K. (1974). Longitudinal study of changes in ego identity status from the freshman to the senior year at college. *Developmental Psychology*, *10*, 387–392.

Waterman, A.S. & Goldman, J.A. (1976). A longitudinal study of ego identity development at a liberal arts college. *Journal of Youth and Adolescence*, *5*, 361–369.

Waterman, A.S., Kohutis, E., & Pulone, J. (1977). The role of expressive writing in identity formation. *Developmental Psychology*, *13*, 286–287.
Waterman, A.S. & Waterman, C.K. (1970). The relationship between ego identity status and satisfaction with college. *Journal of Educational Research*, *64*, 165–168.
Waterman, A.S. & Waterman, C.K. (1971). A longitudinal study of changes in ego identity status during the freshman year at college. *Developmental Psychology*, *5*, 167–173.
Waterman, A.S. & Waterman, C.K. (1972). Relationship between freshman identity status and subsequent academic behavior: A test of the predictive validity of Marcia's categorization system for identity status. *Developmental Psychology*, *6*, 179.
Waterman, A.S. & Whitbourne, S.K. (1982a). Androgyny and psychosocial development among college students and adults. *Journal of Personality*, *50*, 121–133.
Waterman, A.S. & Whitbourne, S.K. (1982b). The Inventory of Psychosocial Development: A review and evaluation. *Journal Supplement Abstract Service*, *11* (Ms. No. 2179).
Waterman, C.K., Beubel, M., & Waterman, A.S. (1970). Relationship between resolution of the identity crisis and outcomes of previous psychosocial crises. Proceedings of the *78th Annual Convention of the American Psychological Association*, 467–468.
Waterman, C.K. & Nevid, J.S. (1977). Sex differences in the resolution of the identity crisis. *Journal of Youth and Adolescence*, *6*, 337–342.
Waterman, C.K. & Waterman, A.S. (1974). Ego identity status and decision styles. *Journal of Youth and Adolescence*, *3*, 1–6.
Waterman, C.K. & Waterman, A.S. (1975). Fathers and sons: A study of ego identity across two generations. *Journal of Youth and Adolescence*, *4*, 331–338.
Weick, K.E. (1964). Reduction of cognitive dissonance through task enhancement and effort expenditure. *Journal of Abnormal and Social Psychology*, *58*, 533–539.
Wells, K. (1980). Gender roles, identity, and psychological adjustment in adolescence. *Journal of Youth and Adolescence*, *9*, 59–73.
Werner, H. (1957). The concept of development from a comparative and organismic point of view. In D.B. Harris (Ed.). *The concept of development.* (pp. 125–148). Minneapolis, MN: University of Minnesota Press.
Whitbourne, S.K. (1986). Openness to experience, identity flexibility, and life changes in adults. *Journal of Personality and Social Psychology*, *50*, 163–168.
Whitbourne, S.K., Jelsma, B.M., & Waterman, A.S. (1982). An Eriksonian measure of personality development in college students: A re-examination of Constantinople's data and a partial replication. *Developmental Psychology*, *18*, 369–371.
Whitbourne, S.K. & Tesch, S.A. (1985). A comparison of identity and intimacy statuses in college students and alumni. *Developmental Psychology*, *21*, 1039–1044.
Whitbourne, S.K. & Waterman, A.S. (1979). Psychosocial development during the adult years: Age and cohort comparisons. *Developmental Psychology*, *15*, 373–378.

Whitbourne, S.K. & Weinstock, C.S. (1979). *Adult development: The differentiation of experience*. New York: Holt, Rinehart and Winston.

Whitbourne, S.K., Zuschlag, M.K., Elliot, L.B., & Waterman, A.S. (1992). Psychosocial development in adulthood: A 22-year sequential study. *Journal of Personality and Social Psychology*, *63*, 260–271.

White, K.M., Speisman, J.C., Jackson, D., Bartis, S., & Costos, D. (1986). Intimacy maturity and its correlates in young married couples. *Journal of Personality and Social Psychology*, *50*, 152–162.

White, R.W. (1959). Motivation reconsidered: The concept of competence. *Psychological Review*, *66*, 297–323.

Wilkerson, J., Protinsky, H.O., Jr., Maxwell, J.W., & Lenter, M. (1982). Alienation and ego identity in adolescents. *Adolescence*, *17*, 133–139.

Yufit, R. (1956). *Intimacy and isolation: Some behavioral and psychodynamic correlates*. Unpublished doctoral dissertation, University of Chicago, Chicago, IL.

Zampich, C.L. (1981). *Ego identity status, intimacy status, and self-disclosure in adult men and women*. Unpublished doctoral dissertation, Rosemead Graduate School of Professional Psychology, Rosemead, CA.

Zimmer, J.M. & Park, P. (1967). Factor analysis of counselor communications. *Journal of Counseling Psychology*, *14*, 198–203.

Author Index

Subject Index

MIX
Papier aus verantwortungsvollen Quellen
Paper from responsible sources
FSC® C105338

If you have any concerns about our products,
you can contact us on
ProductSafety@springernature.com

In case Publisher is established outside the EU,
the EU authorized representative is:
Springer Nature Customer Service Center GmbH
Europaplatz 3, 69115 Heidelberg, Germany

Printed by Libri Plureos GmbH
in Hamburg, Germany